The BioMechanics Method for Corrective Exercise

Justin Price, MA

Creator, The BioMechanics Method

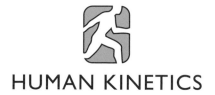

HUMAN KINETICS

Library of Congress Cataloging-in-Publication Data

Names: Price, Justin, author.
Title: The biomechanics method for corrective exercise / Justin Price.
Description: Champaign, IL : Human Kinetics, [2019] | Includes
  bibliographical references and index.
Identifiers: LCCN 2017060221 (print) | LCCN 2017058184 (ebook) | ISBN
  9781492552086 (e-book) | ISBN 9781492545668 (print)
Subjects: | MESH: Exercise Therapy | Musculoskeletal Diseases--rehabilitation
  | Biomechanical Phenomena
Classification: LCC RM701 (print) | LCC RM701 (ebook) | NLM WB 541 | DDC
  615.8/2--dc23
LC record available at https://lccn.loc.gov/2017060221

ISBN: 978-1-4925-4566-8 (print)

The web addresses cited in this text were current as of May 2018, unless otherwise noted.

Senior Acquisitions Editor: Joshua J. Stone; **Senior Developmental Editor:** Amanda S. Ewing; **Managing Editor:** Anne E. Mrozek; **Copyeditor:** Kevin Campbell; **Indexer:** Rebecca McCorkle; **Permissions Manager:** Dalene Reeder; **Senior Graphic Designer:** Joe Buck; **Cover Designer:** Keri Evans; **Cover Design Associate:** Susan Rothermel Allen; **Photograph (cover):** Image with models courtesy of MovieProdigy; Background of dots © Veronaa/Getty Images ; **Photographs (interior):** © Justin Price, unless otherwise noted; F 2.8-2.11, F 3.3, F 3.6-3.8, F 4.2a-b, F 4.4, F 4.7, F 4.8, F 5.3a-c, F 5.6, F 5.9, F 5.10, F 6.4, F 10.6, F 12.4, F 12.6, F 17.7a-b, F 17.12a, F 17.12c, F 18.1, F 18.2, F 18.3a and photos on pages 201, 205 (top L and bottom), 211 (bottom), 218, 227 (top), 230, 247 (top L), 272, 275 (middle), 294, 330, 331 (top), 337 (top), 432 © Human Kinetics; **Photo Production Coordinator:** Amy M. Rose; **Photo Production Manager:** Jason Allen; **Senior Art Manager:** Kelly Hendren; **Illustrations:** © Human Kinetics, unless otherwise noted; **Printer:** Walsworth

The video contents of this product are licensed for private home use and traditional, face-to-face classroom instruction only. For public performance licensing, please contact a sales representative at **www.HumanKinetics.com/SalesRepresentatives**.

Printed in the United States of America

10 9 8 7 6 5 4 3 2 1

The paper in this book was manufactured using responsible forestry methods.

Human Kinetics
P.O. Box 5076
Champaign, IL 61825-5076
Website: www.HumanKinetics.com

In the United States, email info@hkusa.com or call 800-747-4457.
In Canada, email info@hkcanada.com.
In the United Kingdom/Europe, email hk@hkeurope.com.

For information about Human Kinetics' coverage in other areas of the world,
please visit our website: **www.HumanKinetics.com**

E6993

This book is dedicated to our global team of corrective exercise specialists certified in The BioMechanics Method and their devoted and inspirational clients. They create miracles every day by making pain-free movement a reality.

Contents

Part III   Fundamentals of Corrective Exercise   137

Preface

Welcome to *The BioMechanics Method for Corrective Exercise,* the world's premier text on corrective exercise education for fitness professionals. This book is written for fitness professionals for the purpose of teaching you how to address common musculoskeletal imbalances through the use of corrective exercise. Unlike other texts on musculoskeletal and movement dysfunction, this book explains concepts in an easy-to-follow manner using jargon-free language. The content is delivered as a step-by-step process (containing real-world examples and case studies) so that you, the reader, can understand and easily implement these strategies when working with clients.

I have been fortunate enough to be an integral part of the health and fitness industry for almost 30 years. This has given me the wonderful opportunity to observe and assist both clients and professionals as they work toward achieving their personal and career goals. During this exciting and enlightening journey, I have also witnessed a clear change in the landscape of the industry.

Traditionally, the job of fitness professionals has been to provide broad exercise instruction and programming, education, and motivation to a general population looking for athletic or aesthetic improvements. In pursuit of these goals, fitness professionals have guided their clients to perform rather demanding physical activities characteristic of most sporting environments. However, research shows that almost 90 percent of people who currently use personal training services report having temporary or chronic musculoskeletal issues that prevent them from performing even low-level physical activities without experiencing pain (Schroeder and Donlin 2013). Industry studies also show that one of the fastest growing segments of the population joining gyms is the over-55 demographic, yet only about 50 percent of fitness professionals report having the appropriate skills to serve people with muscle or joint pain and other physically limiting musculoskeletal conditions (IHRSA 2017; Schroeder and Donlin 2013). Obviously, a gap in care exists between the abilities of clients and typical fitness service offerings. Clearly, the role of the fitness professional must evolve to meet these needs.

I wrote this book (and created The BioMechanics Method Corrective Exercise Specialist credential) specifically to fill the educational needs of fitness professionals who work with clients experiencing musculoskeletal dysfunction. It provides competency in the areas of musculoskeletal assessment, anatomy, corrective exercise selection, and program design to empower this segment of the health and fitness industry to bridge this gap in care.

The BioMechanics Method is a product of my lifelong dedication to exploring, discovering, creating, teaching, and applying the most effective corrective exercise strategies for assessing and addressing muscle and joint pain. As an internationally recognized expert in the field of corrective exercise, I have had the unique opportunity to provide hands-on corrective exercise education to hundreds of thousands of students in over 50 countries. I have also been privileged to work alongside the most respected medical and health professionals in the field of musculoskeletal rehabilitation, and I have personally helped innumerable clients with both common and unique musculoskeletal challenges. These fantastic experiences have allowed me to gauge trends in the industry, decipher information and methods in complex medical texts and consider their value to the field of corrective exercise, trial thousands of techniques with my own clients, network with esteemed colleagues, and ultimately develop the real-world, practical, and methodical strategies outlined in this text.

I have purposefully presented the content in a manner that is easy for fitness professionals to understand and implement when working with clients. Here are the topics covered:

- Conducting a series of assessments to identify common musculoskeletal imbalances

- Understanding how these common imbalances affect bones and soft tissue structures

- Learning about various types of corrective exercises

- Knowing how to select appropriate exercise strategies for a client's condition

- Designing entire corrective exercise programs to address the underlying cause(s) of muscle and joint pain

Strategies and examples for communicating all of this information effectively to clients—one of the most important and most overlooked facets of developing successful corrective exercise programs—are integrated throughout the text. As an added bonus, there is also material on how to market, promote, and network yourself and your skills appropriately so that you can capitalize financially on your corrective exercise talents. Every procedure, technique, and process is fully illustrated with tables, illustrations, and photographs to enhance your learning experience. In addition, "self-checks" and skill acquisition activities are included in every chapter so you can practice and perfect your assessment, anatomy, program design, and business skills.

The step-by-step nature of the assessment and exercise material ensures that professionals trained and qualified in these techniques are able to identify both the potential causes and the most successful techniques for relieving common musculoskeletal imbalances to swiftly eliminate pain and improve physical function. *The BioMechanics Method for Corrective Exercise* further educates fitness professionals about how malalignments of any kind can create pain, injury, and dysfunction throughout the body. It also enables them to use the results of individual consultations and assessments to pinpoint clients' exercise needs so they can successfully start or return to a regular fitness program. In short, those trained in The BioMechanics Method possess the skills to meet clients' musculoskeletal restoration needs head-on. They represent perfectly the fitness professionals of the future.

ORGANIZATION

The contents of the book are organized in a logical and sequential format and should be read in sequence, beginning with part I, Fundamentals of Structural Assessment. In this section you will learn to perform a cohesive series of verbal, visual, and hands-on assessments for the feet and ankles, knees, lumbo-pelvic hip girdle, thoracic spine and shoulder girdle, and neck and head, as well as how to communicate these assessments effectively to clients. Starting at the beginning of the book is imperative because the results you obtain about a client during the assessment are used as the foundation for the entire corrective exercise process. Understanding your client's skeletal structures from the outset provides the necessary framework and background information you need to understand the detailed functional anatomy and soft tissue information in part II.

Next you will progress to part II, Understanding Muscles and Movement, where you will be introduced to over 100 bones, joints, muscles, and other soft tissue structures and learn how these parts of the body are affected by the musculoskeletal imbalances discussed in part I. The anatomical information in this section also sets the stage for exercise selection by teaching you what myofascial structures may need to be addressed as part of your corrective exercise programs.

In part III, Fundamentals of Corrective Exercise, you will learn about the elements of corrective exercise programs, how to select and adapt exercises to meet the needs of each client, and how to coach each technique. Nonexercise-related strategies to incorporate with corrective exercise programs are also covered in this section.

Part IV, Complete Corrective Exercise Library, contains an array of self-myofascial release, stretching, and strengthening exercises. This comprehensive collection will guide your selection of specific techniques that will constructively address a client's musculoskeletal and physical conditions.

Part V, Corrective Exercise Program Design, provides detailed instruction on developing corrective exercise programs and fostering positive client relationships so that your consultations, individual sessions, and programs prove successful. Part V also contains a valuable case study to help you understand how the various components of the process can be implemented seamlessly when working with clients.

Lastly, to help you capitalize on the corrective exercise skills you learned in parts I through V, part VI, Business of Corrective Exercise, contains information on how to set up a corrective exercise business, with specifics about networking and referral systems, tips for maintaining your scope of practice, and marketing methods for attracting and retaining clients.

The practices outlined in this text have been used and proven successful in real life by both the author and the thousands of The BioMechanics Method Corrective Exercise Specialists around the world trained in these techniques. Your commitment to reading this book and applying the corrective exercise strategies herein will undoubtedly bring continued value to your development as an outstanding fitness professional.

ONLINE VIDEO

As an added bonus, *The BioMechanics Method for Corrective Exercise* includes access to 36 online video clips where I personally demonstrate many of the practices and procedures outlined in the text on a real person. This unique audiovisual component gives you the opportunity to observe the application of some of the musculoskeletal assessment techniques outlined in the text and to follow along as I illustrate how muscle dysfunction can influence movement and posture. The video clips also contain valuable communication techniques, marketing strategies, and exercise cueing tips to further advance your knowledge and skills in successfully applying The BioMechanics Method when working with your own clients. See the next page for how to access the online video.

Go to the online video and watch video P.1. Author Justin Price introduces himself to you and covers information about The BioMechanics Method, this book, and the video clips.

Accessing the Online Video

Throughout *The BioMechanics Method for Corrective Exercise*, you will notice references to online video. This online content is available to you for free upon purchase of a new print book or an ebook. All you need to do is register with the Human Kinetics website to access the online content. The following steps explain how to register.

The online video offers demonstrations by the author of many of the practices and procedures outlined in the text. This unique audiovisual component gives you the opportunity to observe the application of some of the musculoskeletal assessment techniques outlined in the text and to follow along as the author illustrates how muscle dysfunction can influence movement and posture. We are certain you will enjoy this unique online learning experience.

FOLLOW THESE STEPS TO ACCESS THE ONLINE VIDEO:

1. Visit www.HumanKinetics.com/TheBioMechanicsMethodForCorrective Exercise.

2. Click the first edition link next to the corresponding first edition book cover.

3. Click the Sign In link on the left or top of the page. If you do not have an account with Human Kinetics, you will be prompted to create one.

4. After you register, if the online product does not appear in the Ancillary Items box on the left of the page, click the Enter Pass Code option in that box. Enter the following pass code exactly as it is printed here, including capitalization and all hyphens: **PRICE-K9NQ-WR**

5. Click the Submit button to unlock your online product.

6. After you have entered your pass code the first time, you will never have to enter it again to access this online product. Once unlocked, a link to your product will permanently appear in the menu on the left. All you need to do to access your online content on subsequent visits is sign in to **www.HumanKinetics.com/TheBioMechanicsMethodForCorrective Exercise** and follow the link!

Click the Need Help? button on the book's website if you need assistance along the way.

Acknowledgments

I would like to thank all of the dedicated and hard-working professionals at Human Kinetics who contributed to the making of this book. In particular, special thanks go to Amy Tocco, Amanda Ewing, and Joshua Stone for your continued enthusiasm and commitment to seeing this project to fruition. I would also like to express my sincerest gratitude to the amazing team at The BioMechanics Method, with special thanks to Mary, Gene, Robert, Mazza, Gloria, Elizabeth, Jason, and Angel. Without your help, The BioMechanics Method, and this book, would simply not have been possible.

Part I

Fundamentals of Structural Assessment

In part I, you will learn about The BioMechanics Method structural assessment process. This section will teach you how to gather pertinent information about the condition of a client's musculoskeletal system by conducting a series of verbal, visual, and hands-on assessments. You will learn a step-by step process for assessing the feet and ankles, knees, lumbo-pelvic hip girdle, thoracic spine and shoulder girdle, and the neck and head for common musculoskeletal imbalances that can disrupt movement, limit range of motion, and cause muscle and joint pain. In addition to learning methods for assessing specific areas of the body, you will also be taught how musculoskeletal imbalances in one part of the body affect movement and position in other areas. The insight you will gain into how the body works as a series of interrelated parts will inspire you to look beyond clients' symptoms to find the underlying causes of their movement dysfunctions. Furthermore, the knowledge you gain from evaluating the state of a client's musculoskeletal system will help you to understand what muscles and soft tissue structures may be affected by deviations in that system (covered in part II).

Effective communication strategies are emphasized throughout part I to enable you to help clients to understand and appreciate the step-by-step nature of the structural assessment process. These simple strategies will make the assessment process more enjoyable for clients and will strengthen their desire to participate fully with you in the development of corrective exercise programs. Lastly, you will be given detailed instructions on how to record a client's assessment findings and other pertinent information about their musculoskeletal health history on the Client Assessment Diagram (CAD; see the appendix). The CAD will function as an invaluable guide when you begin to design a client's corrective exercise program

CHAPTER 1

The Process of Structural Assessment

A structural assessment is one of the most important tools a fitness professional can use to gather information about the condition and function of a client's musculoskeletal system. The BioMechanics Method structural assessment process is designed to collect this information in an organized, sequential, and logical format. The process involves an initial verbal consultation followed by visual and hands-on assessments of a client's feet and ankles, knees, lumbo-pelvic hip girdle, thoracic spine, shoulder girdle, neck, and head. The results of this structural assessment will provide information about the current state of a client's musculoskeletal system. It will also give you insight into the way the client moves and any dysfunction he or she might exhibit when engaged in daily activities, exercise, and sports. For example, if a structural assessment reveals overpronated feet (i.e., flat feet) when standing, then it is likely that the client's feet will also overpronate during more dynamic activities like walking and running (Bryant and Green 2010).

Before you meet with a client for the structural assessment, a number of matters should be considered to make sure the process runs smoothly. The following guidelines will help you to be proficient and to minimize stress for the client.

INITIAL CONTACT WITH CLIENT

Contact a client before the in-person assessment to answer questions about the appointment. This first exchange, while casual in nature, sets the tone for your ongoing relationship with the client, so it must be done well to help establish your professional credibility. Despite the current popularity of email and texting, you should make this contact via telephone whenever possible, and you should speak with the client directly. The client may feel very anxious about the structural assessment process, and she will likely have questions about such things as what to wear, how long the appointment will last, how much it will cost, and whether she can bring a family member to the appointment. Making contact in person will help you to alleviate these initial anxieties and set up a more encouraging and supportive relationship from the outset (Bryant, Green, and Newton-Merrill 2013). See chapter 22 for more information on client relationships.

To prepare clients adequately for the consultation, give them a basic overview of what to expect. For example, you might say something like, "During the initial session I will be asking you a series of questions about your body, and I will perform a thorough musculoskeletal assessment. This will help us identify any areas of possible dysfunction that might affect your ability to exercise effectively or that might contribute to any aches and pains you feel. I will also happily answer any questions you might have about the process as we go."

Tell clients that the assessment process requires you to view certain areas of their bodies clearly. Therefore, it will be necessary for them to wear assessment-friendly clothing. Advise male clients to wear (or bring to the appointment to change into) shorts and a tank top and female clients to wear shorts and a sports bra or tank top. Also be sure to let clients know they will need to remove their socks and shoes for the assessment.

If clients indicate that they are not comfortable wearing the clothing just described, or if you hear in her voice that she is anxious about wearing such attire, simply find an acceptable alternative that will meet both your needs. A form-fitting T-shirt may suffice for upper body assessments, and running leggings or yoga pants may be worn instead of shorts. Never insist that clients wear clothing that makes them feel uncomfortable.

If a client has never been to your facility, gym, or place of business before, give him accurate directions to the building or meeting area, information about parking, and any other useful information about your premises. Follow up your conversation with an email detailing this information so he can refer to it on the day of the appointment.

Scheduling an initial consultation can be a stressful experience for a client. Do not overwhelm prospective clients with too much information when you first speak on the telephone or in your follow-up email. Keep your instructions concise, clear, and simple. You can elaborate on additional matters when you meet in person (Price 2012).

STRUCTURAL ASSESSMENT PROCESS

The structural assessment process includes the following three elements:

1. A verbal assessment
2. A visual assessment
3. A hands-on assessment

Each part of this process is designed to gather significant information about the client. Complete each element of the process in turn, and do not omit any part.

> Go to the online video to watch video 1.1, where Justin talks about The BioMechanics Method structural assessment process and the importance of the Client Assessment Diagram.

VERBAL ASSESSMENT

The verbal assessment is the first part of the structural assessment process. It is used to acquire health history information about a client's musculoskeletal well-being. The verbal assessment begins informally during the initial contact with the client on the telephone. It continues in a structured format when you meet the client in person for the first visit. The verbal assessment contains questions about musculoskeletal discomfort, past injuries and surgeries, types and intensity of physical activity, occupation, and information the client may have about diagnosed medical conditions that might be affecting her musculoskeletal system. The responses will help you to evaluate her current level of function. It will also provide valuable insight about how the client feels both physically and mentally about her musculoskeletal health. Moreover, the verbal assessment helps you and the client to develop trust and rapport as you progress into the visual and hands-on parts of the assessment process (Price and Bratcher 2010).

The Client Assessment Diagram (CAD) (which will be discussed in detail later in this chapter and is available in the appendix) will guide you through the questions that must be asked during the verbal assessment. There is a space on the CAD for the client's response to each question. You can mark an X on the CAD to indicate areas of the body where the client has experienced pain or dysfunction either now or in the past.

Conduct the verbal assessment in its entirety at the beginning of the appointment so the client can answer all your questions while seated and comfortable. Do not ask clients to fill out the CAD themselves. It is vital that you ask all of the questions and record the information on the CAD yourself. Taking the time to ask each question enables you to encourage feedback, observe body language, and foster an atmosphere of teamwork and communication (Whitworth et al. 2007). Occasionally, clients may be nervous about forgetting something during the verbal assessment. Assure them that you will make a note of any additional information they remember as you are conducting the visual and hands-on assessment.

VISUAL AND HANDS-ON ASSESSMENT

The visual and hands-on assessment portion of the structural assessment process involves visually and manually inspecting each major area of the client's body (Kendall, McCreary, and Provance 2005). These two components of the assessment process are distinct, but they should be carried out simultaneously to make the process more practical and less time consuming. As an inquisitive fitness professional, you may take a keen interest in gathering information about a client's musculoskeletal imbalances, but a nervous client standing before you in tight clothes may not share your level of interest. Therefore, conduct the visual and hands-on assessment quickly and efficiently while also making sure that the client understands each stage of the process.

As the name implies, hands-on assessments will require physical contact between you and the client. Always ask permission before touching a client in any way, and explain what you are going to do before doing it. You should also ask clients to tell you if they feel uncomfortable, do not wish to be touched, or do not wish to continue with an assessment.

You will begin the visual and hands-on assessment at the feet and ankles. This is not because the feet and ankles are more relevant than other parts of the body, but because beginning the assessment here is less intimidating for your client. Once you have completed your assessments for the feet and ankles, you will work your way up the body, performing your assessments on the knees, lumbo-pelvic hip girdle, thoracic spine, shoulder girdle, neck, and head. This foot-to-head approach will allow the client to relax as the process unfolds, enabling him to feel more at ease as you assess each subsequent area of his body (Price and Bratcher 2010).

Go to the online video to watch video 1.2, where Justin explains why the assessment process starts at the feet.

As you conduct the visual and hands-on assessment, you should explain the process and share your findings so the client understands what is happening at each stage. As you assess each body part, record your findings in the appropriate space on the CAD. If a client expresses pain or discomfort at any time during an assessment, stop the assessment immediately and, where appropriate, continue to the next assessment.

As you become more proficient and practiced in performing structural assessments, it will become easier to demonstrate each procedure and to explain the results in simple terms to the client. Your ability to conduct the assessments in an interesting manner will also help to strengthen clients' interest in the process. Then they will begin to appreciate how their own musculoskeletal imbalances are negatively affecting the function of their bodies.

Effective communication during the assessment process can also help with a client's subsequent adherence to a corrective exercise program (Price 2016). Take, for example, a client seeking help to alleviate discomfort in her knees when she exercises. During the structural assessment, you note imbalances in her feet and ankles that could be influencing the discomfort in her knees. As a result, you recommend a series of corrective exercises for the feet and ankles. If you fail to effectively explain during the structural assessment how the foot and ankle imbalances can affect her knees, she may not see the value in doing the exercises. In fact, she may even become annoyed that you are providing the "wrong" exercises since they are for her feet/ankles and not for her painful knees. On the other hand, if you have successfully explained how the imbalances in her feet and ankles can cause her knee pain, she will be more likely to perform the exercises you recommend.

As you evaluate each body part, think about the body as a whole, and try to determine how other structures may be affecting the area you are currently assessing. For example, if you discover a client has an imbalance in his feet and ankles, then consider whether other imbalances elsewhere in his body may be contributing to his foot and ankle problem. The remaining chapters in part I of this text describe in detail how each body area is affected by the other parts. It is critical to understand that each structure in the human body functions as a link in an interconnected chain.

CLIENT ASSESSMENT DIAGRAM

As you progress through the structural assessment process, record all the information you gather about the client. The easiest way to do this is to use the Client Assessment Diagram (CAD), which has been designed for this purpose. The CAD lists all the questions that should be asked and the assessments that should be conducted. It also has space for you to mark when an item has been completed, and it includes areas to record the verbal, visual, and hands-on results for each area of the body. An anatomical figure is provided for you to mark those areas of pain and dysfunction reported by the client during the verbal assessment. Making quick reference marks with an *X* on this figure will allow you to remain focused on what the client is saying and on nonverbal clues the client may reveal as you conduct the assessment. A blank copy of the Client Assessment Diagram can be found in the appendix.

Review of Key Points

The structural assessment process enables fitness professionals to gather pertinent information about a client's musculoskeletal condition in an organized, sequential, and logical format.

- The assessment process consists of three distinct parts:
  1. Verbal assessment
  2. Visual assessment
  3. Hands-on assessment

- The verbal assessment begins with your initial contact on the telephone and continues in a structured format during your first meeting with a client.

- The visual and hands-on assessments are distinct assessments; however, they should be conducted simultaneously to make the process more practical and efficient.

- The visual and hands-on assessment begins with the feet and ankles and moves up the body to the knees, lumbo-pelvic hip girdle, thoracic spine, and shoulder girdle, and it ends at the neck and head.

- The structural assessment process includes protocols that make the experience less stressful for client and assessor alike:
  – Providing information on what to expect during the appointment
  – Providing clear directions to the facility or meeting spot
  – Providing information about what to wear for the assessment
  – Answering any additional questions the client may have about the appointment

- All of the questions and assessments used during the structural assessment process are listed on the Client Assessment Diagram. Spaces are also provided on this form to record your assessment results.

Self-Check

There are a number of obstacles that can make conducting a structural assessment more confusing or stressful than necessary for both you and your client. Consider the following potential problems one might encounter before, during, or after an assessment. Indicate in the space next to each issue who (you, your client, or both) would be affected by each difficulty and what you could do to rectify the problem.

Avoiding Pitfalls During the Structural Assessment Process

Potential issue	Who is affected: you, client, or both	Possible solution
You cannot remember a client's answers to the questions you asked during the verbal assessment		
Client arrives 15 minutes late for the appointment because he could not find parking near the facility		
Client becomes irritated during the assessment process about what you are doing and why you are doing it that way		
Assessor cannot clearly see the structures or areas of the body she is trying to evaluate due to the client's clothing		
Client does not see the point in assessor conducting a whole-body assessment when he only came in for a specific problem (e.g., knee pain)		

CHAPTER 2

Assessing the Feet and Ankles

The foot and ankle complex is very complex indeed. In one foot alone, there are 26 bones, 33 joints, and over 100 ligaments, muscles, and tendons (Gray 1995). Two of the most important functions of the feet and ankles are to keep the body balanced and to ensure that stress is distributed correctly not only through these structures but also throughout the musculoskeletal system (Frowen et al. 2010; Kelikian 2011). If functioning of the foot and ankle complex is compromised during weight-bearing activities, other parts of the body have to compensate to preserve balance, and existing imbalances elsewhere are compounded. The feet and ankles must also adapt to changes in surfaces and terrains (Frowen et al, 2010), so they are continually subjected to stresses from both above and below.

BASIC ANATOMY

The foot and ankle complex can be broken into six parts, three joints of the ankle and three areas of the foot. The joint where the lower leg bones (tibia and fibula) come together at the ankle is the **tibiofibular joint** (figure 2.1). Below the tibia and fibula (and above the talus) is the talocrural joint, also known as the **true ankle joint**. This joint helps the lower leg interact with the foot and ankle and displaces stress downward through to the heel (Snell 2008). The other main joint in the ankle is the **subtalar joint** (below the talus bone). It helps transfer forces forward through to the foot and has great side-to-side movement capabilities to help distribute weight

and pressure and to adapt the body to the terrain or contact surface (Snell 2008).

The three areas of the foot are known as the hindfoot, the midfoot, and the forefoot (figure 2.2). The **hindfoot**, which includes the **calcaneus** (heel bone), is below the ankle and helps absorb shock and distribute forces. It also aids in the transfer of stress through to the midfoot and forefoot. The **midfoot**, which includes the bones in the middle of the foot and is the highest part of the arches of the foot, is also designed to absorb shock. The midfoot also helps dissipate forces through side-to-side movement. The **forefoot**, which includes the metatarsals and the toes, is very flexible; this flexibility serves

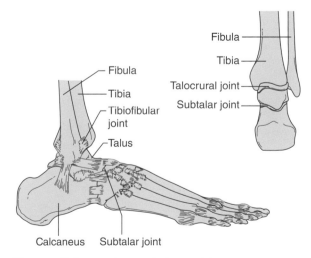

Figure 2.1   Joints of the ankle.

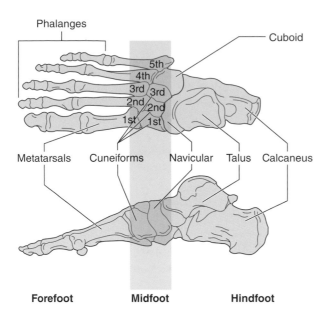

Figure 2.2   Areas of the foot.

to increase the surface area of the foot to improve both balance and the body's interactions with the terrain (Davis, Davis and Ross 2005).

The areas of the foot can also interlock to slow forces down as the foot comes in contact with the ground. This reduces ankle rotation and prevents the system of arches from completely collapsing (Kelikian 2011; Snell 2008). This stabilization function is very important to reducing the risk of injury, and it requires all areas of the foot to function correctly. The foot also sends signals to the brain about the terrain so that future interactions with the ground can be predicted (Price and Bratcher 2010).

As you can see, the feet and ankles are very sophisticated structures, and they can bear a lot of stress. Any injury or malalignment in these structures will be amplified because they never entirely get to rest, especially during weight-bearing activities. Therefore, it is crucial that the foot and ankle complex are healthy and aligned and functioning as well as possible.

COMMON DEVIATIONS

There are two main musculoskeletal deviations that cause pain, injury, and movement dysfunction in the foot and ankle area (Hertel 2002):

- Overpronation
- Lack of dorsiflexion

Pronation is a normal and necessary function that occurs when the foot and ankle roll inward (and forward) toward the midline of the body when the foot makes contact with the terrain. This movement causes the heel to roll inward (eversion), causes the ankle to bend forward (dorsiflexion), causes the lower leg to rotate inward, and causes the foot to move outward slightly (abduction). These movements allow the body to transfer weight forward, from side to side, and in rotation. **Overpronation** occurs when the foot collapses or rolls too far inward for normal function. This excessive movement toward the inside of the body causes the heel and ankle to fall inward, limiting the forward movement of the foot and ankle and causing the arch along the inside of the foot to flatten. It can also make the foot turn too far out to compensate for the excessive transfer of pressure toward the midline of the body that occurs when the foot collapses (Hertel 2002; Lowe 2009). While overpronation occurs at the foot and ankle, it can disrupt movement throughout the entire body (Kendall, McCreary and Provance 2005).

Dorsiflexion occurs at the ankle and is an essential component of pronation. It involves bringing the lower leg over the foot (or vice versa), and it occurs during all weight-bearing activities when the foot is in contact with the ground. Examples include the movement of the lower legs over the feet when squatting, and swinging the leg forward and lifting the foot to clear the ground when walking. Overpronation causes the lower leg, ankle, and foot to collapse in toward the midline of the body too much. This limits proper forward movement of the ankle and results in a **lack of dorsiflexion** (Hertel 2002). When people cannot dorsiflex through a full range of motion, it impairs not only the foot and ankle functions but other movements as well (Cook 2010).

> **Go to the online video to watch video 2.1, where Justin talks about common deviations of the feet and ankles.**

Common foot and ankle imbalances typically occur together, meaning that a person who overpronates almost always lacks dorsiflexion. It is far more common for people to overpronate than to oversupinate. Since the aim of this text is to cover the most common deviations you may see as a fitness professional, oversupination will not be discussed.

ASSESSMENT PROCESS

Having reviewed the structural anatomy of the feet and ankles and the common imbalances clients may have, we now move on to the detailed procedures for assessing these areas of the body. As stated in chapter 1, the foot and ankle assessment process should begin with a verbal assessment.

VERBAL ASSESSMENT

When assessing the feet and ankles, it is important to learn how clients perceive their condition or pain, both in isolation and in relation to other body areas and when performing activities (Price and Bratcher 2010). Ask about the following topics, and write down any pertinent information on the Client Assessment Diagram (CAD) as you conduct the assessment.

1. Ask if the client has ever experienced pain in the feet or ankles, and ask for the specific location of the pain (e.g., is it at the side or front of the ankle, under the heel or the arch of the foot, at the back of the foot on the Achilles tendon, in the toes or on top of the foot). Encouraging verbal descriptions will help you better understand the client and her individual needs (Petty and Moore 2002). For example, if a client has pain on the underside of her foot, it may be a sign that her medial longitudinal arch is stressed. This will prompt you to check for signs of overpronation when you perform the visual and hands-on assessments.

2. Ask if the client has arthritis or any other diagnosed condition that may affect musculoskeletal health. This will help you not only to understand the integrity of the joints and other structures you are assessing, but also to identify factors beyond your control that may affect the success of a corrective exercise program. For example, clients with severe arthritis may still experience aches in the joint, even after you have helped them address their musculoskeletal imbalances. However, do not let a diagnosis of arthritis discourage you from trying to help clients reduce their pain and improve their functional capabilities. Alignment is always the key to reducing stress or pain in the joints, even in cases of arthritis (Miller 1995).

3. Ask about the client's past injuries or surgeries. Note when the injury or surgery took place, what part of the foot or ankle was affected, the diagnosis (if any) that was made by a licensed medical professional, and the name of the physical therapist, doctor, or surgeon who examined the injury or performed the surgery. Gather as much information as possible so you can follow up with the medical professional to gain insight about how the injury or surgery might affect the design, implementation, and success of a corrective exercise program (Petty and Moore 2002).

4. Ask about the client's level of physical activity. Find out how often the person engages in those activities, to what degree of intensity, and for how long. This will help you understand the types and amounts of stress clients place on their bodies (Petty and Moore 2002). For example, if a client with knee pain is an avid runner and she plans to run the same number of miles during her corrective exercise program, this will directly affect her potential success.

5. Ask about the client's job. This will help you to understand the normal physical stresses he experiences (Petty and Moore 2002). A postal carrier will have more stress on his feet and ankles than a computer technician.

6. Ask the client whether her feet or ankles ever prevent her from engaging in an activity or limits what she can do. The answer to this question will help you to understand the underlying motivation for why the client has come to see you (Price and Bratcher 2010). If foot pain is preventing a client from playing tennis, for example, then knowing this from the outset will enable you to relate the benefit of certain exercises to how she can get back to playing tennis if she adheres to the program.

7. Ask if the client's ankle or foot pain coincides with any other pains or symptoms in the body. This will help you to establish causal links between symptoms and activities or circumstances. It also gets clients thinking about how problems in the body can be related. For example, if a client is complaining of ankle pain but also notices that his back hurts when his ankle hurts, then he will be more likely to perform the exercises you design to help align his hips and lower back, knowing that this will also help his ankle feel better.

8. Ask the client what aggravates her condition and what makes it feel better. This will help you to establish the source of the pain. For example, if a client's back pain is worse in the morning, it might be a good idea to evaluate her sleeping position (Petty and Moore 2002). If her pain feels better after she performs an

exercise that she learned in the past, you have the opportunity to review her technique, gather additional clues about a potential cause, and praise her successful adaptation of this beneficial exercise.

Once you have concluded the verbal portion of the assessment, ask the client to remove his shoes and socks for the visual and hands-on assessments.

VISUAL AND HANDS-ON ASSESSMENT

The visual and hands-on portion of the assessment process is used to gain additional information about the condition of a client's feet and ankles. It is also used to confirm or challenge assumptions you might have made during the verbal assessment.

VISUAL ASSESSMENTS

Begin the visual portion of the assessment by asking the client to stand in front of you and facing you. Explain that you will be carefully looking at the condition of his feet and ankles. Specifically, you will be looking for any swelling, calluses, or irregularities between the feet, ankles, and toes.

Evaluate for Overpronation

In order to visually determine the extent and type of pronation in a client's feet, make sure the client is standing on both feet and facing you. Look at the area that runs along the inside of each foot. If the arch is dropped or absent or if a bulge of flesh sticks out on the inside of one or both of the client's feet, this indicates that the client overpronates (see figure 2.3) (Schamberger 2002).

Evaluate for Foot Abduction or Adduction

With the client still standing in front of you, check the position of his feet. Note whether one or both feet are facing forward, if one or both feet are adducted (turned inward "like a pigeon"), or if one or both feet are abducted (turned outward "like a duck") from the midline of the body (see figure 2.4). An abducted or adducted position of the feet may indicate overpronation (Schamberger 2002). For example, a client with an overpronated foot may also abduct her foot when standing because overpronation produces an internal rotation of the lower leg, which causes the knee to turn toward the midline of the body. As a result, she may turn her foot outward to realign the knee to face forward (Price and Bratcher 2010).

Most people who overpronate will abduct rather than adduct their feet. Occasionally, though, you may come across a client who adducts (i.e., turns in) one foot. This problem is usually also caused by overpronation. As previously discussed, when a person overpronates, the foot and ankle move toward the midline of the body. This causes the knee to also move toward the midline. To compensate for this change in knee position, the person will turn the foot outward so that the knee faces forward. However, in clients who are bowlegged or have another congenital condition that affects the alignment and position of their legs, their knees may actually be oriented toward the outside of the body. These clients may overpronate, but they may also turn their feet inward to make their knees face forward.

Check the Big Toes

Calluses, bunions, and crooked toes may also be evidence of common musculoskeletal imbalances in

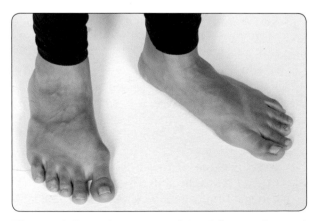

Figure 2.3   Absence of inside arch and ankles rolled inward indicate an overpronated foot position.

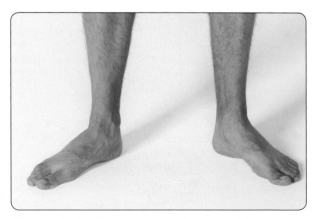

Figure 2.4   Example of abducted foot position.

the feet and ankles, so it is important to ascertain the condition of the client's toes (Arnot 2003). Look at the big toe of each foot to determine if the first joint of that toe is swollen, has a bunion, or looks as though it points away from the midline rather than straight ahead (see figure 2.5). If the big toe on one or both feet is not straight, this may indicate that the client overpronates. When a person overpronates, the foot collapses and weight is transferred toward the centerline of the body. This transfer of weight across the foot before it can pass over the end of the big toe can cause any of the following: irritation on the inside of the big toe (e.g., a callus), inflammation and additional bone growth on the first joint of the big toe (a bunion), or a shift of the big toe toward the other toes (hallux valgus).

Check the Lesser Toes

The term *lesser toes* refers to all toes but the big toes. Structural imbalances of the feet and ankles and certain types of footwear can cause many abnormalities in the lesser toes. These irregularities are often called hammertoes, claw toes, or mallet toes, and they can be very painful (see figure 2.6) (Arnot 2003). To assess a client for these issues, look at the lesser toes to see if they curl up, form a claw, or look as though they are always flexed. Visual abnormalities of the lesser toes may be an indication that the client overpronates because weight is no longer passing correctly over the forefoot and the ends of the toes.

 Go to the online video to watch video 2.2, where Justin demonstrates the visual assessments for overpronation.

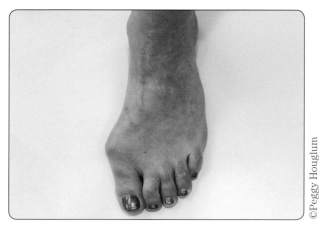

Figure 2.5   Example of hallux valgus and a bunion.

©Peggy Houglum

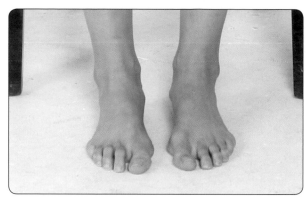

Figure 2.6   Example of irregularities of the lesser toes.

HANDS-ON ASSESSMENTS

Once the visual assessments for the feet and ankles are complete, begin the hands-on portion of the assessment process. Tell the client that you will now be manually evaluating his feet and ankles in order to confirm or refute your visual assessment findings. You will be looking for any irregular joint positions in the ankle and excessive tension in the soft tissue structures of the feet and lower legs. Remember to always ask permission before touching a client or performing any hands-on assessments.

Evaluate the Position of the Talus Bone

The talus bone, which is located in the ankle just below the lower leg bones, helps dissipate some of the side-to-side stresses in the foot and ankle during weight-bearing activities. Evaluating the position of the talus bone will help confirm whether a client overpronates and to what extent (Muscolino 2009).

To assess the position of the talus bone, ask the client to stand facing you with both feet straight and pointed forward. Kneel down and place the thumb and index finger of your right hand on either side of the client's left ankle just below the anklebones (malleolus). You will feel a dimple or indentation on both sides of the ankle. On the inside of the ankle, the dimple is just below and behind the large tendon of the tibialis anterior, the muscle that pulls the foot toward the shin. On the outside of the ankle, the dimple is just below and behind the tendon of the extensor digitorum longus, the muscle that lifts the lesser toes toward the shin (Gray 1995).

When you first begin practicing this assessment, you will find it easier to locate these dimples by asking clients to roll the weight on the foot to the outside (i.e., to supinate) and to pull the foot and the big toe upward using the muscles in the front of the shin.

This will help expose the tendon on the inside of the ankle and highlight the dimpled area where you will place your thumb (see figure 2.7a). Once you have located this position, ask your client to pronate (i.e., roll the weight on the foot to the inside) and pull the lesser toes upward using the muscles in the shin. This will help expose the tendons of the lesser toes on the outside of the ankle and will highlight the dimpled area where you will place your index finger (see figure 2.7b) (Price and Bratcher 2010).

Position your thumb and forefinger and press firmly in the center of the dimples on the inside and outside of the ankle (see figure 2.8). Then ask the client to roll the ankle from side to side in order to raise and lower the arch of the foot (supinate and pronate). As the client rolls the ankle inward, you will feel pressure under your thumb on the inside of the ankle. This is the talus bone pushing into your thumb. As she rolls the ankle outward, you will feel pressure under your forefinger. This is the talus bone moving the other way. Coach your clients to slowly roll the ankle in and out, and stop them in the position when the pressure under your thumb and forefinger feels even.

When you feel even pressure under your thumb and forefinger, instruct your client to hold the foot and ankle in that position. This is the neutral position for the talus bone and the correct position for the foot and ankle in an upright standing position (Magee and Sueki 2011). If the person you are assessing habitually overpronates, then a neutral foot and ankle position will likely feel awkward, as though the weight were all on the outside of the foot. Reassure these clients that it is normal to feel that way because their feet and ankles are used to collapsing under the weight of the body rather than supporting and transferring it correctly.

Now switch hands and use your left thumb and forefinger to assess the position of the talus bone on the client's right foot.

Go to the online video to watch video 2.3, where Justin demonstrates the hands-on assessment for overpronation.

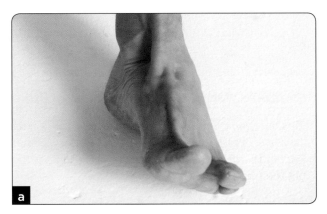 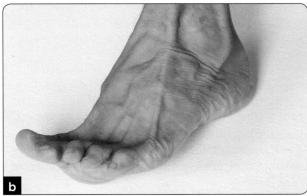

Figure 2.7   *(a)* Dimple on medial side of ankle. *(b)* Dimple on lateral side of ankle.

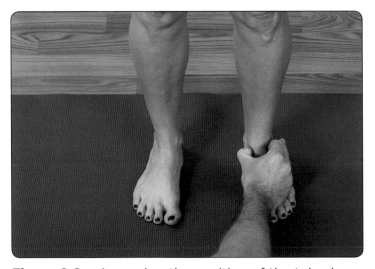

Figure 2.8   Assessing the position of the talus bone.

Once the assessment is done, teach clients visually and kinesthetically how to find the neutral position so they can see and feel what it is like to stand with their feet and ankles in alignment. Teaching them to evaluate themselves enables them to achieve this position on their own. They might even communicate the technique to a friend, colleague, or family member, which could result in another person seeking your help to design a corrective exercise program.

Evaluate the Condition of the Calf Muscles

Musculoskeletal imbalances in the feet and ankles will adversely affect the calf muscles (Kendall, McCreary and Provance 2005). As the foot overpronates, the heel rolls inward, pulling on the Achilles tendon and on the gastrocnemius and soleus, the calf muscles on the back of the lower leg that attach to the heel via that tendon. This excessive pulling causes these muscles to become sore and to lose their flexibility. If these muscles cannot lengthen effectively, then the foot and ankle will not be able to dorsiflex well. This lack of dorsiflexion can compress the structures at the front of the ankle and cause inflammation and irritation of the Achilles tendon (Barnes 1999).

Ask the client to lie down on the floor on her back with her knees bent. Kneel beside the client with one leg forward and lift the lower part of one of the client's legs. Rest the client's foot on your knee and use your thumb and forefinger to squeeze the belly of the client's calf muscle (see figure 2.9). You are looking for the presence of trigger points, nodules, or excessive muscle tension. If you are unsure whether what you are feeling is a tight or tender spot, ask the client to tell you what she is feeling when you squeeze the calf. Repeat the assessment on the other leg. Make a note of any findings, including tenderness, on the CAD.

Evaluate the Condition of the Plantar Fascia

The plantar fascia is a broad, dense, fairly rigid connective tissue that runs the length of the underside of the foot. Forces from the body above and ground reaction forces from below put enormous stress on the plantar surface of the foot during weight-bearing activities such as walking and running (Hyde and Gegenbach 2007). Musculoskeletal imbalances, such as overpronation and lack of dorsiflexion, increase stresses on the plantar fascia. Over time, these can cause the tissue to become overstressed, dysfunctional, and painful (Snell 2008).

To assess the condition of the plantar fascia, ask the client to lie down on the floor on her back with her knees bent. Kneel beside the client with one leg forward and lift the lower part of one of the client's legs. Rest the client's foot on your knee and press your thumbs or fingers into the arches and sole of each of her feet from the heel to the toes (see figure 2.10). Note any tenderness or painful areas, and record them on the CAD. If you are not sure whether you are feeling a tight or tender spot, ask for the client's feedback. The sorest spot for most people will usually be just forward of the heel at the highest part of the arch or just behind the first joint of the big toe (Hobrough 2016).

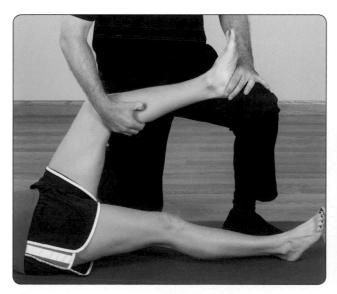

Figure 2.9 Assessing the calf muscle.

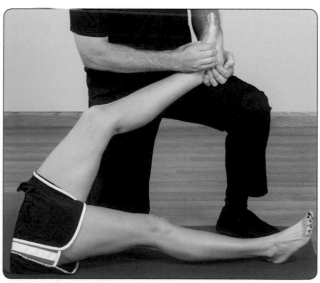

Figure 2.10 Assessing the plantar fascia.

By the end of the foot and ankle assessment, you will have been able to help your clients understand any musculoskeletal imbalances in these areas as well as explain how those imbalances affect their knees. While the assessments you have just completed can reveal specific issues in the feet and ankles, they also begin to demonstrate the interconnectedness of all of the body's parts. This is important because it helps clients to understand that the site of their pain or dysfunction is not always the source of their problem. Therefore, before progressing to the verbal, visual, and hands-on assessments for the knees, briefly sum up your findings about the client's feet and ankles. Make sure you have completed the CAD for this body area, and briefly describe how the feet and ankles relate to the knees (see How the Feet and Ankles Relate to the Knees). Communicating this information to your clients will also help you to move seamlessly into the next part of the assessment process.

HOW THE FEET AND ANKLES RELATE TO THE KNEES

The feet and ankles form the foundation of the human body. As with any structure, the integrity of the foundation affects everything above it, and the weight above has a direct impact on the foundation. Therefore, the condition of the feet and ankles will influence the performance of all weight-bearing activities, such as standing, bending, reaching, squatting, walking, running, and lunging (Schamberger 2002).

When the foot overpronates, it causes the lower leg to roll inward and the heel bone to collapse toward the midline of the body. This collapsing inward of the foot, ankle, and lower leg results in a lack of dorsiflexion—that is, the foot, ankle, and lower leg do not come forward over the foot correctly. Simply put, if the foot and ankle collapse in too much, they cannot come forward enough. Since the soleus and gastrocnemius muscles are attached to the heel bone, this collapsing of the foot and ankle affects the function of these muscles and further limits dorsiflexion (Lowe 2009).

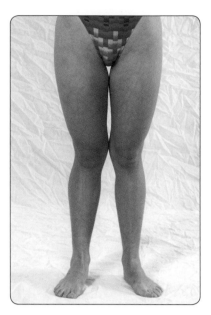

Figure 2.11   Valgus knee position.

The internal movement of the lower leg caused by overpronation also affects the position of the knee, since the bottom of the knee joint sits directly atop the tibia and fibula. Overpronation causes a valgus knee position, that is, an inward displacement of the knee (see figure 2.11) (Johnson and Pedowitz 2007). Excessive inward movement or displacement of the knee joint can result in tracking problems in which the kneecap does not glide smoothly over the femoral groove as it should (Johnson and Pedowitz 2007).

Lack of dorsiflexion in the ankle also directly affects the function of the knee when it is both bending (flexing) and straightening (extending). For example, many weight-bearing activities like squatting and lunging require the ankle to bend forward at the same time the knee is bending (figure 2.12).

Other weight-bearing activities like walking and running require the ankle to bend forward while the knee is straightening (figure 2.13). However, if the foot and ankle complex lacks dorsiflexion, the knee joint must compensate for this lack of movement in the ankle, and pain and injury can result (Cook 2010).

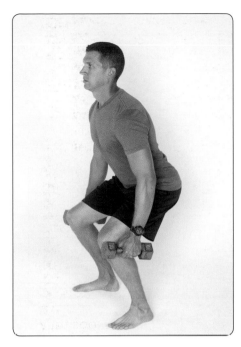

Figure 2.12 Ankle in dorsiflexion when knee is bent.

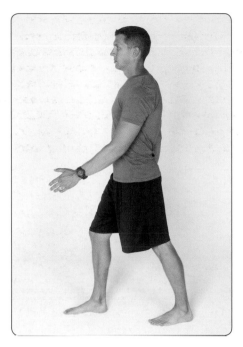

Figure 2.13 Ankle in dorsiflexion when knee is straight.

Assessment Checklist

Before you move on to assess the knees, you must answer the following questions about the feet and ankles:

- ❏ Do you fully understand what type of pain the client is experiencing in her feet and ankles and how this affects their function?
- ❏ Does the client have any arthritis or diagnosed conditions that might affect the success of her program?
- ❏ What makes the client's feet and ankles feel better or worse?
- ❏ Does the foot and ankle pain limit her function in any way?
- ❏ Are other parts of the client's body affected when her feet and ankles hurt?

- ❏ Are the client's feet overpronated?
- ❏ Are the client's feet abducted or adducted?
- ❏ What is the condition of the client's big and lesser toes?
- ❏ What is the condition of the client's calf muscles and plantar fascia?
- ❏ Does the client know how to achieve a neutral foot and ankle position when standing?
- ❏ Do you and the client know how her feet and ankles relate to her knees?

Enter your notes for this part of the assessment on the Client Assessment Diagram (see figure 2.14 for an example).

Feet and ankles	✔	Details
Pain?	✔	lateral R ankle
Arthritis/conditions?	✔	none reported
Function?	✔	limited dorsiflexion both sides
What makes better/worse?	✔	running
Causal links?	✔	medial knee pain R
Visual irregularities?	✔	swelling inside R ankle
Pronated?	✔	R foot O/pronated
Abducted/adducted?	✔	R foot abducted
Condition of toes?	✔	big toes normal, lesser flexed on R
Condition of plantar fascia?	✔	very painful R
Condition of calf muscle?	✔	both sides tight
Client knows neutral?	✔	can achieve

Figure 2.14   Sample of completed foot and ankle assessment on Client Assessment Diagram.

Review of Key Points

Musculoskeletal imbalances in the feet and ankles can be greatly intensiefied by forces transferred both from above and below.

■ The two most common deviations of the feet and ankles are
   1. overpronation and
   2. lack of dorsiflexion.

■ Calluses or bunions on or around the big toe, or a big toe that has moved away from the midline of the body toward the lesser toes, may be visual clues that a person overpronates.

■ Overpronation is far more common than oversupination. Even a foot with an apparent "high arch" can be overpronated. Therefore, you must perform the hands-on assessment of the talus bone; you cannot rely solely on visual clues.

■ Determine your clients' level and type of physical activity in order to understand the amount of stress they place on their feet and ankles. This information, in addition to identifying what activities cause or alleviate pain, can help you to determine what soft tissue structures may be involved.

■ Overpronation contributes to a reduced ability to dorsiflex because as the foot and ankle collapse inward too much, they lose their ability to come forward enough. This also causes the calf muscles to lose their ability to function through a full range of movement.

■ Structural deviations in the feet and ankles directly affect the alignment and function of the knees.

■ Record any pertinent information on the Client Assessment Diagram.

Self-Check

Assess the condition of your own feet and ankles to determine the state of your foundation. Remove your shoes and socks, and check for the following signs of wear and tear.

Do you have...	Yes	No	Where/which side
Bunions			
Tender or sore plantar fascia			
Hammer or claw toes			
Pain in and around the ankle joint			
Valgus position of big toe			
Calluses			
Abducted foot position			
Tight or sore calf muscles			

Now check to see whether you overpronate by using a modified version of the talus bone assessment procedure detailed in the hands-on assessment section Evaluate the Position of the Talus Bone. Reach down with your right hand to assess your right ankle. Repeat assessment on your left ankle with your left hand.

Do you overpronate? _____

Use the talus bone assessment to find a neutral position for your foot and ankle. Assess both sides until you feel confident that you can find the correct position.

Can you find a neutral position for your feet and ankles? _____

Once you can achieve a neutral position in your own feet and ankles, practice the assessment on someone else.

Structural Assessment Skills Test

Perform a complete foot and ankle assessment on another person. Record your findings in the following chart.

Feet and ankles	✔	Details
Pain?		
Arthritis/conditions?		
Function?		
What makes better/worse?		
Causal links?		
Visual irregularities?		
Pronated?		
Abducted/adducted?		
Condition of toes?		
Condition of plantar fascia?		
Condition of calf muscles?		
Client knows neutral?		

CHAPTER 3

Assessing the Knees

The knee is a relatively simple structure whose movement is fairly limited when compared to the other joints of the body. The primary functions of the knee are flexion and extension and linking the upper leg to the lower leg to allow kinetic chain movements. The knee can also move in small degrees of rotation and very minimally from side to side (Hyde and Gengenbach 2007).

The structural integrity of the knees can be compromised when the feet and ankles and the lumbo-pelvic hip girdle are not working correctly. This is because the muscles that help stabilize the knees have origins and insertions in these two areas (Price and Bratcher 2010). Consequently, musculoskeletal issues in the feet and ankles or in the lumbo-pelvic hip girdle can result in the knees bearing the brunt of imbalances in structures above or below them.

BASIC ANATOMY

The main components of the knee joint are the femur, tibia, fibula, patella, menisci, quadriceps tendon, patellar ligament, collateral ligaments (see figure 3.1), and cruciate ligaments (see figure 3.2).

The **patella** (kneecap) is a small bone in the center of the knee. It is attached to the quadriceps muscles of the thigh via the **quadriceps tendon**. As the quadriceps tendon passes over the patella, it morphs into the **patellar ligament**, which then attaches the patella to the **tibia** of the lower leg.

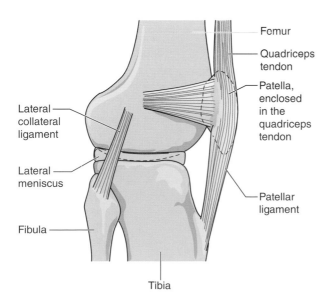

Figure 3.1 Basic anatomy of the knee.

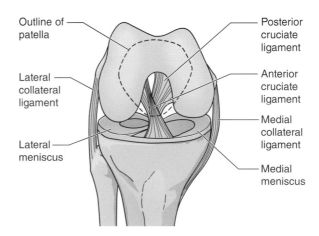

Figure 3.2 Cruciate ligaments of the knee.

(The **fibula** is located beside the tibia on the lateral side of the lower leg.) The correct alignment of the **femur** (upper leg bone) and tibia allows the patella to glide smoothly over the femoral groove at the bottom of the femur (Dimon and Day 2008).

Two C-shaped discs called **menisci** (singular *meniscus*) lie between the femur and the tibia. The menisci are made from cartilage and act as shock absorbers between the bones of the upper leg and the lower leg (Dimon and Day 2008).

The medial and lateral collateral ligaments are on either side of the knee joint. The **medial collateral ligament** acts as a guide rope between the tibia and femur, and the **lateral collateral ligament** acts as a guide rope between the fibula and femur to give side-to-side stability to the knee (Hyde and Gengenbach 2007).

The **anterior** and **posterior cruciate ligaments** are located inside the knee joint; they attach diagonally to the femur and the tibia. The cruciate ligaments provide stability and minimize rotational stress across the knee joint. They also prevent excessive forward or backward movement of the tibia in relation to the femur (Hyde and Gengenbach 2007).

COMMON DEVIATIONS

There are two main deviations that can cause pain, injury, and movement dysfunction in the knee area (Hamel and Knutzen 2003):

- Problems with side-to-side alignment (e.g., a valgus knee)
- Tracking problems during flexion and extension

Side-to-side alignment refers to the alignment of the femur and tibia and the movement and position of these bones in relation to the centerline of the body. Side-to-side alignment problems can occur when the knee collapses in toward the midline of the body (a *valgus* position) or toward the outside of the body (a *varus* position); in these cases the muscles and soft tissue structures cannot properly manage forces on the knee joint. The most common side-to-side alignment imbalance is a valgus position of one or both knees (Hamel and Knutzen 2003). Over time, this condition can cause the kneecap to be pulled laterally so that it no longer moves correctly over the femoral groove. Side-to-side alignment problems typically disrupt function when a person is engaged in dynamic, weight-bearing movements, such as walking, running, squatting, lunging, or going up and down stairs. However, chronic or severe side-to-side alignment issues can also manifest during static activities, such as standing.

Tracking problems of the knee during flexion and extension can occur when the kneecap does not glide smoothly over the bottom of the femur (femoral groove) as it should when the knee bends and straightens. Tracking problems place an abnormal amount of pressure on the underside of the kneecap. Over time, this excessive pressure can cause inflammation and irritation, resulting in pain and dysfunction (Hamel and Knutzen 2003). When the knee bends and straightens (i.e., moves in the sagittal plane), the thighbone above the knee and the tibia and fibula below the knee also move from side to side and rotate to some extent. Therefore, tracking problems during flexion and extension also affect movements in the frontal and transverse planes—that is, from side to side and in rotation.

ASSESSMENT PROCESS

Having reviewed the structural anatomy and common imbalances of the knees, we now turn to the detailed assessment procedures.

VERBAL ASSESSMENT

It is important to learn how clients perceive their condition or pain, both in isolation and in relation to other body areas and activities (Price and Bratcher 2010). Ask about the following topics, and write down any pertinent information on the Client Assessment Diagram (CAD).

1. Ask whether the client has ever experienced knee pain, and ask for the specific location of the pain (Petty and Moore 2002). For example, if the pain is on the medial side of the knee, it may mean that this side is being stressed by the way the client moves, possibly indicating a valgus knee displacement. This will prompt you to check for this imbalance as you move into the visual and hands-on portion of the assessment process.

2. Ask whether the client has arthritis or any other diagnosed condition that may affect the musculoskeletal health of her knees.

3. Ask the client about any past injuries or surgeries. Note when the injury or surgery took place, what was done, the diagnoses, and the name(s) of medical practitioners involved. A procedure such as a total knee replacement will affect both movement and function (Petty and Moore 2002).

4. Ask about the client's level of physical activity. For example, it would be important to know

if the person you are assessing plays sports or runs often. This will help you to gauge the amount of stress he places on his knees during a typical day or week, and it will help you understand whether his knees will be able to rest and recover during a corrective exercise program (Petty and Moore 2002).

5. Ask about the client's occupation (Petty and Moore 2002). It would be important to know if someone is a gardener or a carpet layer who kneels all day long. Kneeling can put a lot of stress on the kneecap. Over time, this could affect the correct functioning of the knee and the ultimate success of a corrective exercise program.

6. Ask the client whether her knees ever prevent her from engaging in an activity or limit what she can do. This will help you to understand why she has come to see you and what she hopes to be able to do after she has regained full function or alleviated her pain (Price and Bratcher 2010).

7. Ask whether the client's knee pain occurs with any other pains or symptoms. This will help the client to understand the body's interconnectedness and will promote adherence to a corrective exercise program (Price and Bratcher 2010). For example, if a client notices that her knee hurts only when she wears a particular pair of shoes, you can use this opportunity to educate her about how foot and ankle movements affect her knees and coach her to choose more appropriate footwear (see Footwear and the Role of Orthotics in chapter 18).

8. Ask the client what aggravates his condition and what makes it feel better. This will help him understand how daily activities can affect the success of his program (Petty and Moore 2002). For example, if riding his bicycle aggravates a client's knees, you can use this opportunity to evaluate the height of his bicycle seat. You may find that raising the seat helps decrease knee flexion reducing stress to his knee.

Once you have concluded the verbal portion of the assessment process, move on to the visual and hands-on assessments.

VISUAL AND HANDS-ON ASSESSMENTS

When assessing the knees, you must have a clear view of the structures you are evaluating. Clients who are not wearing shorts should be asked to pull up their pant legs to reveal the knees and to remain barefooted (following their foot and ankle assessment). Remember to ask permission to touch a client before performing any hands-on assessments.

VISUAL ASSESSMENTS

Begin the assessment by asking the client to stand facing you with her feet hip width apart. Look for swelling on or around the knee(s), and identify any other irregularities, such as muscle size differences and scarring (see figure 3.3) (Magee, Zachazewski, and Quillen 2009). Make a note of any abnormalities on the CAD.

Next, assess for side-to-side alignment. This involves two steps. The first is a static visual evaluation of the position of the center of the kneecap. The second step is a visual evaluation of the center of the kneecap in a dynamic situation, such as during a single-leg squat.

To assess the kneecap in a static position, look at the middle of the client's knee while she is standing in front of you. Draw an imaginary line from the kneecap to the middle of the ankle. Draw another imaginary line from the kneecap to the center of the

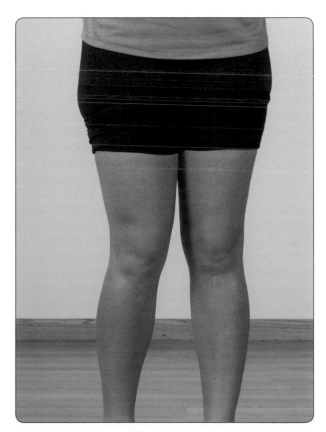

Figure 3.3   Swelling of the knee and scarring are visual irregularities.

front of the client's upper leg (where the quadriceps muscles originate). Note whether the intersection of the two lines at the kneecap deviates too far in or out (see figure 3.4) (Hamel and Knutzen 2003).

The thighbone is naturally angled inward toward the knee. Therefore, the knee joint should be positioned closer to the midline than the center of the hip. This angle of the thighbone in relation to the center of the knee, called the Q angle, is quantified in degrees (see figure 3.5). A Q angle in males of more than approximately 15 degrees is considered abnormal, and a Q angle of more than 18 degrees in females is also considered abnormal (a greater angle is allowed in females due to their wider hips) (Fernandez des-la-Penas, Cleland, and Dommerholt 2016; Frisch 1994). Remember that the purpose of this visual assessment is simply to gauge whether a client's knees appear to deviate excessively inward or outward. The precise Q angle is not vital to this assessment, so the technical protocols for measuring it will not be discussed.

To visually assess the kneecap in a dynamic setting, ask the client to stand on one leg facing you. While the client is in this position, ask her to perform a shallow squat, bending the knee of the standing leg to approximately 30 degrees. As she moves, watch the center of her kneecap, and note whether it moves excessively toward or away from the centerline of her body. It is normal for the knee to move toward the midline of the body as a person squats. In this assessment you are looking for excessive or uncontrolled motion of the knee toward the midline, as shown in figure 3.6.

Do *not* ask clients with severe knee pain to do a single-leg squat. This will add stress to the knee, and it may make their condition worse. Simply perform the static visual assessment to get an idea of the placement of the center of the kneecap.

You can also visually assess the knee for side-to-side alignment problems from behind. Ask the client to stand on one leg facing away from you and to squat to about 30 degrees. Watch the center of the buttock or the sit bone (ischial tuberosity) as she performs this movement. Ideally, as the client squats, the center of her gluteus maximus muscle should lower down just to the side of the center of her heel. There may be an indication of knee alignment problems if the glutes and hip move excessively in a swishing "salsa dance hip" movement away from the centerline of the body (see figure 3.7). If this does happen, the knee will usually move disproportionately toward the centerline to compensate (McLester and St. Pierre 2008).

HANDS-ON ASSESSMENTS

Once the visual assessments for the knees are complete, begin the hands-on portion of the assessment process. Tell the client that you will now be manually evaluating her knees in order to confirm or refute your visual assessment findings. You will be feeling for unusual movements and listening for any irregular sounds as you bend and straighten the knee joint.

Ask the client to lie on the ground on her back. Kneel beside her and coach her to bend one knee.

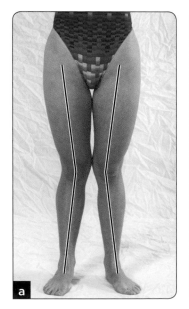 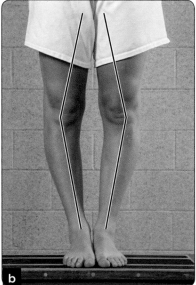

Figure 3.4 Examples of *(a)* valgus and *(b)* varus knee positions.

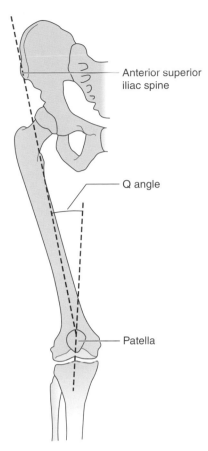

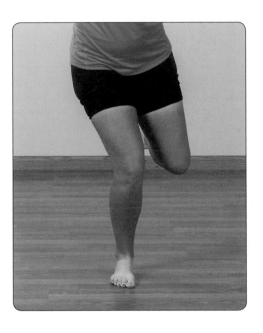

Figure 3.6   Example of valgus displacement of the knee during dynamic assessment.

Figure 3.5   Example of Q angle.

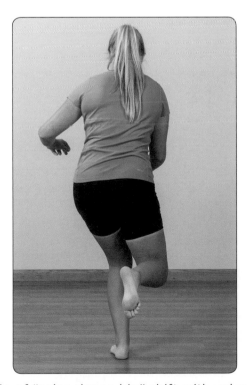

Figure 3.7   Example of "salsa dance hip" shift with valgus knee displacement.

Place one hand on the client's kneecap and use your other hand to bend and straighten the leg two to three times (see figure 3.8). Do not press down excessively on either the kneecap or the lower leg as you perform this assessment. As you bend and straighten the leg, feel the kneecap as it glides over the bottom of the upper leg. If you hear or feel any grinding, crunching, cracking, or popping, then there is probably a tracking issue (Frisch 1994). If the client experiences pain of any kind, stop the assessment immediately.

As you finish the knee assessment process, you can help the client understand how to achieve a neutral position for the knee and explain how better knee alignment can prevent pain and dysfunction not only in the knee itself, but also in the feet and ankles or in the lumbo-pelvic hip area.

TEACHING CLIENTS NEUTRAL POSITION OF THE KNEE

Teaching clients to achieve a neutral position for the knee when standing can help them to better understand how the parts of the body affect each other. Begin by instructing the client to try to attain a neutral foot and ankle position using the technique described in chapter 2 (Evaluate the Position of the Talus Bone). When this position is achieved, the knees should naturally align so that the centers of the client's kneecaps are in line with the second toes (Clippinger 2016). Coach the client to feel what happens to the gluteal muscles as they contract

to rotate the upper and lower leg outward into a more neutral position. You can further help a client align his knees by coaching him to posteriorly tilt his pelvis (i.e., tuck it under) so that the curvature decreases in the lumbar spine. Posteriorly tilting the pelvis will also externally rotate the upper and lower leg, which will also help align the foot and ankle (Kendall, McCreary, and Provance 2005).

Sometimes, a person may not be able to achieve perfect knee-to-foot-and-ankle alignment. This usually happens when the client has severe or long-term alignment problems, bow legs, or another congenital abnormality (Price and Bratcher 2010). Coach these clients to get as close to neutral in the foot, ankle, and knee as possible so that they can feel what it is like (and what muscles and movements are involved) to achieve better alignment.

Before progressing to the verbal, visual, and hands-on assessments for the lumbo-pelvic hip girdle, concisely sum up your findings about the client's knees. Make sure you have completed the CAD for this area, and briefly describe for the client how the knees relate to the structures above and below them (see the next section).

HOW THE KNEES RELATE TO THE FEET AND ANKLES AND THE LUMBO-PELVIC HIP GIRDLE

The knee is the structure that bridges the feet and ankles and the lumbo-pelvic hip girdle. Therefore, any imbalances or malalignments in the structures

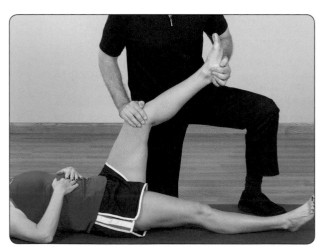
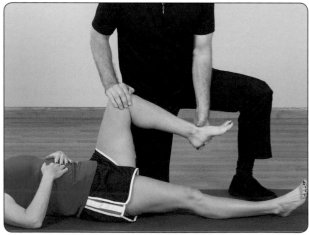

Figure 3.8 Patella tracking assessment.

above or below it will directly affect how the knee feels and functions. For example, during the single-leg squat assessment, you should have noticed that a valgus knee is usually accompanied by overpronation of the foot and ankle complex. This is because as the foot and ankle collapse toward the midline during overpronation, the lower leg also rotates inward excessively, pulling the knee into a valgus position. This movement of the knee also causes the thighbone to rotate inward, affecting the position of the hip socket (where the upper leg articulates with the pelvis). Because of this change in position of the upper leg and hip socket, the pelvis shifts out of alignment by rotating down and forward. This change in position of the pelvis causes the lower back to arch excessively (see figure 3.9) (Kendall, McCreary, and Provance 2005; Price and Bratcher 2010).

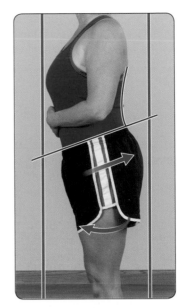

Figure 3.9 Compensations of pelvis caused by excessive inward rotation of upper and lower leg.

Go to the online video to watch video 3.1, where Justin talks about how the feet and ankles relate to the knees and lumbo-pelvic hip girdle.

Assessment Checklist

Before you move on to assess the lumbo-pelvic hip girdle, you must answer the following questions about the knees:

- ❏ Do you know what type of pain the client is experiencing and how it affects the function of her knees?
- ❏ Does the client have arthritis or any diagnosed conditions that might affect the success of her program?
- ❏ What makes the client's knees feel better or worse?
- ❏ Does the client's knee pain limit her function in any way?
- ❏ Are other parts of the client's body affected when her knees are painful?

- ❏ Are there any visual irregularities between the client's knees?
- ❏ Does the client have a valgus position in one or both knees?
- ❏ Are there any problems with the client's kneecap tracking?
- ❏ Does the client know how to achieve a neutral knee and foot position when standing?
- ❏ Do you know how the foot and ankle and lumbo-pelvic hip girdle relate to the knees, and can you explain it to your client?

Make all your notations for this part of the assessment on the Client Assessment Diagram (see figure 3.10 for an example).

Knees	✔	Details
Pain?	✔	medial R
Arthritis/conditions?	✔	none reported
Function?	✔	hurts when standing
What makes better/worse?	✔	sitting for long periods
Causal links?	✔	issues at foot and hip on R
Visual irregularities?	✔	swelling on R
Single-leg squat?	✔	valgus R
Patella tracking?	✔	popping on R
Client knows neutral?	✔	can achieve

Figure 3.10 Sample of completed knee assessment on Client Assessment Diagram.

Review of Key Points

The knee joint is primarily a hinge joint that connects the lower leg and the upper leg. Malalignments or imbalances in the more mobile joints of the feet and ankles or the lumbo-pelvic hip girdle will affect their connection point, the knees.

- The two most common deviations found in the knees are
  1. problems with side-to-side alignment (e.g., valgus knee position) and
  2. tracking problems during flexion and extension.

- Apart from instances of acute trauma, knee pain is usually caused by imbalances in the structures above and below the knee joint. Therefore, the overall health and function of the feet and ankles and the lumbo-pelvic hip girdle directly affect the condition of the knees.

- Placing the feet and ankles into a neutral position when standing will most likely bring the knees into proper alignment. Overpronation of the feet and ankles causes the lower and upper leg to rotate too far inward, moving the knee toward the midline.

- When you learn about the types and intensity of physical activity people engage in, you can better understand the amount of stress they place on their knees. Identifying the activities that cause or reduce pain can help you determine what soft tissue structures may be irritated or dysfunctional.

- Popping or grinding noises that occur when a person sits down, stands up, or otherwise flexes and extends the knee suggest tracking problems.

- Record any pertinent information on the Client Assessment Diagram.

Self-Check

The condition of your knees can act as an early warning system for potential musculoskeletal imbalances in the feet and ankles or in the lumbo-pelvic hip girdle. Assess your own knees, and mark the grade you would give yourself on the following knee health report card.

Possible grades	Description	My grade
Grade A	Kneecap aligned over middle of second toe when standing; appropriate amount of movement toward the midline when squatting; no pain or popping or grinding during any movement	
Grade B	Kneecap nearly aligned over middle of second toe when standing; moderate amount of movement toward the midline of knee when squatting; little or no pain; popping or grinding during flexion/extension is minimal	
Grade C	Kneecap not aligned over second toe when standing, but can be when in neutral foot/ankle position; a little too much movement toward the midline of knee when squatting; occasional pain; slight popping or grinding during flexion/extension	
Grade D	Kneecap not aligned over second toe when standing; find it difficult to bring it into alignment/achieve/maintain neutral foot and ankle position; knee is noticeably shifted toward the middle of body when standing still and squatting; frequent or persistent pain; popping or grinding during movement	
Grade F	Kneecap not aligned over second toe when standing; unable to bring it into alignment/achieve/maintain neutral foot and ankle position; valgus position of the knee standing and even worse when squatting; swelling; constant or persistent pain	

Structural Assessment Skills Test

Perform a complete knee assessment on another person. Record your findings in the Client Assessment Diagram.

Knees	✔	Details
Pain?		
Arthritis/conditions?		
Function?		
What makes better/worse?		
Causal links?		
Visual irregularities?		
Single-leg squat?		
Patella tracking?		
Client knows neutral?		

CHAPTER 4

Assessing the Lumbo-Pelvic Hip Girdle

The lumbo-pelvic hip girdle is where the lumbar spine, pelvis, and hips come together. The hips, pelvis, and lower back are all very complex structures, and at the lumbo-pelvic hip girdle they create an enormously intricate, integrated union of bones, muscles, tendons, ligaments, fasciae, and nerves.

Humans are designed to stand and move about on two legs. The lumbo-pelvic hip girdle is one of the most important features of the body because it provides the structure and support needed to maintain an upright posture. In the lower back, the lumbar portion of the spine features a lordotic curve, which helps to lift the torso and to keep it adjusted over the body's center of gravity. The pelvis adjusts to movements of the upper body and arms and communicates with the lower limbs to aid in propulsion, transmit power, and maintain balance. Several large muscle groups in the lumbo-pelvic hip region work together to help move the lumbar spine, pelvis, and hips in all three planes of motion with great amounts of freedom. While this potential for movement is wonderfully unique to humans, it also puts them at risk of developing compensation patterns, movement dysfunctions, and musculoskeletal imbalances in this area of the body (Schamberger 2002).

BASIC ANATOMY

The main components of the lumbo-pelvic hip girdle are the lumbar spine, the sacrum, the sacroiliac joints, the pelvis, the hip, and the acetabulum (see figure 4.1).

The **pelvis** is a ringlike structure at the base of the spine that is created by the fusion of the ilium, ischium, and pubis bones. These fused bones form either side of the pelvis and are referred to as the left and right innominate bones, or more commonly, the hip bones. The head of the **femur** (upper leg bone) articulates with the pelvis at a deep socket in the hip called the **acetabulum**. The pelvis also articulates with the spine at the **sacroiliac joints**, where the sacrum meets the ilium of the pelvis. The **sacrum** is a triangular series of fused bones at the base of the spine between the lumbar spine and the coccyx (tailbone) (Dimon and Day 2008). The **lumbar spine** is comprised of the five largest vertebrae in the body and is responsible for helping

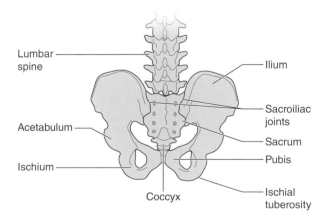

Figure 4.1   Basic anatomy of the lumbo-pelvic hip girdle.

flex, side bend, extend, and rotate the spine (McGill 2016). Many muscles, tendons, and ligaments help hold the structures of the lumbo-pelvic hip girdle together while providing for mobility and movement.

COMMON DEVIATIONS

There are two main deviations that cause pain, injury and movement dysfunction in the lumbo-pelvic hip girdle (Solberg 2008):

- An anterior pelvic tilt
- Excessive lumbar lordosis

When a person is standing in perfect alignment, the pelvis is naturally rotated anteriorly about 10 degrees (Gajdosik et al. 1985; Heino, Godges, and Carter 1990). This means that the front of the pelvis is slightly lower than the back of the pelvis. However, if the pelvis is tilted more than this when standing, the front of the pelvis is too far forward and down, and the back of the pelvis rises too far upward. This excessive forward and downward tilt of the pelvis is called an **anterior pelvic tilt** (see figure 4.2).

Conversely, if the pelvis is too high at the front, then the back of the pelvis will drop. A backward tilt of the pelvis is called a posterior pelvic tilt. Since the purpose of this text is to cover the most common deviations you may encounter as a fitness professional, assessments and other information about the posterior pelvic tilt will not be discussed.

When a person is standing in good alignment, the lumbar spine in the lower back has a slight inward, or lordotic, arch. This is a natural concave curve that can be observed when a person is viewed in profile. **Excessive lumbar lordosis** refers to an excessive curvature (or overarching) of the lumbar spine (see figure 4.3). Excessive lumbar lordosis is problematic because it can lead to movement dysfunction and eventually pain (Houglum 2016).

The lumbar spine, sacrum, and pelvis are linked by the sacroiliac joint and the many strong ligaments that cross and support this joint. Therefore, the position of the pelvis directly affects the position of the sacrum and lumbar spine. Conversely, the position of the lumbar spine and sacrum directly affects the position of the pelvis. If the pelvis tilts too far forward, the lumbar spine will arch excessively. Therefore, an anterior pelvic tilt is almost always accompanied by excessive lumbar lordosis. Similarly, excessive lumbar lordosis is almost always accompanied by an anterior pelvic tilt (Solberg 2008).

ASSESSMENT PROCESS

Having reviewed the structural anatomy of the lumbo-pelvic hip girdle and the common imbalances clients are likely to have in this area, we can now proceed to the detailed assessment procedures.

VERBAL ASSESSMENT

When assessing the lumbo-pelvic hip girdle, it is important to learn how clients perceive their condition or pain, both in isolation and in relation to other body areas and when performing activities (Price and Bratcher 2010). Ask about the following topics,

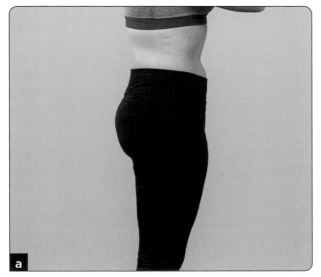 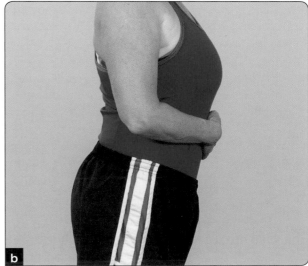

Figure 4.2   Example of (*a*) normal pelvic tilt and (*b*) anterior pelvic tilt.

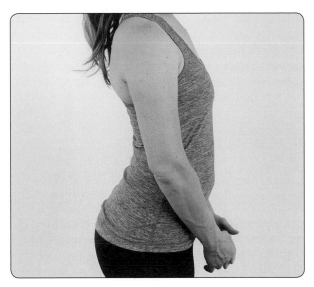

Figure 4.3 Example of excessive lumbar lordosis.

and write down any pertinent information on the Client Assessment Diagram (CAD).

1. Ask if the client has ever experienced pain in the hips, groin, buttocks, or lower back. Encourage specific responses when the person is describing the location and nature of the pain. For example, is the pain on the side or front of the hip? Is it deep in the groin or toward the top of the leg, the top or middle of the buttocks, or the seat of the buttocks? If it is at the base of the spine, is it at the level of the sacroiliac joint or on or near the tailbone? Is it a shooting or a tingling pain? Does it run down the leg? Is there pain in the abdomen? (Petty and Moore 2002). If a client complains of pain on the side of the hip, this may indicate that the leg is not moving correctly in the hip socket, possibly leading to inflammation. Specific clues like this can help guide you toward further examination of the alignment of the leg, hip, and pelvis (Price and Bratcher 2010).

2. Ask whether the client has arthritis or any other diagnosed conditions that may affect the musculoskeletal health of the lumbo-pelvic hip girdle. For example, clients with a diagnosis of disc degeneration may experience pain that could affect the success of their corrective exercise programs (Cramer and Darby 2014). When you know about conditions that may require outside assistance or that are beyond your scope of practice, you have an opportunity to develop referral relationships with like-minded professionals who can help ensure your clients'

long-term success (for more on scope of practice, networks, and referrals, see chapter 28).

3. Ask about the client's past injuries and surgeries. For example, a hip replacement or a lumbar fusion will affect both movement and function (Petty and Moore 2002).

4. Ask about the client's level of physical activity. For example, it would be important to know if a person plays sports or engages in activities such as golf and tennis that put a lot of stress on the hips and spine (Petty and Moore 2002).

5. Ask about the client's occupation. For example, if a person spends much of the day seated in hip flexion with his lower back rounded, this may adversely affect the function of his lumbo-pelvic hip girdle (McGill 2016).

6. Ask the client whether his back or hip problems ever prevent him from engaging in an activity or limit what he can do. This will help you to understand his underlying motivation for coming to see you and what he hopes to be able to do after he has regained full function or alleviated his pain (Price and Bratcher 2010).

7. Ask whether the client's pain coincides with any other pains or symptoms in other areas of the body. This will help the client to understand the body's interconnectedness and may point to possible causes, compensations, and corrections. For example, a client with lower back pain who spends a lot of time at the computer may reveal that when her lower back hurts, her neck also hurts. You can take this opportunity to highlight how her head and neck position directly affects the position of her lumbar spine (learn how the head and neck relate to the rest of the body in chapter 6). You can then tell her that you will be taking a closer look at the condition of her head and neck later in the assessment process (Price and Bratcher 2010).

8. Ask the client what aggravates the pain and what makes it feel better (Petty and Moore 2002). For example, if a client indicates that sitting at work exacerbates his back pain, you can coach him on how to improve his sitting posture (see chapter 18, Static Postural Considerations) to help address this problem.

9. Ask the client if the pain ever wakes him up at night or if he has trouble sleeping because of it. This is important because many lumbo-pelvic hip girdle issues are exacerbated by poor sleeping posture (see chapter 18, Static Postural Considerations) (Price and Bratcher 2010).

Once you have concluded the verbal portion of the assessment process, move on to the visual and hands-on assessments.

VISUAL AND HANDS-ON ASSESSMENTS

When assessing the lumbo-pelvic hip girdle, it is important to have a clear view of the structures you are evaluating. Ask the client to tuck in her shirt so you can see the lumbar spine, pelvis, and hips clearly.

VISUAL ASSESSMENT FOR ANTERIOR PELVIC TILT AND EXCESSIVE LUMBAR LORDOSIS

To visually assess whether a client has an anterior pelvic tilt, ask her to stand in front of you facing sideways. Note how her pants or shorts sit on her hips, and determine if the front of the waistband is lower than the back. The front of the waistband typically rests on the bony protuberance at the front of the pelvis, the anterior superior iliac spine (ASIS). The back of the waistband typically rests on the bony protuberance at the back, the posterior superior iliac spine (PSIS). As such, visually inspecting the client's waistband can provide insight into the position of the pelvis. If the back of the pelvis appears much higher than the front, this may suggest an anterior pelvic tilt (see figure 4.4) (Palmer, Epler, and Epler 1998). On the other hand, if the back of the pelvis appears lower than the front, this indicates that the pelvis has rotated backward. However, most people will have an anterior pelvic tilt.

While the client is still standing side-on, look at the curvature of the lumbar spine to evaluate for excessive lumbar lordosis. You should see a slight curve, or concavity, in the lower back. However, if the curve of the lower back looks markedly arched (like a C or reverse C, depending on which way they are facing), then the client is considered to have excessive lumbar lordosis (see figure 4.5) (Boos and Aebi 2008).

HANDS-ON ASSESSMENT FOR THE LUMBO-PELVIC HIP GIRDLE

Once the visual assessments for the lumbo-pelvic hip girdle are complete, begin the hands-on portion of the assessment process. Tell the client that you will now be manually evaluating his lower back in order to confirm or refute your visual assessment findings. You will be feeling for how much of a curve is in his lower back. Remember to ask permission to touch a client before performing any hands-on assessments.

To manually assess for the presence of excessive lumbar lordosis, ask the client to stand barefoot with his back, buttocks, heels, shoulders, and head against a wall. Before you begin the assessment, you must confirm that all of these structures are touching the wall. Then place your hand, palm down, on the wall and slide it behind the client's lower back (see figure 4.6).

Now evaluate the space between the lower back and the wall. With an acceptable degree of lumbar lordosis, you should only be able to slide your fingers behind the lower back up to and in line with about your second knuckle. If the space between the back

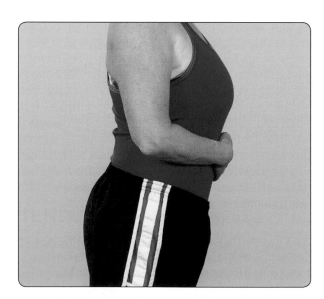

Figure 4.4 Visual assessment for an anterior pelvic tilt.

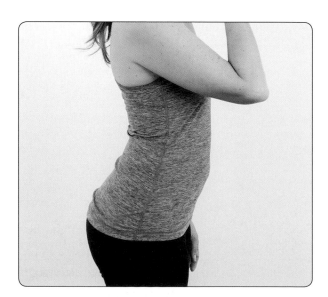

Figure 4.5 Visual assessment for excessive lumbar lordosis.

and the wall is large enough for you to slide your whole hand or arm through, then the client has excessive lumbar lordosis. The greater the space is between the wall and the lower back, the more extreme the deviation or imbalance (Price and Bratcher 2010). The presence of excessive lumbar lordosis will also indicate an anterior pelvic tilt (Kendall, McCreary, and Provance 2005).

Note that if someone has very well-developed gluteal muscles and the base of her spine is not in contact with the wall during the assessment, it will be necessary to make an allowance for the additional space you will find. Use your best judgment to determine whether the lumbar curvature is excessive.

> Go to the online video to watch video 4.1, where Justin demonstrates a hands-on assessment for excessive lumbar lordosis.

You can also assess for excessive lumbar lordosis with the client in a supine position. Ask the client to lie on the floor on his back with his legs straight. Instruct him to keep his knees and toes pointed toward the ceiling. Evaluate the arch in the lumbar spine by sliding your hand under his lower back (see figure 4.7). If you can slide all your fingers or your entire hand into the space between his lower back and the floor, this indicates he has excessive lumbar lordosis (Ward 2016).

It may be difficult to conduct this assessment accurately if the client has an excessive amount of body fat around the midsection. In such cases the excess flesh will fall toward the floor and may pre-

vent you from being able to slide your hand under the lower back. Similarly, if you use a soft assessment surface such as a massage table, the accuracy of the assessment may be affected. If a client has severe lower back pain, you should not ask her to lie on her back with her legs straight because this may aggravate her condition. In such a case, this assessment may be more effective to use as a teaching tool to help the client understand how sleeping with her legs straight may affect her lower back (Price and Bratcher 2010).

As you finish the lumbo-pelvic hip girdle assessment process, you can help the client understand how to achieve a neutral position for this area, and you can explain how better lumbo-pelvic hip girdle alignment can prevent pain and dysfunction not only in the lower back and hips, but also in the feet, ankles, knees, upper back, and shoulders (learn how the lumbo-pelvic hip girdle relates to the thoracic spine and shoulder girdle at the end of this chapter).

TEACHING CLIENTS NEUTRAL POSITION OF THE LUMBO-PELVIC HIP GIRDLE

Use the following strategies to teach your clients to achieve and maintain a neutral position of the pelvis and lumbar spine when they stand.

Instruct the client to stand upright, and place the palms of her hands on the front of her pelvis with her fingers straight. The centers of her palms should rest on the bony protuberances on the front

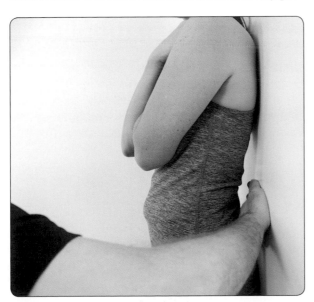

Figure 4.6   Hands-on assessment for excessive lumbar lordosis and anterior pelvic tilt.

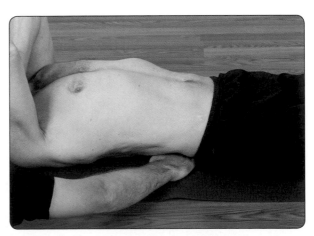

Figure 4.7   Supine assessment for excessive lumbar lordosis and anterior pelvic tilt.

of the pelvis just below the height of (and to the sides of) the navel. Next, she should position her hands so that her fingers are parallel to the floor and close enough together so that the ends of her index fingers and middle fingers are touching (see figure 4.8). Finally, instruct her to look down so that she can see her fingers. If she cannot clearly see both her index fingers and her middle fingers, the pelvis is probably rotated too far forward and downward, putting her fingers out of view. Coach her to tuck the pelvis under (i.e., tilt it posteriorly) until she can see both her index and second fingers clearly. At this point the pelvis will be in a relatively neutral position (Price and Bratcher 2010).

After the client has completed the pelvis adjustment, ask her to stand with her back, buttocks, shoulders, head, and heels touching a wall like she did in the hands-on assessment described previously. Coach her to tilt her pelvis to a neutral position using the palms-on-pelvis technique. This movement will help flatten the lower back to the wall and decrease the excessive arch in the lumbar spine. As she performs this movement, place your hand behind her lower back so that both of you can

feel the space decrease. Coach her to keep tilting her pelvis posteriorly until you can slide only about the first two knuckles of your fingers into the space between the lower back and the wall. As the client tilts her pelvis, her knees should remain straight, and her heels, buttocks, shoulders, and head should remain in contact with the wall. This will result in a relatively neutral position for the entire lumbo-pelvic hip girdle (Price and Bratcher 2010).

Some people may not be able to achieve neutral alignment of the lumbo-pelvic hip girdle. This usually happens in cases where a person has long-term alignment problems or lower back pain or is severely overweight (Price and Bratcher 2010). In such instances, coach clients to get as close to neutral as possible so they can feel what it is like (and what muscles and movements are involved) to achieve better alignment.

Before you move on to the verbal, visual, and hands-on assessments for the thoracic spine and shoulder girdle, briefly sum up your findings about the client's lumbo-pelvic hip girdle. Make sure you have completed the CAD for this area, and briefly describe for the client how the lumbo-pelvic hip region relates to the structures above and below it (see the next section).

HOW THE LUMBO-PELVIC HIP GIRDLE RELATES TO THE FEET, ANKLES, KNEES, AND THORACIC SPINE AND SHOULDER GIRDLE

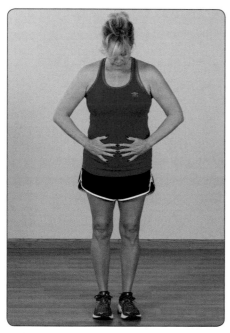

Figure 4.8   Palms-on-pelvis technique for finding a neutral lumbo-pelvic hip position.

In the chapters on assessing the feet, ankles, and knees, you learned that overpronation of the foot and ankle causes these structures to collapse inward with the lower leg toward the midline of the body. The movement of these structures, in turn, also causes the knee to move toward the midline and the upper leg to rotate inward. These positional changes in the feet, knees, and legs cause the top of the upper leg to shift backward where it attaches to the hip socket (see figure 4.9). Since the pelvis houses the hip socket, it must also shift out of alignment—that is, it rotates anteriorly. This

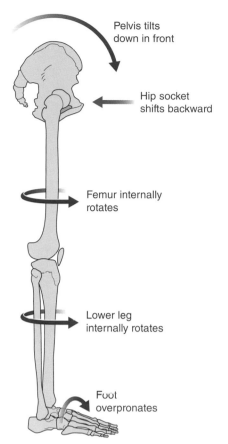

Pelvis tilts down in front

Hip socket shifts backward

Femur internally rotates

Lower leg internally rotates

Foot overpronates

Figure 4.9 How the feet, ankles, knees, and legs affect the position of the hips and pelvis.

causes the lumbar spine to arch excessively (Price and Bratcher 2010).

These compensatory shifts in the lower kinetic chain also affect the position of the thoracic spine and shoulder girdle (Kendall, McCreary, and Provance 2005). Overpronation, a valgus knee position, an anterior pelvic tilt, and excessive lumbar lordosis are all characterized by the feet, ankles, knees, pelvis, and lumbar spine collapsing in and forward. These movements shift the body's center of gravity forward from its optimal position, thereby causing the upper body to tip forward (Whiting and Zernicke 2008). This forward shift is marked by excessive thoracic kyphosis, the thoracic spine rounding forward and collapsing, the shoulder blades protracting forward and elevating on the rib cage and the arms internally rotating (Price and Bratcher 2010).

It is important that you understand these movement patterns and compensations and teach your clients about the interrelatedness of the upper and lower body. This will help you both to better understand the movement patterns and body positions that may be exacerbating their condition or hampering their ability to perform effectively.

Assessment Checklist

Before you move on to assess the thoracic spine and shoulder girdle, you must answer the following questions about the lumbo-pelvic hip girdle:

❏ Do you know what type of pain the client is experiencing and how it affects the function of her hips and lower back?

❏ Does the client have arthritis or any diagnosed conditions that might affect the success of her program?

❏ Does the client have any past injuries or surgeries that might affect the function of her lumbo-pelvic hip girdle?

❏ What makes the client's hips and back feel better or worse?

❏ Does the client's hip or lower back pain limit her function in any way?

❏ Does the client's hip or lower back pain affect her sleep?

❏ Are other parts of the client's body affected when her hips or lower back are painful?

❏ Does the client have an anterior pelvic tilt?

❏ Does the client have an excessive curvature in her lumbar spine?

❏ Does the client know how to achieve a neutral position for the pelvis when standing?

❏ Do you know how the lumbo-pelvic hip girdle relates to the lower kinetic chain and thoracic spine and shoulder girdle, and can you explain it to the client?

Make all your notations for this part of the assessment on the Client Assessment Diagram (see figure 4.10 for an example).

Lumbo-pelvic hip girdle	✔	Details
Pain?	✔	top of R butt near back of hip
Arthritis/conditions?	✔	none reported
Function?	✔	tight after playing tennis
What makes better/worse?	✔	tight in morning after sleeping
Causal links?	✔	R hip—R foot/ankle?
Visual irregularities?	✔	none
Excessive lordosis?	✔	excessive curvature
Anterior rotation?	✔	anterior tilt
Client knows neutral?	✔	can achieve—difficult to maintain

Figure 4.10 Sample of completed lumbo-pelvic hip girdle assessment on Client Assessment Diagram.

Review of Key Points

The lumbo-pelvic hip girdle is the area where the upper half of the body connects to the lower half. It is a multifaceted union of bones, muscles, ligaments, tendons, and fasciae that enables humans to stand upright and move on two legs.

- The two most common deviations found in the lumbo-pelvic hip girdle are
  1. excessive lumbar lordosis and
  2. an anterior pelvic tilt.

- The pelvis is normally rotated anteriorly approximately 10 degrees. This slight forward tilt enables the end of the upper leg to sit properly in the hip socket to enable smooth articulation between the pelvis, lumbar spine, and legs. An excessive anterior pelvic tilt, however, causes the hip socket to shift backward, thereby causing the upper leg to move out of optimal alignment and affecting the positioning of the knees and feet.

- An excessive anterior rotation of the pelvis is almost always accompanied by excessive arching of the lower back. This happens because the lumbar spine and pelvis are linked via the sacroiliac joint.

- It is important to discover the types and intensity of physical activity that a client typically engages in so that you can understand how much stress he places on his lower back and hips. Identifying activities that cause or relieve his pain can help you understand what soft tissue structures may be irritated or dysfunctional.

- The health and function of the feet, ankles, knees, and thoracic spine and shoulder girdle are directly affected by malalignments in the lumbo-pelvic hip girdle.

- Record any pertinent information on the Client Assessment Diagram.

Self-Check

Since the lumbo-pelvic hip girdle is where the upper and lower body connect, everything above and below it are affected by deviations in this area. Stand in front of a mirror and practice trying to tilt the back of your pelvis down to achieve a neutral position for your lumbo-pelvic hip girdle.

As you bring your pelvis and lumbar spine into alignment, look for movements or compensations that occur in other parts of your body. For example, as you tilt your pelvis posteriorly, you might notice your shoulders come forward away from the wall. This may happen because you typically keep your torso upright by overarching your lower back, rather than using the muscles of your upper back and shoulders to remain erect. When you take away this compensation pattern, you may find it hard to keep your shoulders against the wall. Examine each body part, and record what you see or feel in the following chart.

Area of body	What I noticed happened
Feet	
Ankles	
Knees	
Lower back	
Upper back/shoulders	
Neck/head	

Structural Assessment Skills Test

Perform a complete lumbo-pelvic hip girdle assessment on another person. Record your findings in the following Client Assessment Diagram.

Lumbo-pelvic hip girdle	✔	Details
Pain?		
Arthritis/conditions?		
Function?		
What makes better/worse?		
Causal links?		
Visual irregularities?		
Excessive lordosis?		
Anterior rotation?		
Client knows neutral?	✔	

CHAPTER 5

Assessing the Thoracic Spine and Shoulder Girdle

The thoracic spine and shoulder girdle region includes the thoracic portion of the spine, the rib cage, the shoulder girdle, and the upper arms. These components provide functions that are vital to our existence and integral to our movements. The thoracic spine can move forward and backward, side-to-side, and in rotation (Middleditch and Oliver 2005). The rib cage, which attaches to the thoracic spine, is involved in protecting the organs, facilitating breathing, and supporting the structures of the upper body. The shoulder girdle (the means by which the upper arm attaches to the torso with the help of the clavicles and scapulae) articulates with the thoracic spine by means of muscles, tendons, ligaments, bones, and nerves (McMinn 2005).

BASIC ANATOMY

The **thoracic spine** is the part of the spine between the lumbar and cervical segments. It contains the 12 vertebrae in the middle and upper torso area (Middleditch and Oliver 2005). The thoracic vertebrae are medium sized and have more limited movement capabilities than the lumbar vertebrae (McGill 2016). However, they are generally more stable due to their support from the rib cage (Middleditch and Oliver 2005). The **rib cage** is made up of 24 ribs (12 on each side of the thoracic spine) that attach by cartilage to the sternum at the front of the chest and to the sides of each thoracic vertebra at the back. The bottom two sets of ribs do not attach to the sternum and are known as floating ribs (Schenck 1999). The **sternum** is a T-shaped bone at the top and center of the front of the rib cage to which the clavicles (collarbones) attach (Goldfinger 1991). The **clavicle** extends outward from the sternum and across to the acromion to help form the front of the shoulder girdle. The **acromion** is a part of the scapula (shoulder blade) that extends over the top of the **humerus** (upper arm bone), forming the upper border of the shoulder girdle. The **scapula** is a broad, flat bone that sits on the back of the upper rib cage, forming the back of the shoulder girdle. The humerus articulates with the **shoulder joint** via the **labrum**, a ring of cartilage on the edge of the scapula that gives the end of the upper arm a cup-shaped socket in which to sit (Dimon and Day 2008). All the movements of the shoulder are highly complex and depend on precise articulation of all the bones, tendons, ligaments, and fasciae in this area of the body (see figure 5.1).

COMMON DEVIATIONS

There are four main deviations that can cause pain, injury, and movement dysfunction in the thoracic spine and shoulder girdle (Imhoff et al. 2016):

- Excessive thoracic kyphosis
- Protracted shoulder girdle
- Internally rotated arms
- Elevated scapula

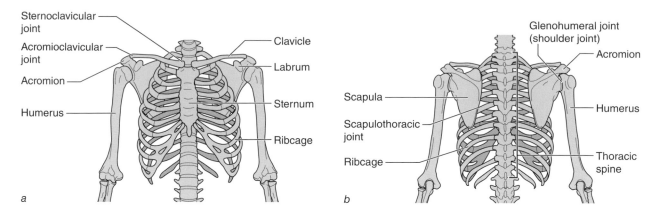

Figure 5.1   Basic anatomy of the thoracic spine and shoulder girdle: *(a)* anterior and *(b)* posterior views.

The thoracic spine naturally has a mild forward-shaped curve called a kyphotic curve. A greater than normal curvature of the thoracic spine is referred to as **excessive thoracic kyphosis**. Excessive thoracic kyphosis disrupts the function of the entire shoulder girdle (Brumitt 2010).

A **protracted shoulder girdle** occurs when the shoulder blades move forward on the rib cage, causing their vertebral borders (the edges closest to the spine) to move away from the spine (Petty and Moore 2002). Protraction of the shoulder blades also protracts the entire shoulder girdle, moving the acromions and collarbones forward and out of alignment (Muscolino 2011). When the shoulder girdle protracts, it affects the position of the glenohumeral joint, causing the upper arm to rotate inward toward the midline of the body. This position of the upper arms in the shoulder joints is referred to as **internally rotated arms** (Solberg 2008).

An **elevated scapula** refers to an atypical, upward position of the shoulder blade as it sits upon the rib cage. Elevated shoulder blades, a protracted shoulder girdle, internally rotated arms, and excessive thoracic kyphosis are inherently linked, and they limit shoulder function and range of motion in the arms, in the upper torso, and throughout the body (Johnson 2012).

 Go to the online video to watch video 5.1, where Justin talks about common deviations of the thoracic spine and shoulder girdle.

ASSESSMENT PROCESS

Having reviewed the structural anatomy of the thoracic spine and shoulder girdle and the common imbalances clients are likely to have in this area, we can proceed to the detailed assessment procedures.

VERBAL ASSESSMENT

When assessing the thoracic spine and shoulder girdle, it is important to learn how clients perceive their condition or pain, both in isolation and in relation to other body areas and when performing activities (Price and Bratcher 2010). Ask about the following topics, and write down any pertinent information on the Client Assessment Diagram (CAD).

1. Ask if the client has ever experienced pain in the mid- to upper back, chest, shoulders, neck, rib cage, or abdomen, and ask for the specific location of the pain. Where on the shoulder does it occur? Is it under the shoulder blade or armpit? On the back or side of the neck? In the middle of one side of the chest? (Petty and Moore 2002). For example, if a client describes pain on the top of her shoulder blade (or on the side or back of her neck), this may indicate that her shoulder blade is elevated on that side, resulting in muscle tightness and tension. Obtaining such detailed information will prompt you to check further during the visual and hands-on assessments.

2. Ask whether the client has arthritis or any other diagnosed condition that may affect the musculoskeletal health of the thoracic spine and shoulder girdle. For example, clients with a diagnosis of arthritis in their acromioclavicular joint (the top of the shoulder) may experience pain and dysfunction that could affect the success of a corrective exercise program (Cramer and Darby 2014). Some conditions may require outside assistance, and this can help you to

develop valuable referral relationships with medical professionals (for more on scope of practice, networks, and referrals, see chapter 28) (Price and Bratcher 2010).

3. Ask about the client's past injuries or surgeries. For example, a torn rotator cuff muscle or a fusion of vertebrae in the thoracic spine may limit movements and functions, and this will affect program design (Petty and Moore 2002).

4. Ask about the client's level of physical activity. Ask whether he plays sports often and, if so, what kind? For example, baseball pitchers experience excessive movement in their throwing arms that can affect shoulder functions (Petty and Moore 2002).

5. Ask about the client's occupation. Does your client work at a computer desk or at a manual labor job? People who work at a computer all day long tend to round their upper backs, protract their shoulder girdles, and internally rotate their arms as they type. Spending lots of time in this posture will affect the alignment of the thoracic spine, the shoulder girdle, and the rest of the body (Price and Bratcher 2010).

6. Ask the client if shoulder and arm or mid-to-upper back pain ever prevents him from engaging in an activity or limits what he can do. This will highlight the activities he feels he is missing out on, and why he is motivated to seek your help (Price and Bratcher 2010).

7. Ask if the client's pain is accompanied by any other pains or symptoms. This will help the client to understand the body's interconnectedness, and it may help you to identify contributing issues or potential solutions. For example, a client who has pain between his shoulder blades after extensive computer work may find that this pain coincides with pain in the back of his neck. You can teach him how imbalances in the upper back can affect the position of the neck and head. (Learn how the thoracic spine and shoulder girdle relate to all other areas of the body later in this chapter). It will also prompt you to take a closer look at the position of his head and neck as you assess that area (Price and Bratcher 2010).

8. Ask the client what aggravates the pain and what makes it feel better (Petty and Moore 2002). If a client indicates, for instance, that driving makes her neck pain worse, you can coach her on improving her sitting and driving posture (see chapter 18, Static Postural Considerations).

9. Ask the client if the pain ever wakes him up at night or makes sleep difficult. For example, if a client tells you that sleeping on his side makes his shoulder or neck pain worse, you can coach him on how to improve his sleeping posture (see chapter 18, Static Postural Considerations) to help address this problem (Price and Bratcher 2010).

10. Ask the client if his pain increases with stress or if he is currently under a lot of stress. Chronic stress responses, such as shrugging the shoulders and rounding the upper back, can have a dramatic effect on the alignment of the thoracic spine and shoulder girdle (Hanna 1988; Price 2015).

Once you have concluded the verbal portion of the assessment process, move on to the visual and hands-on assessments.

VISUAL AND HANDS-ON ASSESSMENTS

When assessing the thoracic spine and shoulder girdle, it is important to have a clear view of the structures you are evaluating. Obviously, the assessment will be more accurate if there are fewer garments obstructing your view, but do not insist that clients remove clothing or wear certain items, such as tank tops, sports bras, or form-fitting shirts, if this makes them feel uncomfortable in any way. You can simply ask them to tuck their shirts into their pants so you can more easily view the structures of the torso and shoulders.

ASSESSMENT FOR EXCESSIVE THORACIC KYPHOSIS

To evaluate whether a client has excessive thoracic kyphosis, ask her to stand in front of you facing sideways. Place your fingers on the back of the client's neck and locate the vertebrae of her cervical spine. Follow the curvature of the spine from the top of the neck to the bottom, and feel each vertebra like the keys of a piano. You will notice that the last vertebra of the neck (C7) protrudes out slightly more than the vertebrae directly above it, perhaps noticeably so in the form of a dowager's hump (see figure 5.2) (Bontrager and Lampignano 2014).

If you are having difficulty locating C7, place your fingers on the base of the client's neck and instruct him to look down at his feet and then back up above his head. As he looks down and up, you will feel that C7 does not move much compared to the vertebrae above it (Kehr and Weidner 1987). Once you have located C7, place the tip of your index finger on this vertebra. Extend your index finger so that it is straight and parallel to the ground (see figure 5.3a).

Now position the index finger of your other hand with your finger straight and parallel to the ground on the indentation on the front of the client's torso between the middle of the collarbones on the top of the sternum (i.e., the jugular notch; see figure 5.3b). When both fingers are in place, evaluate the difference in height between your two fingers (see figure 5.3c).

When a person is in good alignment, your index finger on the front of the client's chest should be about 1-1/2 inches (3.8 cm) lower than your finger positioned on the client's neck since the anatomical position of the spinous process (bony projection off the back) of C7 is about 1-1/2 inches (3.8 cm) higher than the top of the sternum when the thoracic spine is in proper alignment (Bontrager and Lampignano 2014). If your index finger on the front of the client's chest is more than 1-1/2 inches (3.8 cm) lower than your index finger on the neck, it is indicative that the client has excessive thoracic kyphosis. This is because the back of the rib cage attaches to the thoracic spine, and when the thoracic spine rounds forward, the sternum (where the front of the rib cage attaches) drops down and forward. The greater

the difference in height (of more than 1-1/2 inches) (3.8 cm) between your two fingers, the greater the amount of excessive thoracic kyphosis.

EVALUATE THE POSITION OF THE SHOULDER BLADES

When a person is standing with her arms at her sides in good thoracic alignment, the shoulder blades should rest relatively flat and down on the back of the rib cage (Kendall, McCreary, and Provance 2005). You can visually and manually assess the

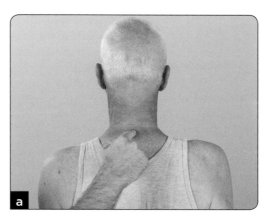

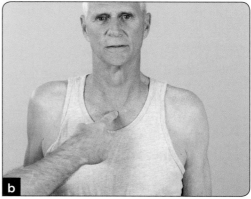

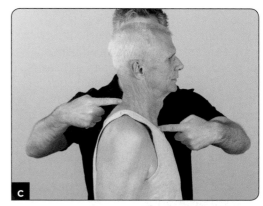

Figure 5.3   (a) Location of spinous process of C7. (b) Location of jugular notch. (c) Assessing for excessive thoracic kyphosis.

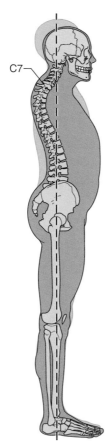

Figure 5.2   Image showing C7 protruding (i.e., a dowager's hump).

client's shoulder blades to evaluate whether they have moved up and away from their correct position, which would denote a protracted shoulder girdle or elevated shoulder blades.

Ask the client to stand facing away from you, and look at the edges of her shoulder blades closest to the spine. If one or both of the shoulder blades appear to stick out away from the body, this indicates a protracted shoulder girdle (see figure 5.4) (Bryant and Green 2010).

To further assess if a client has a protracted shoulder girdle, place your finger(s) on the border of the scapula that is closest to the spine. Evaluate whether the shoulder blades are lying flat to the back of the rib cage. If either scapula sticks out (or you can easily feel the border with your fingers), then either one or both sides of the client's shoulder girdle are likely protracted (see figure 5.5) (Price and Bratcher 2010).

Next, visually and manually assess the height of each scapula. Use your fingers to feel for the top borders of the shoulder blades. Once you have found the top borders, place the forefinger of each hand on this part of the bone and look at your fingers to visually assess the positioning of each scapula. Ideally, the shoulder blades should be at the same height. Make a note of any discrepancies between the shoulder blades or if one appears to be higher than the other one (see figure 5.6) (Rolf 1989).

You can also check to see if one or both shoulder blades are elevated by assessing muscle tension in this area (Petty and Moore 2002). Grasp the upper trapezius muscle on the top of the client's shoulder with your thumb and forefinger. Feel the muscle between your fingertips, and assess any differences in tension between the two sides. Make a note if the muscles in general feel excessively tight or have any

obvious knots (see figure 5.7) (Price and Bratcher 2010). If one or both sides have excessive tension, you can safely assume that one or both shoulder blades are elevated because the tight muscles attach to the scapula.

The position of the shoulder blades may be affected by the presence of scoliosis, depending on the severity of the condition. However, since this text covers only the most common deviations you may encounter as a fitness professional, assessments related to scoliosis will not be discussed.

EVALUATE THE POSITION OF THE ACROMION

To further evaluate the position of the shoulder girdle, ask the client to turn to the side. Note the position of the acromion, the bony protuberance on the top of the shoulder. Ideally, that bony landmark should be in line with the tragus, the fleshy piece of skin that covers up part of the opening at the

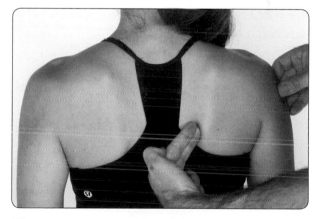

Figure 5.5   Hands-on assessment of scapulae for protracted shoulder girdle.

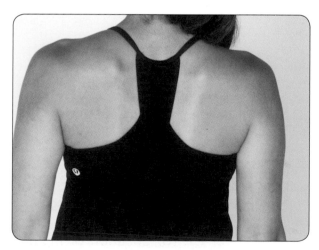

Figure 5.4   Visual assessment of scapulae for protracted shoulder girdle.

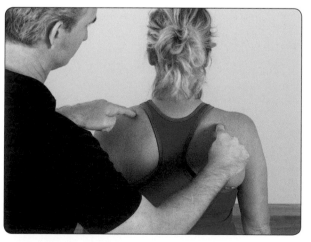

Figure 5.6   Hands-on assessment for elevated scapulae.

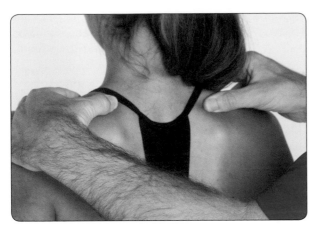

Figure 5.7 Hands-on assessment for muscle tension and elevated scapulae.

front of the ear (Johnson 2016). If the acromion is farther forward than the tragus, it is an indication that the client has a protracted shoulder girdle (see figure 5.8).

EVALUATE THE POSITION OF THE ARMS

Once you have completed your assessment of the shoulder blades and shoulder girdle, visually evaluate the position of the client's arms. You can determine whether a client's arms are rotated too far internally by looking at the position of the fingers, hands, and wrists (Johnson 2016).

Ask the client to let her arms hang by her sides while she stands in a normal, relaxed state. Position yourself directly in front of her and look at her hands. When a person is in proper alignment, the hands and arms should have a slight internal rotation—they should turn in toward the midline of the body about 15 degrees (Betts et al. 2013). If only the thumbs, forefingers, and some of the middle fingers are visible, then the arms are in correct alignment (see figure 5.9).

However, if you can see all of the client's fingers and the backs of her hands, then her arms are considered to be excessively internally rotated (see figure 5.10) (Betts et al. 2013).

Go to the online video to watch video 5.2, where Justin demonstrates the visual assessment for internally rotated arms.

TEACHING CLIENTS NEUTRAL POSITION OF THE THORACIC SPINE AND SHOULDER GIRDLE

As with the lumbo-pelvic hip girdle, one of the keys to correcting dysfunctions in the thoracic spine and shoulder girdle is to teach clients how to achieve and

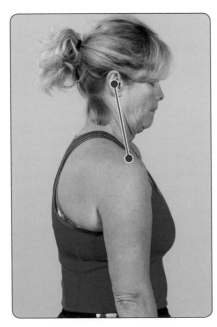

Figure 5.8 Acromion-to-tragus visual assessment for protracted shoulder girdle.

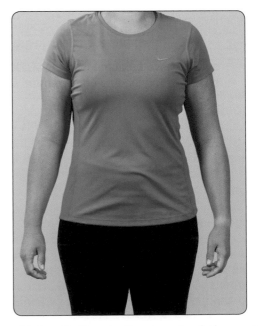

Figure 5.9 Optimal alignment of the arms when standing.

maintain a neutral position for the thoracic spine, shoulders, and arms when standing. You can coach them using the following strategies.

Ask the client to stand against a wall and to pull the thoracic spine upright until his shoulders touch the wall. As he does this, have him retract his shoulder blades so that his arms rotate outward. Coach him not to shrug his shoulders or arch his lower back as he performs these movements with the torso, shoulders, and arms (see figure 5.11). You can check to see if he has "cheated," using the lower back to lift the torso, by sliding your hand into the space between the lower back and the wall to check for excessive lumbar lordosis (see chapter 4, Assessing the Lumbo-Pelvic Hip Girdle). You should also coach the client to avoid compensating in other ways, such as by bending his knees or moving his feet or hips away from the wall.

Achieving and maintaining a neutral standing position for the thoracic spine and shoulder girdle will be difficult for most clients. However, encouraging them to try will help them to understand how far they are from neutral and what muscles they must activate to achieve it.

Before you move on to the verbal, visual, and hands-on assessments for the neck and head, briefly sum up your findings about the client's thoracic spine and shoulder girdle. Make sure you have com-pleted the CAD for this area, and briefly describe for the client how the thoracic spine and shoulder girdle relate to the structures above and below them.

HOW THE THORACIC SPINE AND SHOULDER GIRDLE RELATE TO ALL OTHER AREAS OF THE BODY

As the thoracic spine rounds forward and the kyphotic curve increases, the lordotic curve in the lumbar spine also tends to increase to help maintain balance (Kendall, McCreary, and Provance 2005). This causes the pelvis to rotate forward and the leg to rotate internally, producing a valgus knee displacement and overpronation of the foot and ankle complex (see figure 5.12) (Price and Bratcher 2010).

Excessive thoracic kyphosis is also accompanied by a protracted shoulder girdle, elevated shoulder blades, and internally rotated arms. These imbalances in the thoracic spine and shoulder girdle consequently affect the position of the neck and head since the head is attached to the neck, which

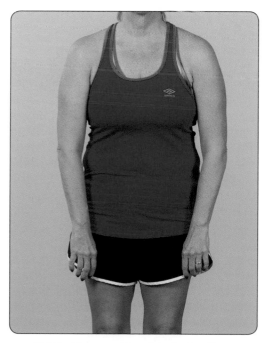

Figure 5.10 Example of internally rotated arms.

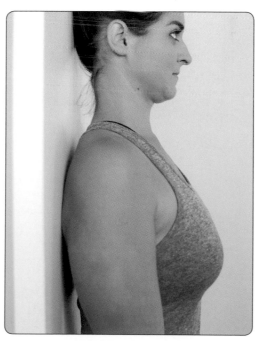

Figure 5.11 Neutral position of thoracic spine and shoulder girdle.

is in turn attached to the thoracic spine (Palmer, Epler, and Epler 1998). When the thoracic spine and shoulders collapse, the head and neck follow and fall forward also. As the head collapses down and forward, the neck arches backward and upward to maintain balance and to enable the eyes to focus on the horizon (see figure 5.13) (Palmer, Epler, and Epler 1998). Over time, this collapsing forward of the head and overarching of the cervical spine can place undue stress and strain on the structures of the neck and upper back.

It is important that you understand these patterns of movement and teach your clients about how problems in one part of the body produce compensations elsewhere. This will help both parties to better understand movement patterns and positions that may be exacerbating clients' conditions or hampering their ability to perform effectively.

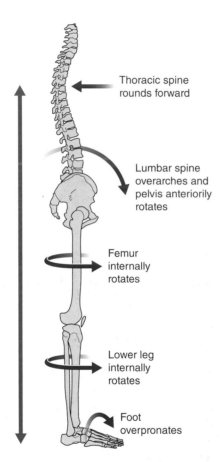

Figure 5.12 How overpronation or excessive thoracic kyphosis affects the knees and lumbo-pelvic hip girdle.

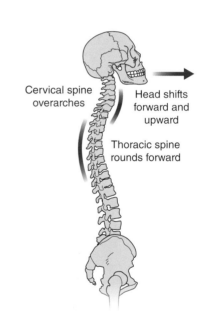

Figure 5.13 How excessive thoracic kyphosis affects the position of the neck and head.

Assessment Checklist

Before you move on to assess the neck and head, you must answer the following questions about the thoracic spine and shoulder girdle:

❑ Do you know what type of pain the client is experiencing and how it affects the function of his upper back, shoulders, and arms?

❑ Does the client have any arthritis or diagnosed conditions that might affect the success of his program?

❑ Does the client have any past injuries or surgeries that might affect the function of his thoracic spine and shoulder girdle?

❑ What makes the client's upper back and shoulders feel better or worse?

❑ Does the client's upper back and shoulder pain limit his function in any way?

❑ Does the client's upper back and shoulder pain affect his sleep?

❑ Are other parts of the client's body affected when his upper back and shoulders are painful?

❑ Does the client have excessive thoracic kyphosis?

❑ Does the client have a protracted shoulder girdle?

❑ Does the client have elevated shoulder blades?

❑ Does the client have internally rotated arms?

❑ Does the client know how to achieve a neutral position for the thoracic spine and shoulder girdle when standing?

❑ Do you know how the thoracic spine and shoulder girdle relate to the rest of the body, and can you explain it to the client?

Make all your notations for this part of the assessment on the Client Assessment Diagram (see figure 5.14 for an example).

Thoracic Spine/Shoulder Girdle	✔	Details
Pain?	✔	top of R shoulder sometimes
Arthritis/conditions?	✔	none reported
Function?	✔	pain after long periods of computer use
What makes better/worse?	✔	computer mousing, sleeping, stress
Causal links?	✔	is torso affecting low back?
Excessive kyphosis?	✔	yes
Protracted/elevated scapula?	✔	more on R
Internally rotated arms?	✔	more on R
Muscle tension?	✔	R side
Client knows neutral?	✔	can achieve—watch for lumbar cheat

Figure 5.14   Sample of completed thoracic spine and shoulder girdle assessment on Client Assessment Diagram.

Review of Key Points

The thoracic spine and shoulder girdle comprises the middle and mid-upper part of the spine, the rib cage, the shoulder girdle, and the arms. These structures are intrinsically involved in nearly every movement the body makes, and they also protect vital organs, such as the heart and lungs.

- The four most common deviations found in the thoracic spine and shoulder girdle are
  1. excessive thoracic kyphosis,
  2. protracted shoulder girdle,
  3. elevated scapula, and
  4. internally rotated arms.

- The thoracic spine naturally contains a slight kyphotic curve. However, an excessive curvature in the thoracic region can cause compensatory movements in the lumbar and cervical regions of the spine. Therefore, the lower back, hips, and neck are adversely affected by excessive thoracic kyphosis.

- It is important to learn the types and intensity of physical activity that a client typically engages in so that you can understand how much stress she places on her shoulders, arms, and upper back. This information, in addition to identifying which activities cause or alleviate her pain, can help you determine which soft tissue structures may be irritated or may need to be addressed in a corrective exercise program.

- Chronic stress can affect the upper body as the thoracic spine rounds forward into a protective or defensive posture. Asking clients about their stress levels can help you to determine if stress might be affecting their musculoskeletal health.

- Internally rotated arms and an elevated or protracted scapula can affect the function of the shoulder girdle and arms, which can create problems for both exercise and activities of daily living.

- Record any pertinent information on the Client Assessment Diagram.

Self-Check

To help you feel how excessive thoracic kyphosis affects the functions of the thoracic spine and shoulder girdle, perform the following movements. Try each movement first with your upper back rounded into an excessively kyphotic position. Then correct your posture and repeat the same movement. Note the quality and the range of motion you achieve when you perform each movement in both the bad posture trial (A) and the good posture trial (B).

MOVEMENT 1

Trial A: Bad Posture

Round your upper back and shoulders. Try to lift your arms over your head and back toward your ears while still keeping your upper back and shoulders rounded forward. Make a mental note of how high you can lift your arms back to your ears.

Trial B: Good Posture

Now correct your posture in your thoracic spine and shoulder girdle and try to lift your arms again. You will notice that your arms can go much higher and farther back to your ears when your thoracic spine is upright in the correct position.

MOVEMENT 2

Trial A: Bad Posture

Round your upper back and shoulders. Try to rotate your torso to the right and then to the left while still keeping your upper back and shoulders rounded forward. Make a mental note of how far you can rotate to the right and to the left.

Trial B: Good Posture

Now correct your posture and try to rotate your torso to the right and then to the left again. You will notice that you can rotate much farther when your thoracic spine is positioned correctly.

MOVEMENT 3

Trial A: Bad Posture

Round your upper back, stretch out your arms to your sides, and try to rotate your arms outward and behind you so that the palms of your hands point to the ceiling. Be sure to keep your upper back and shoulders rounded forward as you perform the movement. Make a mental note of how far your arms and shoulders rotate back.

Trial B: Good Posture

Now correct the posture in your thoracic spine and try the same movement again. You will notice that you can rotate your palms, arms, and hands much farther and pull your arms back more easily when your thoracic spine is in correct alignment.

Structural Assessment Skills Test

Perform a complete thoracic spine and shoulder girdle assessment on another person. Record your findings in the following Client Assessment Diagram.

Thoracic spine and shoulder girdle	✔	Details
Pain?		
Arthritis/conditions?		
Function?		
What makes better/worse?		
Causal links?		

Thoracic spine and shoulder girdle	✔	Details
Excessive kyphosis?		
Protracted/elevated scapula?		
Internally rotated arms?		
Muscle tension?		
Client knows neutral?		

CHAPTER 6

Assessing the Neck and Head

The weight of the human head is typically between 9 and 12 pounds. It accounts for about 8 percent of the average person's body mass (Louw 2007). Head position affects the alignment of the musculoskeletal system all the way down to the toes because the body must be constantly adjusting to keep the head balanced. When the head moves too far forward, the effect is significant. When the head moves even one inch ahead of the body's center of gravity, for example, its effective weight for the rest of the body doubles (Eriksen 2004). Therefore, optimal alignment of the neck and head complex is essential for whole-body musculoskeletal health.

BASIC ANATOMY

The neck and head comprise the cervical spine and the skull (see figure 6.1). The **skull** provides the general framework for the head and has two main components: the cranium and the mandible. The **cranium** contains several bones held together by sutures, or immobile joints. The bones that make up the cranium include the occipital, two parietal bones, two temporal bones, the frontal, the sphenoid, and the ethmoid (Adds and Shahsavari 2012). The **mandible**, also known as the jawbone, is connected to the cranium via the temporomandibular joint. The skull sits on top of the **atlas bone**, which is the first vertebra of the cervical spine (C1). The **cervical spine**, also known as the neck, has seven small vertebrae and a mild lordotic curve that arches the neck backward to help keep the head upright and the eyes level (Clippinger 2007). As the head moves forward, backward, and from side to side, the neck moves accordingly, communicating with the head through a complex system of nerves, muscles, tendons, ligaments, and fasciae.

COMMON DEVIATIONS

There are two main deviations that can cause pain, injury, and movement dysfunction in the neck and head (Muscolino 2011):

- A forward position of the head
- Excessive cervical lordosis

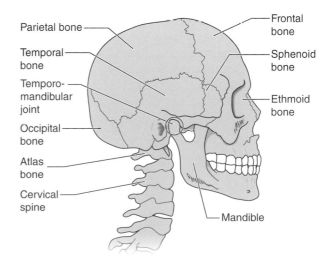

Figure 6.1 Basic anatomy of the neck and head.

When in perfect alignment, the head should be naturally balanced atop the spine, torso, and lower body. A **forward position of the head** refers to a projection of the head that places it too far forward of the body's plumb line or center. The farther the head moves forward of the thoracic spine and shoulder girdle, the more the neck has to arch (or the head has to tip up and back) to keep the eyes level (Palmer, Epler, and Epler 1998). A malaligned head position can disrupt the entire musculoskeletal system, as well as sensory systems such as the eyes and ears (Jones 2011).

The cervical spine naturally contains a slight lordotic curve. **Excessive cervical lordosis** refers to an increased curvature of the neck that accompanies a forward head position. Excessive cervical lordosis is problematic because it can compress discs or nerves in the neck and cause pain or dysfunction in this area, as well as in the upper torso, head, and arms (Kendall, McCreary, and Provance 2005).

ASSESSMENT PROCESS

Having reviewed the structural anatomy of the neck and head and the common imbalances clients are likely to have in this area, we can now proceed to the detailed assessment procedures.

VERBAL ASSESSMENT

When assessing the neck and head, it is important to learn how clients perceive their condition, both in isolation and in relation to other body areas and when performing activities. Ask about the following topics, and write down any pertinent information on the Client Assessment Diagram (CAD).

1. Ask if the client has ever experienced pain, headaches, or tension in the neck or head, and ask about the specific location and nature of the pain (Petty and Moore 2002). For example, many people suffer headaches as a result of muscle tension that compresses nerves in the neck and shoulder. Corrective exercises can help alleviate headaches caused by this problem.

2. Ask whether the client has arthritis or any other diagnosed condition that may affect the musculoskeletal health of the neck and head. For example, a client with a diagnosis of arthritis in the facet joints of the neck (joints between the vertebrae) may experience pain and dysfunction that could affect the success of a corrective exercise program (Shen and Shaffrey 2010).

Knowing about such conditions may give you an opportunity to network with other health care providers to manage the issues.

3. Ask about the client's past injuries or surgeries. For example, a fusion of two or more cervical vertebrae may affect movements and functions and program design (Petty and Moore 2002).

4. Ask about the client's level of physical activity. Ask whether he plays sports, and if so, which ones? Someone who rides a bicycle for exercise may have significant stresses on his neck because he must round his shoulders over the handlebars while his neck arches backward to keep his eyes focused ahead (Petty and Moore 2002).

5. Ask about the client's occupation. Does the client sit for prolonged periods in front of a computer? If so, where is the monitor in relation to where he sits—for instance, must he look sideways to see it? Does the job require him to look down a lot, bend over a table, or look over his shoulder for sustained periods? Over time, repetitive work positions can lead to shoulder, back, and neck pain (Price and Bratcher 2010).

6. Ask whether neck or head pain ever prevents the client from engaging in an activity or limits what he can do. This will highlight the activities he feels he is missing out on, and it will help you to understand his underlying motivation for seeking your help (Price and Bratcher 2010).

7. Ask if the client's pain coincides with any other pains or symptoms. This will ultimately progress both parties' understanding of the body's interconnectedness and will help you to identify causes and solutions for the person's musculoskeletal issues. For example, a client who experiences headaches after standing for many hours may also notice that this pain coincides with lower back pain and her choice to wear high-heeled shoes. You can then teach her about how her choice of footwear can affect the position of her lower back and neck and cause pain (Price and Bratcher 2010).

8. Ask the client what aggravates his condition and what makes it feel better (Petty and Moore 2002). For example, if a client tells you that sitting and watching television makes his neck pain worse, you can coach him on how to improve his posture when seated (see chapter 18, Static Postural Considerations).

9. Ask whether the client's pain ever makes sleeping difficult. For example, if a client tells

you that sleeping on her stomach makes her neck pain worse, you can coach her on how to improve her sleeping posture (see chapter 18, Static Postural Considerations) to help address this problem (Price and Bratcher 2010).

10. Ask the client if his pain increases with stress or if he is currently under a lot of stress. Chronic stress responses, such as gritting or grinding the teeth, can cause headaches, tension, and jaw pain, and it can affect the alignment of the neck and head. The temporomandibular joint can also be affected by alignment issues in the neck and head as a result of chronic stress, which can manifest as painful popping or grinding when a person opens or closes his jaw (Grimsby and Rivard 2008).

Once you have concluded the verbal portion of the assessment process, move on to the visual and hands-on assessments.

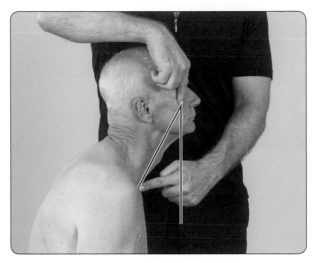

Figure 6.2   Example of forward head position.

VISUAL AND HANDS-ON ASSESSMENTS

When assessing the neck and head, it is important to get a clear view of these structures. Ask clients to remove hats and to tie their hair away from their necks if necessary. Remember to ask permission to touch a client before performing any hands-on assessments.

EVALUATE THE POSITION OF THE HEAD

To evaluate whether a client's head is forward of its optimal position in relation to the rest of the body, ask the person to sit on a gym ball or on the edge of a chair with the feet and head facing forward, then look at him from the side. From this position, locate the part of his cheekbone that protrudes outward the most, just below the eye. Place one of your index fingers on this part of the client's cheekbone and your other index finger directly below it on the client's collarbone. With your index fingers positioned in this way, stand directly over your fingers and look down to assess the position of your index fingers in relation to each other (see figure 6.2). Ideally, they should be vertically aligned, that is, with one directly below the other (Chek 2001; Palmer, Epler, and Epler 1998; Price and Bratcher 2010). If the index finger on the client's cheekbone is ahead of the one on his collarbone, the head is

too far forward for optimal alignment (Chek 2001; Price and Bratcher 2010).

EVALUATE FOR EXCESSIVE CERVICAL LORDOSIS

To evaluate whether the curve in a client's neck is excessive, ask the client to stand with his back to a wall with his heels, buttocks, and shoulders touching the wall. Have him straighten his legs and tilt his pelvis posteriorly to decrease the arch in his lower back to find a neutral position (see the section Hands-On Assessment for the Lumbo-Pelvic Hip Girdle in chapter 4 for more information on how to coach a client into this position).

While he is holding this position, ask him to touch the wall softly with the back of his head. (While the back of the head will be in contact with the wall, it is not necessary to have the head pulled back firmly.) Make sure he does not arch his lower back as he pulls his head back; this is a common movement compensation.

Next, with the back of the client's head gently touching the wall, assess his line of sight by drawing an imaginary line from the corner of his eye through the center of his eyeball and out into the room. If the neck is arched backward and the eye socket is tilted upward, this imaginary line will not be parallel to the floor and indicates that the client has excessive cervical lordosis (see figure 6.3) (Johnson 2016; Price and Bratcher 2010).

TEACHING CLIENTS NEUTRAL POSITION OF THE NECK AND HEAD

As with every other structure in the body, there is a neutral position that is optimal for the neck and head. The ability to achieve and maintain neutral positions is the key to helping eliminate pain and dysfunction (Griffin 2015). When we teach clients to attain a neutral neck and head position, it is important to ensure that they do not cheat in positioning other areas of the body to achieve the desired neck and head posture.

Instruct the client to stand with her heels, buttocks, back, and shoulders against a flat wall. Next, have her tilt her pelvis (without bending her knees) so that only two of your knuckles will fit between her lower back and the wall (see the section Hands-On Assessment for the Lumbo-Pelvic Hip Girdle in chapter 4). Then ask her to pull her head and shoulders back to the wall without arching her lower back or neck. The head and neck are in neutral positions when the back of the head is gently touching the wall, the shoulders are aligned under the tragus of the ear, and there is only a two-knuckle space between the client's lower back and the wall (see figure 6.4) (Kendall, McCreary, and Provance 2005; Price and Bratcher 2010). For an example of optimal alignment of the entire body in a standing position, see figure 6.5.

HOW THE HEAD AND NECK RELATE TO THE REST OF THE BODY

When the head moves forward from its optimal position, the thoracic spine and shoulders round forward to accommodate this shift and the resulting effective increase in the weight of the head. As this happens, the neck typically arches backward excessively to keep the eyes level and in line with the horizon (Palmer, Epler, and Epler 1998). This forward shift in the thoracic spine, shoulders, and head subsequently causes compensatory shifts in the pelvis and lower back. Specifically, the lower back arches excessively in an attempt to keep the body upright and balanced, and the pelvis rotates anteriorly (Kendall, McCreary, and Provance 2005). This shift in the pelvis and lower back causes the hip socket to move backward and the legs and hips to internally rotate, resulting in further compensations all the way down to the feet as the knees move toward the midline and the feet and ankles overpronate (see figure 6.6) (Price and Bratcher 2010).

Go to the online video to watch video 6.1, where Justin talks about what areas of the body are the most important to assess.

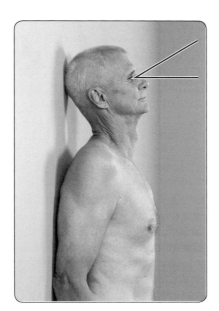

Figure 6.3   Example of excessive cervical lordosis.

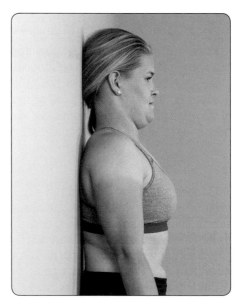

Figure 6.4   Neutral position for the neck and head.

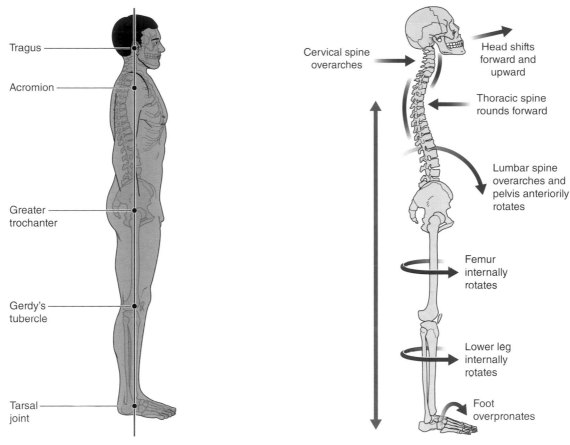

Figure 6.5 Optimal alignment for the body when standing.

Figure 6.6 How a forward head position affects alignment throughout the body.

Assessment Checklist

Before you complete your assessment of the neck and head, you must answer the following questions:

- ❏ Do you know what type of pain the client is experiencing and how it affects the function of her upper back, shoulders, neck, and head?
- ❏ Does the client have arthritis or any diagnosed conditions that might affect the success of her program?
- ❏ Does the client have any past injuries or surgeries that might affect the function of her neck and head?
- ❏ What makes the client's neck and head feel better or worse?
- ❏ Does the client's neck and head pain limit her function in any way?

- ❏ Does the client's neck and head pain affect her sleep?
- ❏ Are other parts of the client's body affected when her neck and head are painful?
- ❏ Does the client have a forward head?
- ❏ Does the client have excessive cervical lordosis?
- ❏ Does the client know how to achieve a neutral position for the neck and head?
- ❏ Do you know how the neck and head relate to the rest of the body, and can you explain it to the client?

Make all your notations for this part of the assessment on the Client Assessment Diagram (see figure 6.7 for an example).

Structural Assessment Skills Test

Perform a complete neck and head assessment on another person. Record your findings in the following Client Assessment Diagram.

Neck and head	✔	Details
Pain?		
Arthritis/conditions?		
Function?		
What makes it better/worse?		
Causal links?		
Visual irregularities?		
Forward head?		
Excessive neck curvature?		
Client knows neutral?		

Part II

Understanding Muscles and Movement

In part II, you will learn how to use the results of your assessment findings to gain insight into which muscles (and other soft tissues) are contributing to or are affected by the structural imbalances you have identified. An in-depth understanding of functional anatomy is critical to your success because it helps you to focus on the specific soft tissue problems that underlie most musculoskeletal imbalances.

Part II will introduce you to more than 100 muscles, ligaments, and tendons. Information is presented on muscle locations, origins and insertion points, movement actions, and how all these elements are interconnected through fascial networks. You will also learn how dysfunction, weakness, or restrictions in these structures can contribute to the common musculoskeletal imbalances you learned about in part I. You will also learn how muscles perform in relation to gravity and ground reaction forces. This will help you to understand how the body moves in real-life settings so that you can design effective corrective exercise programs that not only alleviate pain, but also help clients to get back to enjoying those physical activities they love.

Learning the technical and anatomical details about major muscles and how they work can be overwhelming. However, the following chapters will guide you through this process using easy-to-understand language, imagery, and real-life examples. Major muscles of the body are grouped by area of the body, such as the feet and ankles, lumbo-pelvic hip area, or the upper back and shoulder region. Each muscle is illustrated, with its origin and insertion points described, and its primary actions are described both from a traditional anatomy standpoint (i.e., when it contracts) and a functional standpoint (i.e., when it lengthens under tension). Explanations of the movements that each muscle helps the body perform, and examples of how that muscle works during activities such as walking, running, and squatting, are also provided. Lastly, each muscle description contains helpful tips to enhance your comprehension and to improve your ability to work with clients.

It is important to remember that part II does not discuss all the muscles in the human body, and the information should not be seen as a substitute for medical advice. These chapters are intended simply to give you an overview of the location and function of many important muscles involved in the most common musculoskeletal imbalances and their effect on movement.

keep people grounded, the structures of the body must also work hard against this downward pull to remain upright. If we could not do this, we would be crushed like aluminum cans against the ground. One of the most important parts of the human body is the skeletal system, which provides a strong, unyielding frame to support the body's resistance to the pull of gravity.

The human body is also equipped with soft tissue systems (muscles, ligaments, tendons, and fascia) whose role is to help the skeleton move. As you know from traditional anatomy, when muscles contract, they bring bones together. As we will discuss in later chapters, muscles also lengthen to slow bones and joints as they move apart. Soft tissue structures also help minimize stress on the skeletal system from gravity (Siegfried 2016). If you were standing upright and were in perfect structural alignment, for example, your skeletal system, along with the ligaments, would keep you erect; your center of gravity would be balanced over a solid foundation, and your muscles would not need to work much against the force of gravity. However, if you were to lean forward as if to pick up a pencil on the floor, your center of gravity would shift forward, and the muscles on the back of your torso would lengthen (with tension in them) to help slow down the movement of your skeleton as you reach toward the ground (Price 2014).

HOW GROUND REACTION FORCES AFFECT MOVEMENT

Ground reaction forces are explained by Newton's third law of motion, which states that for every action there is an equal but opposite reaction. Simply put, when force is applied by one object to another object (for example, by your body coming into contact with the ground through your foot when you walk), the ground returns the same amount of force through the foot to the body in the opposite direction (Ayyappa 1997).

What this means for our musculoskeletal system is that in addition to dealing with the constant pull of gravity, the body must also contend with the resulting shock that is created and transferred back into the system every time any part of you comes in contact with another object or surface. Muscles, tendons, ligaments, and fascia help regulate this stress from ground reaction forces by lengthening and stretching in order to slow the transmission of energy as it travels through the body to the joints and underlying skeletal system (Myers 2008; Price 2010).

The amount of force exerted on the bones, joints, ligaments, tendons, muscles, and fascia by gravity and ground reaction forces is remarkable. If every component of the musculoskeletal system is in perfect working order, the body can withstand tremendous pressure without any negative effects. However, if any of the elements are not functioning at their best, then musculoskeletal imbalances that can affect movement and performance may develop over time. To help people to identify and overcome musculoskeletal imbalances, a fitness professional must understand how the body and its soft tissue structures work both individually and together to resist gravity and absorb ground reaction forces. This will enable you to choose appropriate corrective exercises to correct imbalances and retrain a client's musculoskeletal system to effectively deal with these constant forces of nature (Price and Bratcher 2010).

OVERVIEW OF THE MUSCULOSKELETAL SYSTEM

Before we go into the functions of specific muscles and other soft tissues in depth, an overview of all the major structures of the musculoskeletal system will be presented, briefly describing how they work together to facilitate movement. Understanding the anatomy of individual muscles, especially where they originate and insert, will help you to link together chains of muscles and fascia from the feet to the head. As you begin to see the body as an integrated chain of bones, ligaments, tendons, muscles, and fascia, you will better appreciate how musculoskeletal dysfunction in one part of the body can have its roots elsewhere. The remainder of part II will examine the purposes of individual muscles (and other soft tissue structures) and their role in some of the most common musculoskeletal imbalances.

BONES

At birth, the human body contains about 300 bones (Marshall 2010). As we grow and age, some of these bones, such as those in the head, pelvis, and sacrum, fuse together. As a result, an adult has approximately 206 bones. The exact number can differ from person to person due to the fact that some people are born with extra bones, such as ribs (Gray 1995). Bones provide the internal framework for the body (see figure 7.1). They also protect vital organs and nerves, and together with muscles, ligaments, tendons, and fascia they comprise the musculoskeletal system.

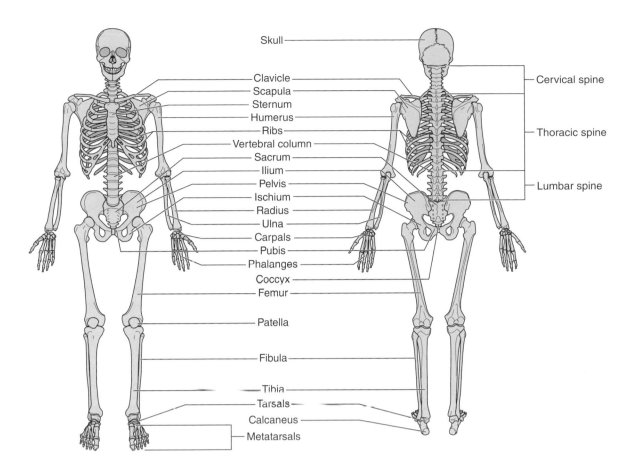

Figure 7.1   The human skeleton system.

Bones are made of hard, inflexible tissue that contains mainly calcium and collagen (Gray 1995). There are five types of bones in the body: long, short, flat, sesamoid, and irregular. The long bones are so named because they are usually longer than they are wide. They are designed to provide mobility. Examples of long bones include the femur in the upper leg, the humerus in the upper arm, the metatarsals in the feet, and the metacarpals in the hands (Dimon and Day 2008). A short bone is usually about as wide as it is long. Short bones are designed to provide support and stability. Examples include the tarsal bones toward the back of the foot, such as the navicular bone and the cuneiforms (Dimon and Day 2008). Flat bones are generally flat and help protect the body and its vital organs. They also provide surface area for muscular attachment (Dimon and Day 2008). Examples of flat bones include ribs, the bones of the skull, the scapula, and the pelvis (Price and Bratcher 2010). Sesamoid bones are usually embedded in tendons, and their function is to protect the host tendon (Gray 1995). The patella is an example. Irregular bones have an irregular shape and cannot be classified as any other type of bone. The vertebrae, the sacrum, and the mandible (jawbone) are examples of irregular bones (Gray 1995).

Bones are usually covered in smooth cartilage at either end to help prevent the two ends from rubbing together and to protect the joint space. Since cartilage is a firm, rubbery tissue, it also helps aid in shock absorption; it serves this function between the intervertebral discs of the spine (Gray 1995). The joint spaces between bones contain synovial fluid, a clear substance that is secreted to help lubricate the joint and keep it mobile (Dimon and Day 2008). Some bones have rounded edges called condyles that protrude from the ends of the bone to enable smooth articulation between bones, particularly at a joint (Gray 1995).

LIGAMENTS

The word *ligament* comes from the Latin word *ligare*, which means to "bind or tie." Ligaments are tough bands of connective tissue that join bones together at a joint like the knee. Ligaments provide

Review of Key Points

The musculoskeletal system is comprised of an intricate arrangement of several different types of bones and soft tissue structures that work in concert to control movement, deal with the constant pull of gravity, and dissipate ground reaction forces.

- Traditional anatomy texts emphasize the functions of muscles as contracting to bring bones together. However, muscles also help regulate the transfer of energy through the body by elongating, or working eccentrically.

- Bones occur in five main types to provide shape, support, and protection for our bodies: long bones, short bones, flat bones, sesamoid bones, and irregular bones.

- Ligaments are a type of connective tissue that connects bones together and helps provide stability and mobility for our joints.

- There are three types of muscle in the human body: smooth, cardiac, and skeletal.

- There are over 650 skeletal muscles in the human body. They apply force to bones to help create and regulate movement.

- Tendons are a type of connective tissue that binds muscle fibers together to enable individual muscles to attach to bone. It is the attachment of muscles to bones via tendons that enable muscles to produce movement.

- Fascia connects everything together in the body. Since fascia is interconnected and wrapped around every part, any restrictions or irritations in the fascia can affect the functioning of structures both in the immediate area and in other areas of the body.

- The human muscular system works in a fashion similar to bungee cords in that muscles and soft tissue structures must lengthen under tension, and at the right rate, to help slow movement and prevent injury. Muscles and soft tissue structures also use potential energy stored in them as they lengthen under tension to produce powerful movements when they contract.

Self-Check

Fill in the letter that best describes each musculoskeletal structure.

a. Connective tissue that attaches bones to other bones

b. Calcified tissue that gives support to our bodies

c. Specialized fibers that produce movement

d. Three-dimensional connective tissue that wraps around and throughout the body

e. Connective tissue that attaches muscles to bones

_____ Tendon

_____ Ligament

_____ Bones

_____ Muscles

_____ Fascia

CHAPTER 8

Functional Anatomy of the Feet and Ankles

The feet and ankles act as shock absorbers when the body interacts with a contact surface, and they help the body adapt to the terrain. They also contain several key soft tissues and muscles that help resist gravity and dissipate ground reaction forces (Davis, Davis, and Ross 2005; Frowen et al. 2010).

BONES AND JOINTS

The many bones and joints in the foot and ankle complex provide framing and unyielding support for the foot and ankle and help form its shape and structure (Dimon and Day 2008). The soft tissues assist the skeletal structures in maintaining the shape of the foot and ankle when it is placed under stress during exercise and other weight-bearing activities. By controlling movement, these soft tissues protect the underlying skeletal structures from damage, and they also provide feedback to the body about the nature of the contact surface (Page, Frank, and Lardner 2010).

SOFT TISSUE STRUCTURES

Here we describe several key soft tissue structures so that you can understand how they help with and influence movement. These structures are in part supported by (and intricately linked with) the muscles of the feet and ankles, and therefore they can be negatively affected by musculoskeletal imbalances.

ARCHES OF THE FEET

There are three arches in the feet (figure 8.1) made of a combination of bones, muscles, fascia, ligaments, and tendons:

1. The medial longitudinal arch
2. The lateral longitudinal arch
3. The transverse arch

The two longitudinal arches run along the sides of the foot from the heel to the toes. These two arches are intricately designed to help displace the weight of the body as it comes forward over the foot and to dissipate ground reaction forces as they travel back up to the body. The foot is also arched transversely (across the foot) to enable it to interact softly with the ground as weight is displaced from side to side and to provide additional stability and mobility to the foot so it can adapt to the terrain of the contact surface. The arches of the feet also lift the structures of the foot up and away from the ground to help protect these areas from injury (Clemente 2011).

The medial longitudinal arch is the prominent, big arch that runs along the inside of the foot from the heel to the base of the big toe. It is formed by the bones, ligaments, tendons, muscles, and fascia on the medial side of the foot. This arch is an excellent shock absorber, and it helps dissipate weight and force forward and toward the midline of the body (Dimon and Day 2008).

SLINGS OF THE FEET

Most of the muscles described in this chapter originate on the lower leg (or just above the knee, as in the case of the gastrocnemius) and wrap under the arches on either side of the foot or from around the back of the foot. These muscles act as slings that pull up on the feet and ankles, giving them tremendous support (Snell 2008). This sling support mechanism is very important in helping the body to interact with contact surfaces and in helping to regulate the transfer of weight forward and from side to side.

To help you better understand how the muscles of the feet and ankles act as slings, just imagine pulling a sock on over your foot. As you pull it up your leg, the sock pulls on the underside of your foot, creating tension on the sole of your foot. This pulling action supports the foot during the entire time you are pulling up the sock. The muscles of your lower leg, feet, and ankles work in a very similar fashion. They all wrap under and around your foot to ensure that your foot has support and does not collapse under your body weight (Price and Bratcher 2010).

MUSCLES

Now that we have examined the general functions of the foot and ankle muscles, we will discuss the details of certain key muscles in this area of the body. These include:

- Flexor hallucis longus
- Abductor hallucis
- Peroneus longus
- Tibialis posterior
- Tibialis anterior
- Soleus
- Gastrocnemius

Flexor Hallucis Longus

Muscle specifics: A long muscle that originates on the outside of the fibula on the back of the lower leg. It travels down and across the back of the lower leg and wraps around the inside of the anklebone. It then runs the length of the underside of the foot and inserts near the tip of the big toe on the plantar surface (Gray 1995).

Muscle action(s): Pushes the big toe down (i.e., flexes the big toe), pushes down the foot and ankle (i.e., plantar flexion) and rolls the ankle to the outside (i.e., inverts the ankle) (Clippinger 2007).

Real-life movements: The bungee cord action of the flexor hallucis longus helps support the medial longitudinal arch. In supporting this arch it directly helps to slow down overpronation of the foot and thereby increases ankle dorsiflexion. The potential energy stored in the muscle during these movements then helps the ankle and foot to plantar flex and helps the foot to push off powerfully in movements like walking and running.

Real-life movement example: Involved in supporting the foot and resisting overpronation in weight-bearing activities such as walking, squatting, lunging, jogging, and running.

Helpful tips: The flexor hallucis longus acts like a brake to help prevent the foot and ankle from overpronating.

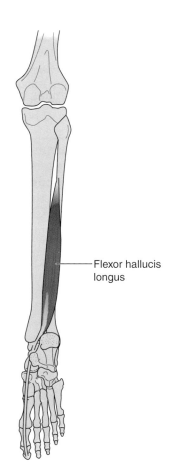

Flexor hallucis longus

Abductor Hallucis

Muscle specifics: A relatively small muscle on the underside of the foot. It is located on the medial side of the foot and travels from the heel bone to the first bone of the big toe (Gray 1995).

Muscle action(s): Pulls the big toe up and away from the rest of the toes and foot (i.e., abducts and flexes the big toe) (Muscolino 2010).

Real-life movements: The bungee cord action of the abductor hallucis helps keep the big toe straight and pointing forward to help support the medial longitudinal arch. This action helps the foot and ankle to resist overpronation and encourages better dorsiflexion.

Real-life movement example: Involved in helping maintain the structural integrity of the foot; ensures that the big toe spreads out to increase the surface area of the foot during weight-bearing activities such as walking, squatting, lunging, jogging, and running.

Helpful tips: The abductor hallucis works in conjunction with the flexor hallucis longus to support the medial longitudinal arch and to ensure that the big toe is aligned and working correctly.

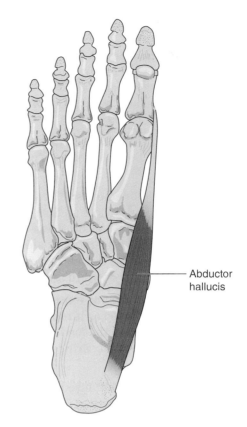

Abductor hallucis

Peroneus Longus

Muscle specifics: A part of the peroneal group of muscles that originate on the outside of the lower leg. The peroneus longus muscle travels down the leg, wraps behind the ankle and under the foot, and inserts at the base of the big toe (Gray 1995).

Muscle action(s): Helps roll the foot and ankle inward (eversion) and pushes the foot downward (plantar flexion) (Golding and Golding 2003).

Real-life movements: The bungee cord action of the peroneus longus helps support all the arches of the foot because it wraps under the outside, travels across the middle, and terminates toward the medial side. It also plays a vital role in helping the foot to accept weight and decelerate forces from both above and below.

Real-life movement example: Involved in helping maintain the integrity and strength of the arches of the feet during weight-bearing activities such as standing, walking, and running.

Helpful tips: The peroneus longus acts like a stirrup running beneath the foot to help hold up the arches.

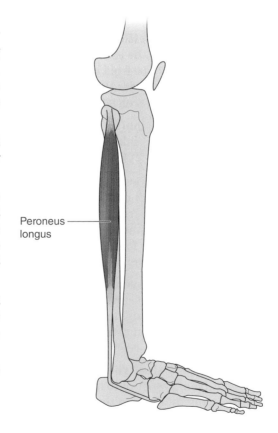

Peroneus longus

EFFECT OF FOOT AND ANKLE MUSCLES ON THE MOST COMMON MUSCULOSKELETAL DEVIATIONS

The muscles just described play a vital role in mitigating the two most common deviations of the foot and ankle. They provide strength and support to absorb shock and transfer the body's mass forward, side-to-side, and in rotation during weight-bearing activities. They also store potential energy to help with propulsion and to create powerful athletic movements. However, when musculoskeletal deviations affect the feet and ankles, they cannot perform these crucial tasks correctly. The foot and ankle structures can become strained and stressed, and musculoskeletal compensation patterns elsewhere in the body can become exacerbated, making everyday activities and exercise problematic and painful.

To illustrate how the foot and ankle muscles help prevent overpronation and lack of dorsiflexion, consider what happens when a person is walking. During a normal gait cycle, the feet and ankles work together to help stabilize the body's center of gravity and displace the weight of the body as it travels over the foot (Chinn and Hertel 2010). This helps to maintain an upright position and forward momentum. When a person begins walking, the outside of the heel connects with the ground first. At this point in the gait cycle, the ankle is inverted and weight is on the outside of the foot and heel. As weight is transferred forward into the foot and it makes full contact with the ground, the ankle rolls inward (pronates) and bends forward (dorsiflexes) to transfer weight over the entire foot (Donatelli and Wooden 2010).

These movements are critical to helping ensure that the foot and ankle muscles act like bungee cords to decelerate stresses. As the foot and ankle pronate, the muscles that support the arches of the foot lengthen under tension as the insertion points of these muscles (under the foot) move away from their points of origin (on the lower leg). This creates potential energy, which is then used to help roll the foot and ankle back out and to push the foot down and off the ground to complete the gait cycle. This motion becomes problematic when the foot and ankle overpronate. When the muscles that limit pronation do not work correctly or lengthen effectively, the bungee cord effect is lost. Consequently, no tension is created in the muscles to prevent the foot and ankle from overpronating. This results in the ankle failing to bend forward (dorsiflexing) enough to transfer weight correctly over the foot (Donatelli and Wooden 2010).

Here are two examples of how the bungee cord action of specific muscles controls both overpronation and dorsiflexion.

EXAMPLE ONE: TIBIALIS ANTERIOR AND TIBIALIS POSTERIOR

As the foot pronates, the medial longitudinal arch flattens out slightly and the toes move forward and away from the heel. This causes the insertion point of the tibialis anterior (in the midfoot area just behind the toes) to pull away from its origin point on the front of the tibia. This pulling motion creates tension and activates the bungee cord effect that helps to support the medial longitudinal arch and decelerate the foot, ankle, and lower leg as they roll inward. The tibialis posterior, which runs from beneath the foot, up and across the back of the leg to its origin high on the back of the tibia, also lengthens as the foot pronates. Its bungee cord effect prevents the lower leg from internally rotating too quickly over the foot. The actions of these two muscles help coordinate the timing of the lower leg's internal rotation and ensure that the foot pronates at the appropriate rate. Since the movement of the lower leg also affects the position and timing of the knee as it moves medially, these muscles also indirectly affect knee position and function.

EXAMPLE TWO: SOLEUS AND GASTROCNEMIUS

After the heel has made contact with the ground during the gait cycle, weight is transferred forward as the lower leg and knee move over the foot. The soleus originates high on the back of the lower leg and is attached to the back of the heel by the

Achilles tendon. As the knee and ankle bend, the movement of its insertion point away from its origin point enables the bungee cord feature to help control both dorsiflexion and knee flexion. As the gait cycle continues, the foot remains in contact with the ground as the leg extends behind the body. During this movement, the gastrocnemius lengthens like a bungee cord, and the tension in the muscle slows down the lower leg as it continues to move forward over the foot and the knee as it straightens.

Go to the online video to watch video 8.3, where Justin talks about how dysfunction of the calf muscles can affect the most common imbalances.

If the calf muscles and other muscles of the foot and ankle (such as the anterior and posterior tibialis discussed in example one) do not prevent the foot from overpronating, then the foot and ankle collapse, and the lower leg rotates inward too quickly instead of coming forward over the foot as it should. This disruption of the forward motion of the lower leg over the foot is why overpronation and a lack of dorsiflexion are inherently linked. Moreover, when any of the other muscles of the feet and ankles discussed in this chapter are not working correctly, overpronation and lack of dorsiflexion can result. This can lead to the structures of the foot and ankle becoming stressed, compensation patterns developing elsewhere in the body and, over time, pain or injury.

Review of Key Points

The muscles and soft tissue structures of the feet and ankles play an important role in helping to support and balance the body while it interacts with a contact surface.

- Most of the muscles vital to the function of the foot and ankle complex come down from the lower leg, wrap around the ankle, and attach on the underside of the foot. They act like a sling support system to control the movement of the foot and ankle in all three planes of motion and engage as weight is transferred over the feet and ankles during weight-bearing activities.

- The feet contain a system of arches that displace body weight and dissipate ground reaction forces when they interact with a contact surface. The arches also help to provide propulsion during the gait cycle.

  - Medial longitudinal arch
  - Lateral longitudinal arch
  - Transverse arch

- The muscles in the feet and ankles are like bungee cords in that they develop more tension as they lengthen. This elastic property of muscles enables them to slow down forces on the foot and ankle joints and to store potential energy to facilitate movement.

- The Achilles tendon is a strong and resilient soft tissue structure that attaches the soleus and gastrocnemius muscles to the heel. Tension on the Achilles tendon when the foot dorsiflexes helps to decelerate forces on the foot and ankle and to generate power for propulsion.

- When the muscles and other soft tissue structures of the feet and ankles are healthy and functioning well, they can help prevent overpronation and lack of dorsiflexion.

Self-Check

Perform each of the common activities and movements listed in the following chart. During each activity, try to visualize when the muscle listed next to it is lengthening like a bungee cord. Place a check mark in the box next to each activity or muscle pairing when you can visualize or feel the bungee cord feature activate.

Movement	Muscle	Able to visualize
Standing with your feet hip width apart and rocking backward and forward	Flexor hallucis longus	❏
Walking slowly	Flexor hallucis longus	❏
Single-leg squat	Tibialis anterior	❏
Squatting	Soleus	❏
Walking slowly	Gastrocnemius	❏
Standing with your feet shoulder width apart and rocking from side to side	Peroneus longus	❏
Walking backward	Gastrocnemius	❏
Going down stairs	Tibialis posterior	❏
Jogging	All the muscles of the feet and ankles	❏

CHAPTER 9

Functional Anatomy of the Knees

The knee is the largest joint in the body (Schlossberg and Zuidema 1997). Its primary purpose is to link the upper leg to the lower leg with a hinge joint. Although the knee can move in all three planes of motion, its main functions are flexion and extension (Hyde and Gengenbach 2007). The knee, therefore, plays a vital role in all weight-bearing activities that involve forward, backward, and vertical movement.

BONES AND JOINTS

The knee joint is where the tibia and fibula connect with the femur to enable articulation between the lower and upper leg (Dimon and Day 2008). The kneecap is located in the center of the knee joint; it connects to the upper leg via the quadriceps tendon and to the lower leg via the patellar ligament. Two discs of cartilage, the medial and lateral menisci, provide a layer of cushioning between the bones of the lower leg and the femur.

SOFT TISSUE STRUCTURES

Several key soft tissue structures in the knees are discussed next so that you can understand how they help with and influence movement. These structures are supported in part by the muscles of the knees, and therefore can be negatively affected by musculoskeletal imbalances.

COLLATERAL AND CRUCIATE LIGAMENTS

There are four major ligaments in the knee joint that connect the lower leg bones with the femur and help stabilize movement. The medial collateral ligament connects the tibia and femur, and the lateral collateral ligament connects the fibula and femur. The primary function of these ligaments is to provide side-to-side support to the knee. Inside the knee joint are the anterior cruciate ligament (ACL) and the posterior cruciate ligament (PCL), which connect the tibia and femur in a crisscross fashion. The primary function of these ligaments is to help stabilize the knee from front to back, side to side, and in rotation (Hyde and Gengenbach 2007).

ILIOTIBIAL BAND

The iliotibial band (IT band) is a dense strip of connective tissue that runs along the lateral side of the thigh (see figure 9.1). It originates from the fibers of the gluteus maximus and tensor fasciae latae muscles and serves to connect these muscles to the lower leg (Clippinger 2007). Because of its origins above the knee and attachment below it, the IT band has a direct impact on knee function. Specifically, the IT band works in conjunction with the gluteus maximus and tensor fasciae latae to help decelerate internal rotation of the leg. However, when the gluteus maximus becomes deconditioned as a result of musculoskeletal imbalances, it cannot do this effectively. This results in the IT band overworking and experiencing excessive tension and stress, often resulting in pain.

MUSCLES

There are many muscles in the upper and lower leg that help stabilize and mobilize the knee. In chapter 8 you learned that some of the muscles of the lower leg that affect the foot and ankle also affect the knee (e.g., the soleus and the gastrocnemius). In this chapter, you will learn about muscles in the upper leg that originate above the knee (and attach either to the knee or just below it) and directly affect its function (Gray 1995). The muscles identified in this chapter are the following:

- Vastus lateralis
- Vastus intermedius
- Vastus medialis
- Rectus femoris
- Gluteus maximus
- Semimembranosus
- Semitendinosus
- Biceps femoris
- Adductor magnus
- Adductor longus
- Adductor brevis
- Pectineus
- Gracilis

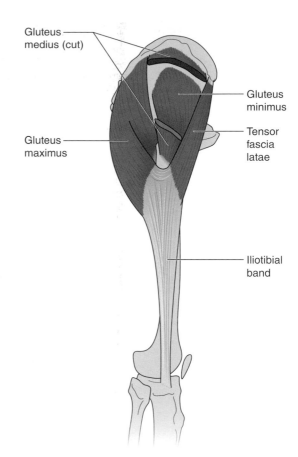

Gluteus medius (cut)

Gluteus minimus

Gluteus maximus

Tensor fascia latae

Iliotibial band

Figure 9.1   Iliotibial band.

Vastus Lateralis (Quadriceps Group)

Muscle specifics: A large quadriceps muscle that originates near the top of the leg on the femur, travels down the outside of the thigh, and inserts at the kneecap by way of the quadriceps tendon (Kulkarni 2012).

Muscle action(s): Straightens the knee (i.e., knee extension) and helps hold the kneecap in place (Gray 1995).

Real-life movements: The "bungee cord" action of the vastus lateralis helps slow down the knee as it bends when the foot comes in contact with the ground during closed-chain movements such as squatting. The lengthening of this muscle as the knee bends stores potential energy, which is then used to help the knee straighten.

Real-life movement example: Acts like a bungee cord to decelerate force transferred through the knee during movements like lunging or bending down in preparation for a jump. Tension created in the muscle when the knee bends is then used to help straighten the knee and enable the person to jump higher.

Helpful tips: As the knee bends during a squat, it creates tension in the vastus lateralis muscle. This tension helps pull the kneecap tight to help it track and move correctly, thereby providing protection and stability for the knee joint.

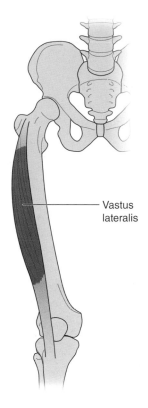

Vastus lateralis

Vastus Intermedius (Quadriceps Group)

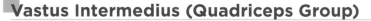

Muscle specifics: A large quadriceps muscle that lies beneath the rectus femoris muscle on the front of the upper leg. It originates on the femur near the top of the thigh, travels down the middle of the front of the thigh, and inserts at the kneecap by way of the quadriceps tendon (Kulkarni 2012).

Muscle action(s): Straightens the knee (knee extension) and helps to hold the kneecap in place (Gray 1995).

Real-life movements: The bungee cord action of the vastus intermedius helps decelerate flexion of the knee as it bends. The lengthening of the muscle as the knee bends stores potential energy, which is then used to help the knee straighten.

Real-life movement example: Acts like a bungee cord to decelerate force transferred through the knee during movements like squatting down to pick up a heavy weight. Tension created in the muscle when the knee bends is used to straighten the knee to help a person stand back upright.

Helpful tips: Performing leg extensions while seated on a machine in the gym may not adequately prepare the quadriceps muscles for their more functional purpose of decelerating the knee as it bends when the foot is in contact with the ground.

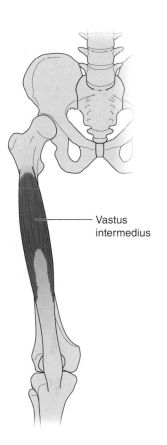

Vastus intermedius

Vastus Medialis (Quadriceps Group)

Muscle specifics: A large quadriceps muscle that lies toward the midline of the body on the front of the thigh. It originates near the top of the femur, travels down the medial side of the front of the thigh, and inserts at the kneecap via the quadriceps tendon (Kulkarni 2012).

Muscle action(s): Straightens the knee (knee extension) and holds the kneecap in place (Gray 1995).

Real-life movements: The bungee cord action of the vastus medialis helps decelerate flexion of the knee. The lengthening of the muscle as the knee bends stores potential energy, which is then used to help the knee straighten.

Real-life movement example: Acts like a bungee cord to slow down the knee as it bends during movements like squatting down to hit a low volley in tennis. Tension created in the muscle when the knee bends is used to straighten the knee to help the person hit the ball as they return to a standing position.

Helpful tips: The muscle fibers of the quadriceps group come down the front, outside, and inside of the upper leg, and they all tie together at the quadriceps tendon, which helps hold the kneecap in place.

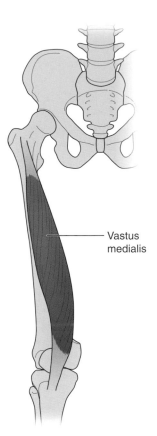

Vastus medialis

Rectus Femoris (Quadriceps Group)

Muscle specifics: A large quadriceps muscle on the front of the leg. It originates on the pelvis on a bony protuberance at the front of the pelvis, travels down the front of the thigh, and inserts at the kneecap by way of the quadriceps tendon (Kulkarni 2012).

Muscle action(s): Straightens (extends) the knee, brings the leg toward the trunk (i.e., flexes the hip joint), and helps hold the kneecap in place (Gray 1995).

Real-life movements: The bungee cord action of the rectus femoris helps decelerate flexion of the knee. Since the rectus femoris is the only quadriceps muscle that originates from the pelvis, it also helps slow down extension of the hip and leg as the muscle lengthens.

Real-life movement example: Acts like a bungee cord to decelerate the knee as it bends in movements like lunging forward. Due to its origin on the front of the pelvis, it also helps decelerate the hip and leg as it extends—for example, when the leg travels behind the body during walking or running. Tension created in the muscle when the knee bends or the hip extends is then used to straighten the knee or flex the hip.

Helpful tips: The rectus femoris muscle assists the hip flexor group of muscles in slowing down extension of the hips and legs. People with tight hip flexors may experience problems with their rectus femoris as it tries to overcompensate for dysfunctional hip flexors.

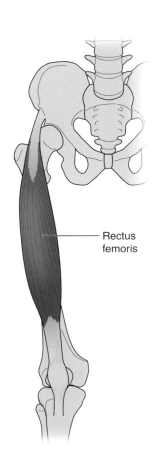

Rectus femoris

Gluteus Maximus

Muscle specifics: A large superficial muscle on the back of the hips and pelvis. It originates on the back of the pelvis, at the base of the spine (i.e., sacrum and coccyx), and on the thoracolumbar fascia of the lower back. It runs across the back of the hips and pelvis and has a small insertion on the upper femur. However, the larger portion of the gluteus maximus muscle blends into the IT band, which inserts below the knee on the outside of the tibia (Clippinger 2007).

Muscle action(s): Pushes the hips forward (i.e., extends the hip and leg) and outwardly rotates the leg (Gray 1995).

Real-life movements: The bungee cord action of the gluteus maximus helps decelerate hip flexion (i.e., bending of the hips) and internal rotation of the leg.

Real-life movement example: Acts like a bungee cord to decelerate hip flexion in activities such as bending your hips to sit or squat down. Also helps to slow the internal rotation of the leg during weight-bearing activities like walking, lunging, and squatting when the foot pronates and the ankle and leg rotate in to help the body to transfer weight.

Helpful tips: The gluteus maximus attaches to the lower leg via the IT band. It is an important muscle that, when working properly, helps to slow down pronation and displacement of the leg toward the midline of the body. People who overpronate and their knees move medially will typically have weak gluteus maximus muscles and irritated IT bands.

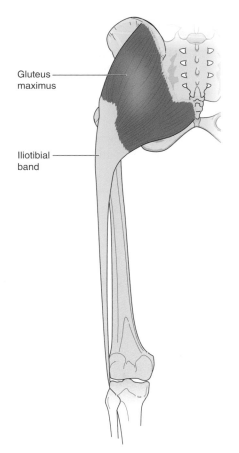

Gluteus maximus

Iliotibial band

Semimembranosus (Hamstring Group)

Muscle specifics: A hamstring muscle on the back of the leg. It originates on the ischial tuberosity of the pelvis (i.e., the "sit bone"), travels down the back of the upper leg, crosses the knee joint, and inserts on the medial side of the tibia (Agur and Dalley 2013).

Muscle action(s): Bends (flexes) the knee and pushes (extends) the hips forward. Also helps with inward rotation of the lower leg when the knee is bent (Gray 1995).

Real-life movements: The bungee cord action of the semimembranosus helps decelerate the knee as it straightens and the hips as they bend. As this muscle lengthens, tension is created, which is then used to help extend the hips.

Real-life movement example: Acts like a bungee cord to decelerate flexion of the hips during movements such as bending over to touch your toes with your legs straight. Since the semimembranosus inserts at the tibia, it also helps control movement of the lower leg during weight-bearing activities like walking and running.

Helpful tips: The semimembranosus is the most medial of the three hamstring muscles, and it helps protect the knees, hips, and lower back from excessive stress.

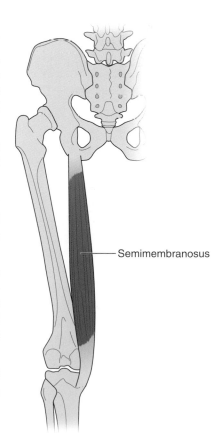

Semimembranosus

Semitendinosus (Hamstring Group)

Muscle specifics: A hamstring muscle on the back of the leg. It originates on the ischial tuberosity of the pelvis (i.e., the "sit bone"), travels down the back of the upper leg, crosses the knee joint, and inserts on the medial side of the tibia a little lower down than the semimembranosus (Agur and Dalley 2013).

Muscle action(s): Bends (flexes) the knee and pushes (extends) the hips forward. It also helps with inward rotation of the leg when the knee is bent (Gray 1995).

Real-life movements: The bungee cord action of the semitendinosus muscle helps decelerate flexion of the hips when the knee is relatively straight. This motion helps load the muscle with potential energy that is then used to help extend the hips when a person stands erect.

Real-life movement example: Acts like a bungee cord to decelerate flexion of the hips during movements such as bending forward at the waist to pat a dog or tie your shoe laces. Since the semitendinosus inserts at the tibia, it also helps control the rotation of the lower leg during weight-bearing activities like walking and running.

Helpful tips: The semitendinosus muscle works in concert with the semimembranosus muscle to help minimize stress to the knees, hips, and lower back.

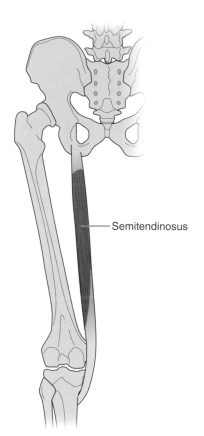

Semitendinosus

Biceps Femoris (Hamstring Group)

Muscle specifics: A hamstring muscle on the back of the leg. It has two origin points: The long head originates on the ischial tuberosity of the pelvis (i.e., "the sit bone"), and the short head originates lower down on the femur. The muscle travels down the back of the upper leg, crosses the knee joint, and inserts on the outside of the fibula and tibia (Agur and Dalley 2013).

Muscle action(s): Both the long head and the short head of the biceps femoris are responsible for bending the knee (knee extension), and the long head also helps extend the hips. Both heads help with outward rotation of the leg when the knee is bent (Gray 1995).

Real-life movements: The bungee cord action of the biceps femoris helps decelerate flexion of the hips and extension of the knee. It also helps decelerate internal rotation of the lower leg.

Real-life movement example: Acts like a bungee cord to decelerate hip flexion during movements such as bending over at the waist to touch your toes or pick a flower. It also helps control internal rotation of the lower leg during weight-bearing activities like walking and running.

Helpful tips: All of the hamstring muscles work in concert like guide ropes coming up from the lower leg to help control movement of the hips, pelvis, and lower back during weight-bearing activities.

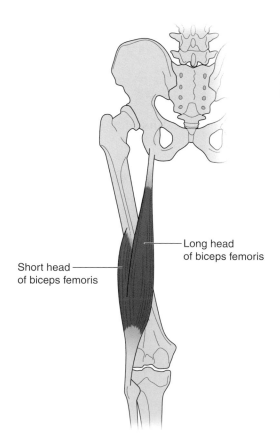

Long head of biceps femoris

Short head of biceps femoris

Adductor Magnus (Adductor Group)

Muscle specifics: A large adductor muscle in the upper leg. It is divided into two parts, an adductor portion on the inside of the thigh and a hamstring portion on the back of the leg. Both portions originate at the base and front of the pelvis (ischium and pubis), fan diagonally across to the leg, and insert in many areas just behind the midline of the femur nearly all the way down to the knee (Antevil, Blackbourne, and Moore 2006).

Muscle action(s): Moves the hip and leg toward the midline of the body (i.e., adducts the hip and leg). In addition, the hamstring portion of the muscle pushes the hip forward (extends the hip), while the adductor portion helps lift the leg forward (hip flexion) (Antevil, Blackbourne, and Moore 2006).

Real-life movements: The bungee cord action of the adductor magnus helps decelerate abduction of the leg away from the midline of the body. The muscle also stores potential energy as a person walks to assist with both hip flexion and extension (depending on which part of the muscle is emphasized during the movement).

Real-life movement example: Acts like a bungee cord to decelerate the leg as it moves outside the pelvis (and the pelvis as it moves inside the leg) as weight is transferred from one leg to the other, as when getting in and out of a car. The adductor portion of the muscle also helps to slow down the leg as it travels behind the body when walking or running, and the hamstring portion helps slow down hip flexion during movements like bending over to tie your shoelaces.

Helpful tips: To feel the bungee cord effect of this muscle as the hip extends and then prepares to flex, stand in a split stance. Place your hand on the inside of the upper thigh of the leg that is behind you. Raise that heel off the ground and lower it again to feel the muscle shorten and lengthen.

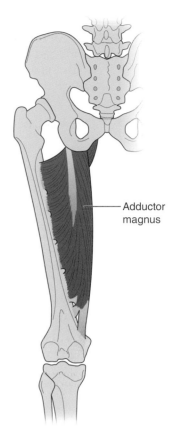

Adductor magnus

Adductor Longus (Adductor Group)

Muscle specifics: An adductor muscle of the inner thigh. It originates on the front of the pelvis near the bottom of the pubis, crosses over diagonally to the thigh, and inserts on the inside of the femur about halfway down the upper leg (Antevil, Blackbourne, and Moore 2006).

Muscle action(s): Pulls the leg toward the midline of the body (i.e., adducts the leg) and outwardly rotates the leg. It also helps to flex the hip and leg (Gray 1995).

Real-life movements: The bungee cord action of the adductor longus helps decelerate the hip and leg as they move away from the midline of the body (i.e., abduct) during weight-bearing activities. It also helps slow down the hip and leg as they travel into extension.

Real-life movement example: Acts like a bungee cord to decelerate movement of the leg to the side of the body during actions like lunging to the side; it has the same effect on movement of the trailing leg behind the body when a person lunges forward.

Helpful tips: All the adductors work together to help the hip flexors to slow down hip and leg extension. During hip extension, the leg also internally rotates. The adductors also play a role in slowing down the internal rotation of the leg when it travels behind the body into extension.

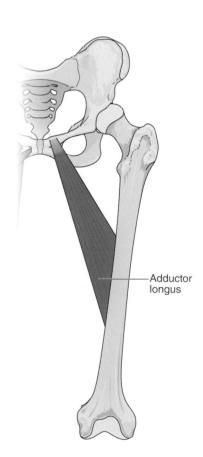

Adductor longus

Adductor Brevis (Adductor Group)

Muscle specifics: A small adductor muscle that originates on the front of the pelvis near the bottom of the pubis, fans diagonally across to the leg, and inserts on the upper part of the femur (Antevil, Blackbourne, and Moore 2006).

Muscle action(s): Brings the leg toward the midline (adduction) and flexes the hip and leg (Gray 1995).

Real-life movements: The bungee cord action of the adductor brevis helps decelerate movement of the hip and leg away from the midline of the body (i.e., abduction). It also slows down hip extension during gait when the trailing leg is on the ground and travels behind the body.

Real-life movement example: Acts like a bungee cord to assist with many movements of the hip and leg complex when the pelvis has to travel over and forward of the leg, such as what happens during activities like walking, running, and going up stairs.

Helpful tips: The tension created in the adductor muscles during hip extension (and the accompanying internal rotation of the leg) creates potential energy for lifting the leg off the ground, flexing the hip, and externally rotating the leg to help swing it forward for the next phase of gait.

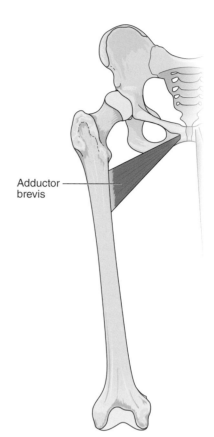

Adductor brevis

Pectineus (Adductor Group)

Muscle specifics: A small adductor muscle that originates on the front of the bottom of the pelvis near the top part of the pubis, runs across diagonally to the leg, and inserts near the top of the femur slightly toward the back (Clippinger 2007).

Muscle action(s): Brings the hip and leg toward the midline (adduction), outwardly rotates the leg, and assists in hip flexion.

Real-life movements: The bungee cord action of the pectineus helps decelerate the hip and leg as they move away from the midline (abduct), and it slows down hip and leg extension (and the accompanying internal rotation of the leg) during weight-bearing activities.

Real-life movement example: Acts like a bungee cord to slow down the hip and leg complex as it moves away from the midline and behind the body when the leg is in contact with the ground during weight-bearing activities such as walking, lunging, or working out on an elliptical machine.

Helpful tips: Exercise equipment such as the Thigh Master and similar machines primarily work the adductors in a concentric manner. However, to develop strong and healthy muscles that function well, the adductors must be strengthened using exercises that lengthen the muscle, such as what happens when lunging or stepping from side to side.

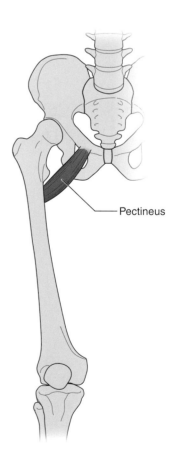

Pectineus

Gracilis (Adductor Group)

Muscle specifics: A long adductor muscle that originates on the front of the bottom of the pelvis on the medial part of the pubis, runs on an angle all the way down the inside of the upper leg, and inserts on the medial side of the tibia just below the knee (Antevil, Blackbourne, and Moore 2006).

Muscle action(s): Adducts, flexes, and externally rotates the hip and leg. Due to its attachment just below the knee, it also helps flex the knee (Gray 1995).

Real-life movements: The bungee cord action of the gracilis helps decelerate the hip and leg as they move away from the midline (hip and leg abduction); it also helps decelerate internal rotation of the leg and extension of the hip and leg. Since it attaches to the lower leg, it also helps stabilize the knee as the leg moves into extension.

Real-life movement example: While similar to the other adductor muscles, the gracilis is distinct in that it crosses the knee joint and attaches to the tibia. Consequently, the gracilis provides stability to the knee during activities where the trailing leg moves into extension, such as climbing a ladder or steep hill or when ice skating.

Helpful tips: All the adductor muscles work together to help stabilize the pelvis on top of the legs during weight-bearing activities.

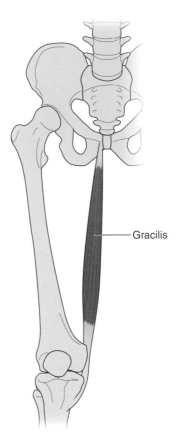
Gracilis

EFFECT OF KNEE MUSCLES ON THE MOST COMMON MUSCULOSKELETAL DEVIATIONS

The muscles described in this section play a vital role in mitigating the two most common deviations of the knee: side-to-side alignment problems and tracking problems during flexion and extension. They directly strengthen and support the knee and decelerate forces on the knee by controlling the body's weight as it is transferred over the feet, ankles, legs, and pelvis (Price and Bratcher 2010).

When considering the real-life functions of the muscles that surround the knees, it may be helpful to visualize these soft tissue structures as strings of a puppet that hang down from the pelvis and upper leg, attaching to various parts of the upper leg, knee, and lower leg. The positioning of these "strings" and their appropriate movement control the bones that affect the knee (the femur, kneecap, tibia, and fibula) and stabilize, decelerate, and accelerate the knee in all planes of motion.

Here are three examples of how the bungee cord feature of specific muscles and muscle groups can prevent the two most common deviations of the knee.

EXAMPLE ONE: GLUTEUS MAXIMUS AND THE ADDUCTORS

The gluteus maximus and the adductor group of muscles both help prevent side-to-side displacement of the knee (as well as overpronation of the foot and ankle complex).

When a person is walking, part of the gait cycle involves the leg swinging forward and the foot striking the ground. When this happens, the insertion point of the gluteus maximus on the leg is pulled away from its origins on the back of the pelvis and the base of the spine. As the gait cycle continues and pressure is transferred into the foot, the leg rotates inward, pulling the insertion point of the gluteus maximus even farther from its origin points. This motion creates tension in this muscle (and in the iliotibial band) that slows the internal rotation of the leg and the movement of the knee toward the midline of the body and prevents a valgus knee position, tracking problems, and overpronation at the foot and ankle (see figure 9.2).

As the gait cycle continues, the knee and leg straighten as the leg travels behind the body into extension. As the leg travels behind the pelvis, the heel remains in contact with the ground, the foot pronates, and the leg rotates inwardly. The adductor muscles, which attach mostly to the medial sides of the upper and lower leg bones, lengthen and decelerate hip extension and internal rotation of the leg. As they lengthen, they also slow the pelvis as it shifts inside the leg and toward the midline during weight transfer. Effective lengthening of the adductors, therefore, is vital to minimizing stress on the pelvis, hips, knees, feet, and ankles (see figure 9.3).

EXAMPLE TWO: THE QUADRICEPS

The quadriceps play an important part in preventing tracking problems of the knee. The quadriceps muscles attach to the kneecap via the quadriceps tendon. As the knee bends, the quadriceps lengthen, creating tension in these muscles, the quadriceps tendon, and the patellar ligament, which helps to pull the kneecap tight to the knee so it can track correctly over the femoral groove (at the bottom of the femur) (see figure 9.4). As the knee straightens, the pressure on the kneecap is reduced, enabling the knee to straighten.

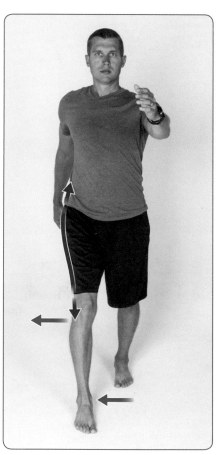

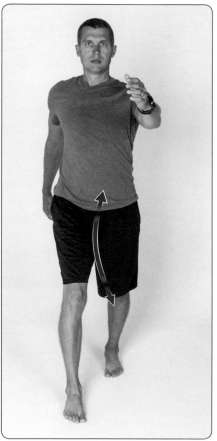

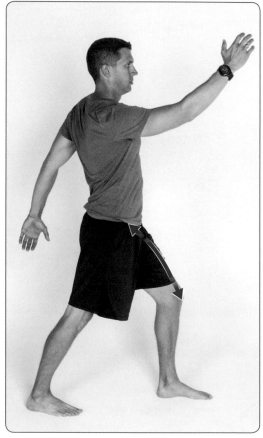

Figure 9.2 Example of the bungee cord action of the gluteus maximus slowing down the internal rotation of the leg.

Figure 9.3 Example of the bungee cord action of the adductors as they slow down the leg going behind the body and the pelvis shifting inside the trailing leg.

Figure 9.4 Example of the bungee cord action of the quadriceps helping hold the kneecap in place as the knee bends.

EXAMPLE THREE: THE HAMSTRINGS

The hamstrings help prevent side-to-side alignment problems of the knee. These muscles run like guide ropes from the base of the pelvis, down the back of the leg, and attach to either side of the lower leg. When the hip is flexed and the leg is relatively straight (such as what happens when bending over to touch one's toes), the hamstrings lengthen under tension to control side-to-side movement of the knee and prevent valgus or varus imbalances (see figure 9.5). They also work in a bottom-up fashion (from insertion point to origin) by lengthening to control the pelvis as the base of it rotates away from the knee (i.e., an anterior pelvic tilt).

When all the muscles that cross the knees are working correctly, then the bones that meet at the knee joint can move in a controlled manner, and deviations or movement imbalances in the knees can be reduced.

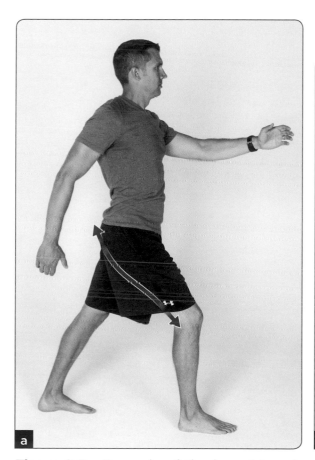
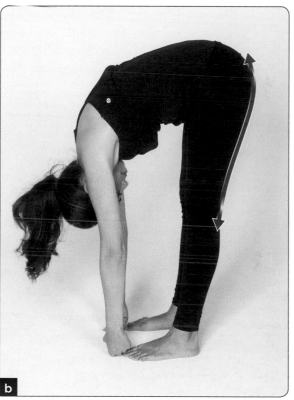

Figure 9.5 Example of the hamstrings lengthening to (a) slow down the pelvis as it anteriorly rotates and (b) control side-to-side motion of the knee.

Review of Key Points

The knee joint is controlled and affected by muscles in the lower and upper leg. The muscles that cross the knee both produce movement and slow down movement to protect the knee joint and its soft tissue structures from unnecessary stress.

- Although the knee joint is a hinge joint, it has the capability to move in all three planes of motion.

- The quadriceps group consists of four muscles on the front of the upper leg that lengthen under tension to slow down forces on the knee as it bends. As they lengthen, they also help pull the kneecap tight on the femoral groove so that it tracks correctly.

- The gluteus maximus has attachments on the femur and the tibia, which enables it to slow down hip flexion and internal rotation of the upper and lower leg. A weak gluteus maximus is less able to prevent excessive inward rotation of the leg and overpronation of the foot. Therefore, the gluteus maximus is an important muscle to target in a corrective exercise program to address these common imbalances.

- The position and attachment sites of the hamstring muscles enable them to help control movement of the torso as a person bends forward and to slow down the knee as it straightens and moves from side to side during the gait cycle.

- Unlike most of the other muscles in the upper leg, which generally run parallel to the femur, the adductor group runs diagonally from the pelvis to the femur. Their prime job is to help stabilize the pelvis as it moves from side to side and to decelerate the leg as it internally rotates and extends.

- The only adductor muscle that does not attach to the femur is the gracilis. It attaches to the medial side of the top of the tibia, which means it has a direct impact on knee function.

Self-Check

There are many distinct groups of muscles in the upper leg that cross the knee joint and affect knee function. For the actions that follow, try to describe what each muscle or muscle group is doing during that movement to help minimize unnecessary stress on the knee or to enable the movement to happen correctly. An example is provided.

MOVEMENT: Getting out of a car

Gluteus maximus: Stabilizes the knee and helps extend the hips to help you stand up out of the seat.

Quadriceps: Ensure that the knee tracks correctly and help extend the knees to stand.

Adductors: Stabilize the pelvis over the leg that is still inside the car as you begin to stand and lift the other leg in preparation for stepping out of the car.

Hamstrings: Slow down hip flexion so you do not lean too far forward when you try to stand up.

MOVEMENT: Stepping sideways over a puddle

Gluteus maximus:

Quadriceps:

Adductors:

Hamstrings:

MOVEMENT: Sitting down on a chair

Gluteus maximus:

Quadriceps:

Adductors:

Hamstrings:

MOVEMENT: Bending down to pick up a penny

Gluteus maximus:

Quadriceps:

Adductors:

Hamstrings:

CHAPTER 10

Functional Anatomy of the Lumbo-Pelvic Hip Girdle

The lumbo-pelvic hip girdle is composed of the lumbar spine, pelvis, and hips. The robust bones, strong ligaments, and large muscles of this area provide support and balance for the entire body. They also supply mobility to both generate and transfer forces from the lower kinetic chain to the upper kinetic chain and vice versa during all dynamic weight-bearing activities (Gamble 2013).

BONES AND JOINTS

The lumbo-pelvic hip girdle includes the bones of the pelvis (ilium, ischium, and pubis), the lumbar segment of the spine, and the sacrum and coccyx (figure 10.1). It also has two very important articulations where the bones of the spine, leg, and pelvis come together: the sacroiliac joint and the acetabulum. The sacroiliac joint is where the sacrum meets the back of the pelvis (ilium). The acetabulum is a cup-shaped depression in the pelvis formed where the ischium, ilium, and pubis meet that accommodates the end of the femur to create the hip socket. Many ligaments help hold the bones of the pelvis, spine, and femur in place to enable the myriad of movements possible in the lumbo-pelvic hip region (Clark and Lucett 2011).

SOFT TISSUE STRUCTURES

Here we discuss several key soft tissue structures in the lumbo-pelvic hip girdle so that you can understand how they assist with and influence movement. They are supported by the muscles of the torso and legs, and therefore can be negatively affected by musculoskeletal imbalances in these areas.

THORACOLUMBAR FASCIA

The thoracolumbar fascia, also sometimes called the lumbodorsal fascia, is a collection of three layers of fascia that help tie down, connect to, and bind with many of the ligaments and big, strong muscles of the lower back, pelvis, and rib cage (figure 10.2). This system of fascia helps provide extra stability and creates localized tension around the pelvis and lower back by pulling tight when muscles of the lumbo-

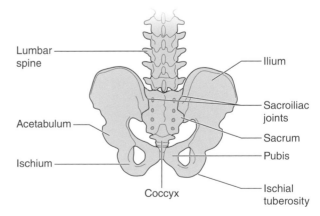

Figure 10.1 Anatomy of the lumbo-pelvic hip girdle.

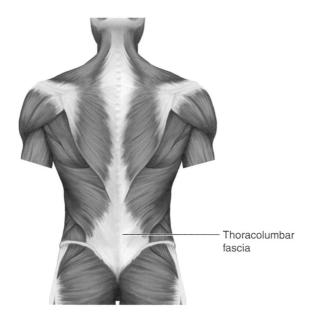

Figure 10.2   The thoracolumbar fascia.

pelvic hip girdle lengthen and contract. Although the thoracolumbar fascia provides sturdiness and support, it is also flexible and thus permits the many movements that are required of the lumbo-pelvic hip girdle (Middleditch and Oliver 2005).

To appreciate how the thoracolumbar fascia provides extra stability to this region, imagine the difference between pumping air into a balloon and pumping air into a soccer ball. As air is pumped into the balloon, it expands and does not provide much resistance against the air going in. On the other hand, the leather casing of a soccer ball provides much more resistance and creates more tension on the outside of the ball as it inflates. This is similar to how the dense connective tissue of the thoraco-lumbar fascia works. As muscles of the lumbo-pelvic hip girdle contract, the membrane surrounding them, the thoracolumbar fascia, becomes taut like the outer membrane of the soccer ball. This adds stability to the lumbo-pelvic hip girdle (Price and Bratcher 2010).

The attachments of the thoracolumbar fascia to muscles and structures across the lower back also contribute to its stabilizing features when these muscles or structures move (Middleditch and Oliver 2005). For example, the thoracolumbar fascia has attachments to the back of the pelvis. Therefore, when the back of the pelvis is engaged in movement (e.g., during a posterior pelvic tilt), it pulls on the thoracolumbar fascia, and tension is created across and throughout the tissue, helping stabilize the area.

LIGAMENTS

There are many ligaments in the lumbo-pelvic hip area that help provide stability and help transfer forces through the joints of the hips, pelvis, and spine (figure 10.3) (Muscolino 2011). These ligaments not only provide local stability to the lumbo-pelvic hip region, but because they share connective tissue with many large muscles, they also help transfer tension across some of the most important joints in the body, such as the sacroiliac joint. For example, the sacrotuberous ligament spans from the base of the spine (the sacrum) across to the ischial tuberosity of the pelvis (see figure 10.4). In most people this ligament is a direct continuation of the tendon of the biceps femoris (a hamstring muscle). Consequently, it links the lower body directly to the spine by way of the hamstrings, since the hamstrings originate on the ischial tuberosity and run down the back of the leg, attaching just below the knee (Gray 1995). When the hamstring group lengthens under tension, it not only slows the hips as they flex, but it also provides stability and support to the sacroiliac joint and spine by way of the sacrotuberous ligament (Myers 2008).

MUSCLES

Many muscles originate in the lumbo-pelvic hip girdle. This chapter examines those muscles that originate from the pelvis and spine (Gray 1995). They include the following:

- Gluteus minimus
- Gluteus medius
- Tensor fasciae latae (TFL)
- Spinalis
- Longissimus
- Iliocostalis
- Quadratus lumborum
- Rectus abdominis
- Internal obliques
- External obliques
- Psoas major
- Iliacus

Note: While the gluteus maximus muscle originates from the lumbo-pelvic hip region and affects the function of this area, it also has great influence on movements of the leg and knee. The gluteus maximus muscle is described in detail in chapter 9.

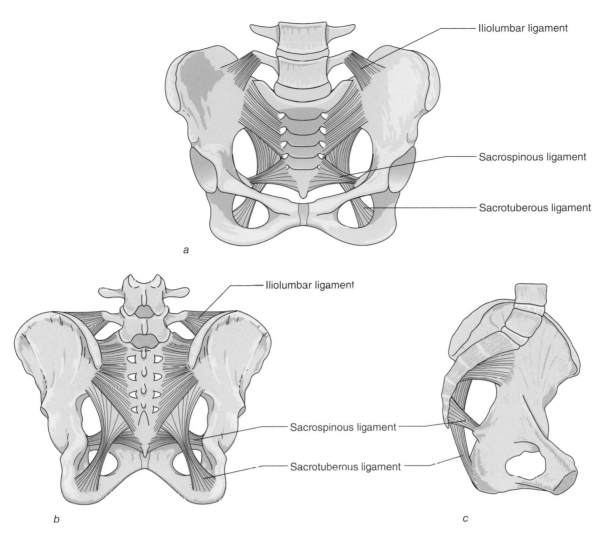

Sacrospinous ligament

Sacrotuberous ligament

Iliolumbar ligament

Iliolumbar ligament

Sacrospinous ligament

Sacrotuberous ligament

a

b

c

Figure 10.3 Ligaments of the lumbo-pelvic hip region: *(a)* anterior view, *(b)* posterior view, and *(c)* left view of medial section through the pelvis.

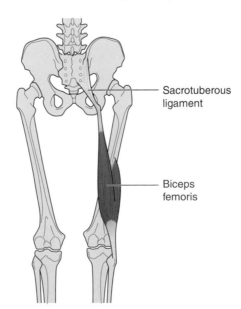

Sacrotuberous ligament

Biceps femoris

Figure 10.4 The sacrotuberous ligament connects with the biceps femoris, thus linking the lower body directly to the spine.

Gluteus Minimus (Abductor Group)

Muscle specifics: A deep abductor muscle that originates on the side of the pelvis on the outside of the ilium, fans down across the side of the pelvis, and inserts on the top of the outside of the femur (Gray 1995).

Muscle action(s): Moves the hip and leg away from the midline (i.e., abducts the hip and leg). The fibers toward the front of the muscle also help to internally rotate the hip and leg (Muscolino 2011).

Real-life movements: The bungee cord action of the gluteus minimus helps to decelerate the pelvis as it shifts over and outside the leg when the foot is in contact with the ground (i.e., when the leg adducts and externally rotates).

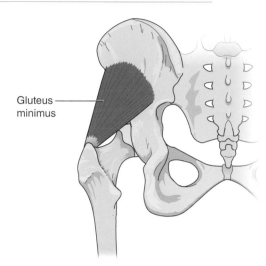

Gluteus minimus

Real-life movement example: Acts like a bungee cord to help slow the side-to-side movements of the hip and the external rotation of the leg when the foot first strikes the ground during activities like walking and running. Tension created in this muscle during these side-to-side movements is then used to help pull the hip back toward the midline of the body and to internally rotate the leg to help transfer weight to the other side.

Helpful tips: The gluteus minimus and gluteus medius work together to help decelerate the hip as it moves toward the outside of the body during all weight-bearing activities.

Gluteus Medius (Abductor Group)

Muscle specifics: A fan-shaped muscle of the buttocks that originates on the side and back of the pelvis just below the iliac crest, runs down the side of the pelvis, and inserts at the top of the femur on the outside surface (Gray 1995).

Muscle action(s): Moves the hip and leg away from the midline (i.e., abducts the hip and leg). The fibers toward the back of the muscle help to rotate the leg outward, while the fibers toward the front of the muscle help to rotate the leg inward (Muscolino 2011).

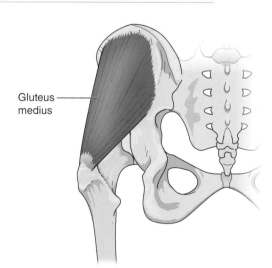

Gluteus medius

Real-life movements: The bungee cord action of the gluteus medius helps to decelerate the pelvis as it shifts over and outside the leg when the foot is in contact with the ground (i.e., adducts the hip and leg). The fibers toward the front of this muscle also help slow down outward rotation when lengthened, while the fibers toward the back help slow down inward rotation of the hip and leg when lengthened.

Real-life movement example: Acts like a bungee cord to help slow down hip and leg adduction during activities such as walking, running, side-shuffling, and salsa dancing, where the knee moves toward the midline and the hip moves toward the outside. The gluteus medius also helps to slow down the leg as it moves into internal and external rotation (depending on the parts of the muscle that are lengthening) during all dynamic weight-bearing activities.

Helpful tips: The gluteus medius is one of the best lateral stabilizing muscles of the hip and leg complex.

Tensor Fasciae Latae (Abductor Group)

Muscle specifics: An abductor muscle that originates on the side of the pelvis on the iliac crest, runs down the side of the pelvis, and merges with the iliotibial band, which continues all the way down the side of the thigh and inserts on the outside of the tibia (Gray 1995).

Muscle action(s): Moves the hip and leg away from the midline (i.e., abducts the hip and leg). The fibers toward the back of the muscle help with hip extension and outward rotation of the leg. The fibers toward the front of the muscle help with hip flexion and inward rotation of the leg (Muscolino 2011).

Real-life movements: The bungee cord action of the tensor fasciae latae helps decelerate the hip and leg as they move toward the midline (i.e., as they adduct). The front portion of the muscle helps slow down outward rotation and extension of the hip and leg when lengthened. The back portion of the muscle helps slow down inward rotation and flexion of the hip and leg.

Real-life movement example: Acts like a bungee cord to help slow down hip and leg adduction during activities such as walking, running, or hula dancing, where the knee moves toward the midline and the hip moves toward the outside. The tensor fasciae latae also helps to slow down flexion and extension of the hips during activities like jumping over hurdles, and it controls internal and external leg movements during weight-bearing activities.

Helpful tips: Tensor fasciae latae tightness or dysfunction can cause pain in the lower back, in the side of the hips, and in the side of the knee.

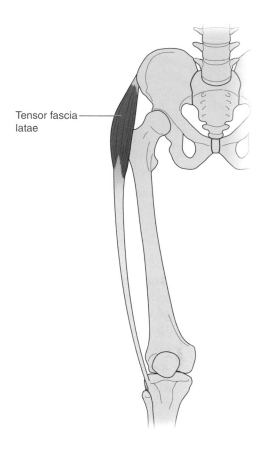

Tensor fascia latae

Spinalis (Erector Spinae Group)

Muscle specifics: An erector spinae muscle that is divided into three parts. The bottom part originates from the top portion of the lumbar spine and the bottom of the thoracic spine, runs up along the thoracic spine, and inserts on the spinous processes near the top of the thoracic spine. The two upper segments run from the top of the thoracic spine to the top of the neck and from the bottom of the cervical spine to the top of the neck (Gray 1995).

Muscle action(s): Arches the spine and head backward (i.e., extends them) and bends the spine and head to the side when the fibers on only one side of the spine contract (Cramer and Darby 2014).

Real-life movements: The bungee cord action of the spinalis helps decelerate the spine and head as they bend forward (i.e., into flexion) and to the side (when the fibers on only one side of the spine elongate).

Real-life movement example: Acts like a bungee cord in conjunction with the other erector spinae muscles to help slow down the spine as it bends forward and from side to side, like when leaning over the counter to wash dishes or cook.

Helpful tips: The spinalis muscle is the erector muscle that lies closest to the spine.

Spinalis

Internal Obliques (Abdominal Group)

Muscle specifics: Abdominal muscles that originate at the back of the torso from the sides of the thoracolumbar fascia and ilium of the pelvis, wrap up and around to the front and side of the torso, and insert in the connective tissue on the midline of the abdominals and the bottom three ribs (Gray 1995).

Muscle action(s): Help bend the spine forward (i.e., flex the spine) and rotate the torso. They also assist in abdomen compression and in side bending of the spine when the fibers on only one side contract (Clippinger 2007).

Real-life movements: The bungee cord action of the internal obliques helps decelerate the spine as it arches backward (i.e., extends), rotates, and side bends. During these movements, the muscle also stores potential energy to assist with spine flexion and rotation in the opposite direction.

Real-life movement example: Works in a traditional sense to help flex, rotate, and side-bend the spine (e.g., to produce power to chop wood). Acts like a bungee cord to slow down extension, rotation, and side bending of the spine in activities like golf, tennis, and turning around in the car to get something from the back seat.

Helpful tips: The abdominal muscles all work together to help slow down extension, rotation, and side bending of the spine. They are multifunctional muscles and should be exercised in a multifunctional manner.

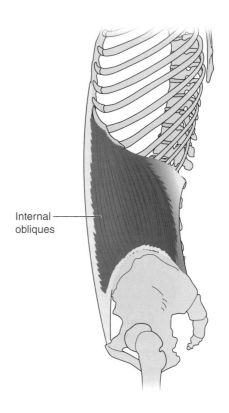

Internal obliques

External Obliques (Abdominal Group)

Muscle specifics: Abdominal muscles that originate from the sides of the lower eight ribs, travel down and slightly across the front of the torso, and insert at the middle of the abdomen on the linea alba and the sides and front of the pelvis (Gray 1995).

Muscle action(s): Help bend the spine forward (i.e., flex the spine) and rotate the torso. They also assist with side bending of the spine (when the fibers on only one side are contracted) and abdominal compression (Clippinger 2007).

Real-life movements: The bungee cord action of the external obliques helps decelerate the spine as it arches backward (extends), rotates, and side bends.

Real-life movement example: Acts like a bungee cord in conjunction with the internal obliques to slow down extension, side bending, and rotation of the torso in movements such as swinging the arms and rotating the torso when walking, running, and taking a backswing in golf. Furthermore, these muscles store potential energy during these movements to produce powerful movements in the opposite direction (e.g., a follow-through in a golf swing).

Helpful tips: The movement produced in the torso by the rotary action of the obliques helps increase blood supply to the abdominal fascia, helping to keep it healthy, flexible, and functional.

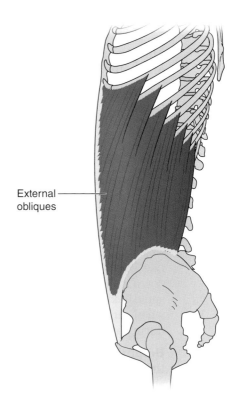

External obliques

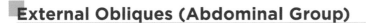

Psoas Major (Hip Flexor Group)

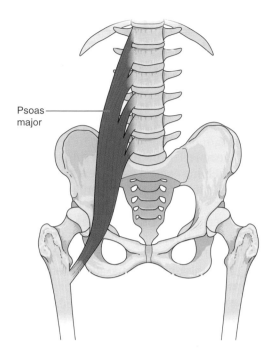

Psoas major

Muscle specifics: A hip flexor muscle that originates on the sides of all the lumbar vertebrae and last thoracic vertebrae, travels across the pelvis, and inserts on the inside of the top of the femur toward the back (Gray 1995).

Muscle action(s): Flexes the hip and leg and outwardly rotates the hip and leg. It also helps stabilize the lumbo-pelvic hip girdle when a person is standing (Gray 1995).

Real-life movements: The bungee cord action of the psoas major helps decelerate extension and internal rotation of the hip and leg. This action enables the muscle to store potential energy, which is then used to help the leg externally rotate as the hip flexes.

Real-life movement example: Acts like a bungee cord to slow down the leg as it moves behind the pelvis during activities like walking and running. The lengthening of this muscle creates potential energy that is used to help swing the leg forward and bend the hip during these activities.

Helpful tips: Tight hip flexors can pull the lumbar spine forward, causing (and exacerbating) excessive lumbar lordosis and an anterior pelvic tilt.

 Go to the online video to watch video 10.1, where Justin talks about how the psoas major muscle works in real-life.

Iliacus (Hip Flexor Group)

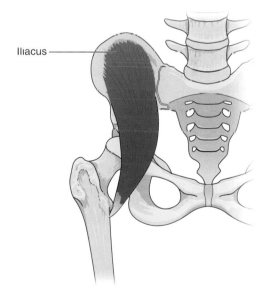

Iliacus

Muscle specifics: A hip flexor muscle that originates on the inside of the front of the pelvis near the top and travels down the pelvis and across the hip socket before inserting on the inside of the top of the femur toward the back (Gray 1995).

Muscle action(s): Flexes and outwardly rotates the hip and leg (Gray 1995).

Real-life movements: The bungee cord action of the iliacus helps decelerate the extension and internal rotation of the hip and leg.

Real-life movement example: Acts like a bungee cord to help slow down the hip and leg as the leg travels behind the body (i.e., into extension); it also slows the internal rotation of the leg during activities like walking, running, and climbing stairs. The lengthening of this muscle also creates potential energy to subsequently help lift the leg forward and rotate it outward (i.e., flex the hip).

Helpful tips: The iliacus connects with the muscle fibers of the psoas major as it crosses the hip socket, ensuring that the leg and pelvis work together as the hip and leg flex, extend, and rotate.

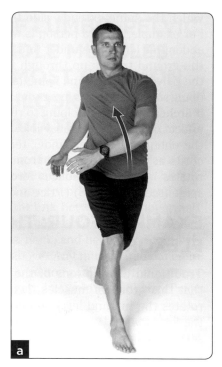
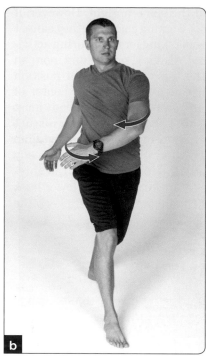

Figure 10.8 Example of the obliques lengthening to decelerate *(a)* side flexion of spine and *(b)* rotation of spine.

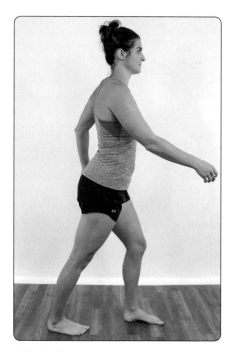

Figure 10.9 Excessive lumbar lordosis (and associated anterior pelvic tilt) caused by tight hip flexors.

when the foot is on the ground. However, if the hip flexors cannot lengthen effectively, it causes the lower back to overarch as the leg extends (see figure 10.9). Since the hip flexors originate from the lumbar spine and pelvis and attach to the top of the femur, chronic shortening (or dysfunction) of these muscles results in the lumbar spine being pulled forward toward the leg, exacerbating the common imbalance of excessive lumbar lordosis (and accompanying anterior pelvic tilt).

The inability of the hip flexors to lengthen effectively causes problems during all weight-bearing activities, but especially those that require the hip and leg to go into extension because more flexibility is required of the hip flexors to help regulate extension movements (Price and Bratcher 2010).

Go to the online video to watch video 10.2, where Justin talks about how dysfunction of the psoas muscle can affect the most common imbalances.

Review of Key Points

The muscles and other soft tissues of the lumbo-pelvic hip region provide wonderful stability to the hips, pelvis, and lumbar spine. They also play a key role in helping with locomotion by facilitating great degrees of movement in the legs and torso.

- The thoracolumbar fascia is a broad, dense, and multilayered fascial system that covers the bones, muscles, and soft tissues of the lower back, pelvis, and spine. It provides incredible support and stability for the lumbo-pelvic hip area.

- Many important ligaments help tie the lumbo-pelvic hip region together. The sacrotuberous ligament, for example, binds the sacrum to the pelvis, but it also connects the legs (via the hamstrings' origin point) to the base of the spine. This cooperation between the hamstrings and the spine that results from this ligament (and others) enables the hips, legs, and spine to work together to control flexion and extension.

- The abductors lengthen to slow down hip and leg adduction when force is being transferred to the weight-bearing leg during gait.

- The erector spinae muscles help lift the spine upright, but they also work in a lengthening fashion to slow the spine down as it bends forward and from side to side.

- The abdominal muscles help flex, side bend, and rotate the spine. They are commonly conditioned to perform these movements using concentric exercises such as sit-ups or crunches. However, since their function is also to help slow down spine rotation, side flexion, and extension as they lengthen, they should also be strengthened with exercises that require eccentric movements.

- The hip flexor muscles contract to swing the leg forward when walking, but they also work in a lengthening fashion to slow down hip and leg extension. Musculoskeletal deviations such as overpronation, a valgus knee, or an anterior pelvic tilt affect the alignment of the leg in the hip socket, thereby affecting the ability of the hip flexors to lengthen and load correctly.

Self-Check

Your understanding of the bungee cord concept of how muscles lengthen to slow movement (and subsequently store potential energy to produce movement) should be improving. The loading and unloading of muscles in this way ensures that joints experience less stress from the forces of nature and that movement is more effective and efficient.

Try to think of a movement for each of the following muscles where the muscle works to help slow down gravity, rotary forces, or both. For example, if someone were to bend over and pick up a coin, the spinalis muscle would help slow down the spine as it rounds forward against the force of gravity.

Muscle	Movement example	Force it slows down (gravity, rotation, or both)
Internal obliques		
Iliocostalis		
Rectus abdominis		
Psoas major		
Iliacus		
Gluteus medius		
External obliques		

CHAPTER 11

Functional Anatomy of the Thoracic Spine and Shoulder Girdle

The thoracic spine is the middle portion of the spinal column that articulates with the rib cage. The shoulder girdle connects and moves with this area of the body through muscles, tendons, ligaments, and joints (McMinn 2005).

BONES AND JOINTS

The thoracic spine and shoulder girdle is comprised of the many bones of the upper torso and the 12 vertebrae of the thoracic spine. The scapulae sit on the back of the rib cage (which is formed by 24 bones that attach to either side of each of the thoracic vertebrae). The acromion extends outward from the top of the shoulder blade (via the spine of the scapula) (see figure 11.1) (Middleditch and Oliver 2005).

The sternum is a broad, flat bone located on the front of the chest where the ribs come together to form the front of the rib cage. The clavicle bones attach to and extend outward from the top of the sternum (i.e., the sternoclavicular joint) to help form the upper part of the shoulder girdle with the acromion (i.e., the acromioclavicular joint). The end of the humerus articulates with the labrum and glenoid cavity to form the main shoulder joint (i.e., the glenohumeral joint) (Siegel 2002). All of the movements of the shoulder girdle are highly complex and depend on perfect coordination of all

the bones, muscles, tendons, ligaments, and fascia in that area.

SOFT TISSUE STRUCTURES

Several soft tissue structures in the thoracic spine and shoulder girdle assist with and influence movement. This area also contains other soft tissue structures that assist with essential life functions, such as breathing, that can be negatively affected by musculoskeletal imbalances.

DIAPHRAGM

The thoracic diaphragm is a dome-shaped muscle that extends across the bottom of the rib cage (figure 11.2). Unlike other skeletal muscles, the diaphragm is a membrane surrounded by muscle fibers that separates the thoracic cavity of the torso (which contains the heart and lungs) from the abdominal cavity (which contains the digestive organs). It can expand and contract like other muscles and, along with the intercostals, it is the main muscle used for breathing (Rhoades and Bell 2009).

Breathing in (inhaling) causes the diaphragm and the intercostal muscles of the rib cage to contract, resulting in an increase of space in the thoracic cavity. This increase allows the lungs to expand into the empty space that has been created by the

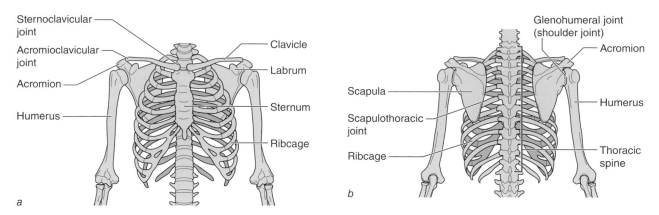

Figure 11.1   Anatomy of the thoracic spine and shoulder girdle: *(a)* anterior and *(b)* posterior views.

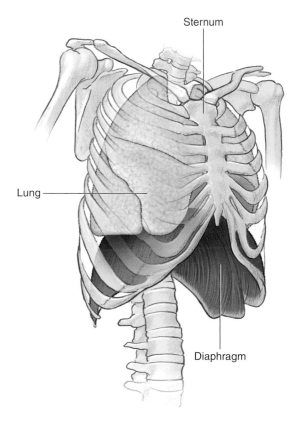

Figure 11.2   Thoracic diaphragm.

contraction of those muscles. Once the lungs have filled with air, the diaphragm and intercostal muscles relax. This reduces the amount of space available in the thoracic cavity and forces air back out of the lungs (exhalation) (Rhoades and Bell 2009).

In addition to its role in breathing, the diaphragm helps increase intra-abdominal pressure when contracted by pushing down on the contents of the abdomen during movements that require expulsion such as coughing, sneezing, urination, and defecation (West 2000). This pressure increase during inhalation further helps to stabilize the lumbar spine for lifting heavy loads, and it increases blood supply to the organs, keeping them healthy (Middleditch and Oliver 2005).

INTERCOSTAL MUSCLES

The group of muscles that lies between the ribs and facilitates breathing is called the intercostals (figure 11.3). There are 22 individual intercostal muscles, 11 internal and 11 external. The external intercostals expand the rib cage when they contract, allowing the lungs to intake air. The internal intercostals, which are located underneath the external intercostals, compress the rib cage to expel air from the lungs (Singh 2005).

Common musculoskeletal imbalances in the thoracic spine and shoulder girdle can have adverse effects on the way a person breathes. For example, excessive thoracic kyphosis causes the rib cage to collapse forward and down, which chronically compresses the ribs, intercostals, and diaphragm and makes it more difficult to draw in air. Since we need air to survive, breathing may be initiated by other structures when imbalances exist; for example, the upper rib cage and shoulders may shrug upward to allow the lungs to expand. This dysfunctional adaptation can lead to muscle fatigue and musculoskeletal compensation patterns developing in the shoulders and neck. Therefore, the thoracic spine and shoulder girdle must be aligned and functioning correctly to facilitate the act of breathing (Karageanes 2005).

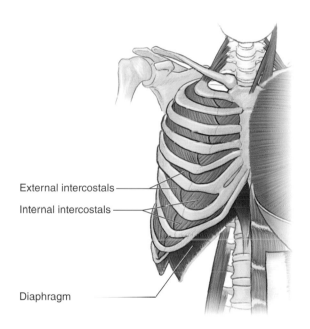

External intercostals
Internal intercostals
Diaphragm

Figure 11.3 Intercostal muscles.

MUSCLES

There are many muscles that originate from the thoracic spine, rib cage, and shoulder girdle (Gray 1995). The muscles discussed in this chapter are the following:

- Latissimus dorsi
- Pectoralis major
- Pectoralis minor
- Rhomboids (minor and major)
- Serratus anterior
- Trapezius (upper fibers)
- Trapezius (middle fibers)
- Trapezius (lower fibers)
- Subscapularis
- Supraspinatus
- Infraspinatus
- Teres minor
- Biceps brachii

Latissimus Dorsi

Muscle specifics: A broad muscle on the back of the torso that sweeps upward and across from either side of the lower back to the top of the arm. It originates from the spinous processes of the bottom five thoracic vertebrae and the lumbar vertebrae, the top and sides of the pelvis, the thoracolumbar fascia, the bottom four ribs, and the bottom edge of the shoulder blade and inserts at the top of the arm on the humerus toward the front (Gray 1995).

Muscle action(s): Brings the arm downward behind the body and rotates it inward. When the arms are fixed, the latissimus dorsi helps to move the trunk and pelvis toward the arms (Gray 1995).

Real-life movements: The bungee cord action of the latissimus dorsi decelerates the arm as it moves up and away from the body. It also helps decelerate the trunk as it moves away from the arms when they are fixed. Due to its origins on the lower thoracic and lumbar spine and the fascia of the lower back, it also helps to stabilize the spine.

Real-life movement example: Works in traditional anatomy terms to pull the arms down and toward the body during movements like swinging the arms when walking, chopping downward with an ax, or swimming. Acts like a bungee cord to help slow down the arms and torso as they move away from each other during movements like climbing down from a tree.

Helpful tips: People who have chronically shortened latissimus dorsi muscles typically have internally rotated arms and a protracted shoulder girdle.

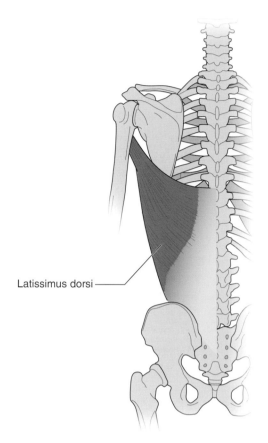

Latissimus dorsi

Pectoralis Major

Muscle specifics: A muscle that fans across the chest on the front of the upper torso. It originates from the fascia of the external obliques, the cartilage of the first six ribs, and the sternum and medial half of the clavicle. It attaches to the front of the upper arm on the humerus (Di Giacomo, Pouliart, Costantini, and De Vita 2008).

Muscle action(s): Lifts the arm up and across the body and helps rotate the arm inward (Di Giacomo, Pouliart, Costantini, and De Vita 2008).

Real-life movements: The bungee cord action of the pectoralis major decelerates the arm as it moves down and away from the midline of the body. It also helps slow down the arm as it rotates outward.

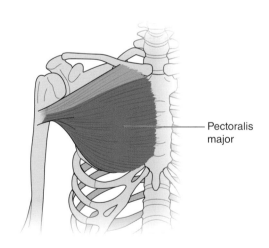

Pectoralis major

Real-life movement example: Acts like a bungee cord to slow down the arm(s) during movements such as taking a forehand backswing in tennis or reaching behind you to grab something from the back seat of a car.

Helpful tips: During prolonged computer use, the arms must come forward and across the body to type on the keyboard. This action can chronically shorten the pectoralis major muscle over time.

Pectoralis Minor

Muscle specifics: A muscle on the front, upper portion of the torso. It originates from the anterior portions of the third, fourth, and fifth ribs and inserts on the coracoid process of the scapula (Di Giacomo, Pouliart, Costantini, and De Vita 2008).

Muscle action(s): Pulls the shoulder blade down and forward. If the shoulder blade is fixed, the pectoralis minor also assists with breathing by elevating the third, fourth, and fifth ribs (Di Giacomo, Pouliart, Costantini, and De Vita 2008).

Real-life movements: The bungee cord action of the pectoralis minor helps stabilize the shoulder blade against the rib cage when the shoulder blade retracts and the arm is taken behind the body.

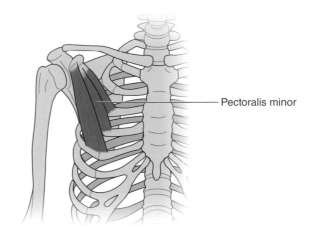

Pectoralis minor

Real-life movement example: Acts like a bungee cord to help slow down (and stabilize) the shoulder blade as the shoulder girdle is put under stress during such movements as taking a backswing in golf.

Helpful tips: A chronically tight pectoralis minor can protract the scapula, raising the vertebral border and bottom of the shoulder blade away from the rib cage.

Rhomboids (Minor and Major)

Muscle specifics: Muscles on the back of the torso between the spine and the shoulder blades. Both rhomboid minor and major originate from the upper thoracic spine (and last cervical vertebrae and nuchal ligament for rhomboid minor), travel on a downward angle to the shoulder blade, and insert on the edge of the shoulder blade closest to the spine (Rockwood and Matsen 2009).

Muscle action(s): Moves the shoulder blades closer to the spine (i.e., retracts them) (Rockwood and Matsen 2009).

Real-life movements: The bungee cord action of the rhomboids helps slow down movements of the shoulder blades away from the spine (i.e., protraction of the shoulder blades).

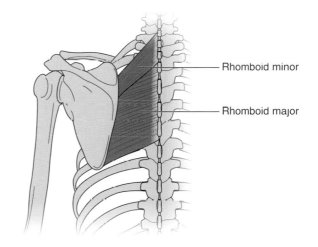

Rhomboid minor

Rhomboid major

Real-life movement example: Work in a traditional sense during all movements that involve pulling the shoulder blades toward the spine, like rowing. Act like bungee cords to help slow down the shoulder blades as they move away from the spine, such as when lowering a box to the ground or when the arms swing forward when walking.

Helpful tips: People with a protracted shoulder girdle usually have chronically lengthened rhomboid muscles that cannot contract effectively.

Serratus Anterior

Muscle specifics: A muscle that wraps around the sides of the upper torso. It originates on the front of the rib cage from the top eight ribs, travels under the shoulder blade, and attaches to the border of the scapula closest to the spine (Clippinger 2007).

Muscle action(s): Stabilizes the shoulder blade and keeps it flat to the rib cage as it moves away from the spine so the vertebral edge does not protrude outward (Clippinger 2007).

Real-life movements: The bungee cord action of the serratus anterior decelerates the shoulder blade as it moves toward the spine (retracts) to help stabilize the entire shoulder girdle.

Real-life movement example: Acts like a bungee cord to help slow down the shoulder blades as they move toward the spine during closed-chain movements of the arms, such as push-ups and crawling.

Helpful tips: The serratus anterior works as an antagonist to the rhomboid muscles.

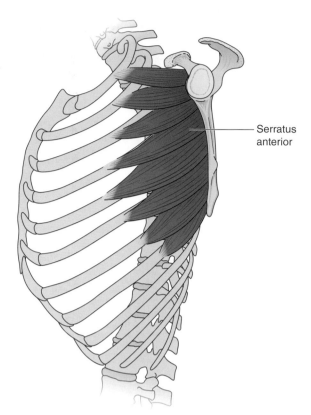

Serratus anterior

Trapezius (Upper Fibers)

Muscle specifics: One portion of a large triangular muscle on the back of the torso. The upper fibers of the trapezius originate on the base of the skull, the nuchal ligament on the back of the neck, and the bottom of the cervical spine, travel in a downward sweeping motion, and insert on the outside edge of the clavicle, the acromion, and the spine of the scapula (Palmer, Epler, and Epler 1998).

Muscle action(s): Elevates the shoulder blades. When the shoulder blades are fixed, it helps extend the neck and head by pulling the base of the skull closer to the top of the shoulder blades (Palmer, Epler, and Epler 1998).

Real-life movements: The bungee cord action of the upper trapezius decelerates the shoulder blades as they depress. The lengthening action of this part of the trapezius muscle also helps decelerate the neck and head as the head tips down and forward into flexion.

Real-life movement example: Acts like a bungee cord to slow the downward movement of the shoulder blades during activities such as lowering a box from a high shelf. The bungee cord feature of the upper fibers also activates when nodding the head forward or looking down during activities like texting.

Helpful tips: All three portions of the trapezius muscle perform different functions to help control the shoulder blades as they move up and down and in and out.

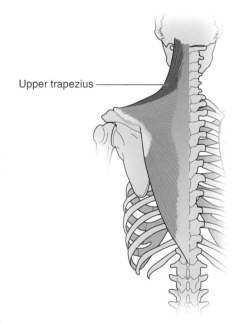

Upper trapezius

Trapezius (Middle Fibers)

Muscle specifics: One portion of a large triangular muscle on the back of the torso. The middle fibers of the trapezius originate on the last cervical vertebra and upper part of the thoracic spine, run outward toward the shoulder blade, and attach to the top of the spine of the scapula (Palmer, Epler, and Epler 1998).

Muscle action(s): Pulls the shoulder blades toward the spine, retracting them (Palmer, Epler, and Epler 1998).

Real-life movements: The bungee cord action of the middle fibers of the trapezius decelerates the shoulder blades as they move away from the spine.

Real-life movement example: Acts like a bungee cord to help slow the movement of the shoulder blades as they travel away from the spine during activities such as bending over and lowering a weight to the ground or trying to hold a rope at arm's length during a game of tug-of-war.

Helpful tips: The middle fibers of the trapezius work in concert with the rhomboids to stabilize, decelerate, and retract the shoulder blades.

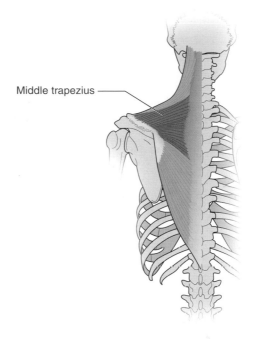

Middle trapezius

Trapezius (Lower Fibers)

Muscle specifics: One portion of a large triangular muscle on the back of the torso. The lower fibers of the trapezius originate from the middle and lower thoracic spine, travel upward and outward to the shoulder blade, and insert near the top of the shoulder blade on the spine of the scapula (Palmer, Epler, and Epler 1998).

Muscle action(s): Pulls the shoulder blade downward (i.e., depresses it) (Palmer, Epler, and Epler 1998).

Real-life movements: The bungee cord action of the lower fibers of the trapezius decelerates the shoulder blade as it moves upward.

Real-life movement example: Acts like a bungee cord to decelerate the upward movement of the shoulder blades during activities like the downward phase of pull-ups or throwing a medicine ball over and behind your head.

Helpful tips: Typically, the lower fibers of the trapezius are chronically lengthened and weak in people who have elevated shoulder blades.

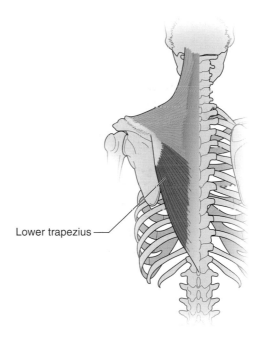

Lower trapezius

Subscapularis (Rotator Cuff Muscle)

Muscle specifics: One of four rotator cuff muscles of the shoulder. It originates on the underside of the shoulder blade on the edge closest to the spine, runs under the scapula and armpit, and inserts on the front of the humerus (Clippinger 2007).

Muscle action(s): Responsible for inward rotation of the arm and taking the arm behind the body (adduction and extension). It also helps secure the head of the humerus in the shoulder joint (i.e., the glenohumeral joint) (Maffulli and Furia 2012).

Real-life movements: The bungee cord action of the subscapularis decelerates the arm as it moves forward, out, and away from the body. This muscle also helps stabilize the glenohumeral joint.

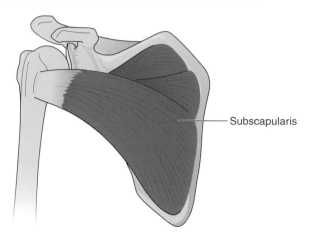
Subscapularis

Real-life movement example: Works in a traditional sense by rotating the arm inward and behind you, like when you tuck the back of your shirt into your pants. Acts like a bungee cord to slow the arm as it swings forward of the body like when clapping your hands and also helps stabilize the arm in the glenohumeral joint in movements like push-ups.

Helpful tips: Injuries to the rotator cuff muscles are common among baseball pitchers, tennis players, weightlifters, volleyball players, and other athletes who place the shoulder girdle and arms under a lot of continued stress.

Supraspinatus (Rotator Cuff Muscle)

Muscle specifics: One of four rotator cuff muscles of the shoulder. It originates on the top edge of the shoulder blade closest to the spine, travels across the top of the shoulder blade, tucks underneath the acromion, and inserts on the top of the humerus toward the outside (Clippinger 2007).

Muscle action(s): Raises the arm out to the side away from the body (i.e., abduction). Also helps to hold the head of the humerus in the glenohumeral joint (Maffulli and Furia 2012).

Real-life movements: The bungee cord action of the supraspinatus decelerates movements of the arm as it is lowered to the side of the body. It also helps stabilize the head of the humerus in the glenohumeral joint.

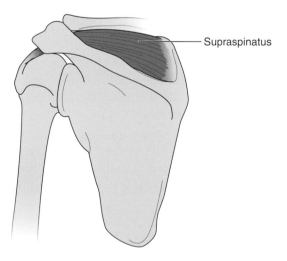
Supraspinatus

Real-life movement example: Works in a traditional sense during movements like lifting the arm to wave goodbye. Acts like a bungee cord and shoulder joint stabilizer in activities that require the slowing down of the arm while lowering an object, such as returning the hand to your side after waving farewell.

Helpful tips: The supraspinatus is the most often injured of the four rotator cuff muscles because the tendon of this muscle passes under a bone, the acromion, in a highly mobile area of the shoulder girdle.

Infraspinatus (Rotator Cuff Muscle)

Muscle specifics: One of four rotator cuff muscles of the shoulder. It originates from the edge of the shoulder blade nearest the spine, runs upward across the shoulder blade, and inserts on the top of the upper arm near the outside of the humerus (Gray 1995).

Muscle action(s): Outwardly rotates the arm. It also helps stabilize the arm in the glenohumeral joint (Maffulli and Furia 2012).

Real-life movements: The bungee cord action of the infraspinatus decelerates internal rotation of the arm. It also helps stabilize the head of the humerus in the glenohumeral joint.

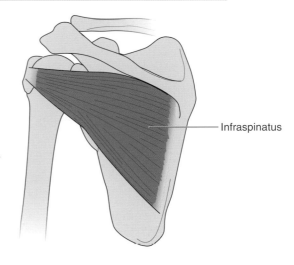

Infraspinatus

Real-life movement example: Works in a traditional sense to help rotate the arm outward during movements like reaching diagonally behind you into the back seat of a car. Acts like a bungee cord to slow down the arm as it internally rotates in activities where the arm swings forward and across the body, such as when walking or when hitting a topspin forehand shot in tennis. It also helps stabilize the arm in the glenohumeral joint when performing an exercise like the seated row.

Helpful tips: People who always have their arms forward and internally rotated, such as long-distance drivers or those with computer jobs, likely have chronically lengthened infraspinatus muscles.

Teres Minor (Rotator Cuff Muscle)

Muscle specifics: One of four rotator cuff muscles of the shoulder. It originates from the outside edge of the shoulder blade and inserts on the outside of the humerus near the top (Gray 1995).

Muscle action(s): Outwardly rotates the arm. It also helps stabilize the arm in the glenohumeral joint (Clippinger 2007).

Real-life movements: The bungee cord action of the teres minor helps slow down the arm as it moves forward and internally rotates. It also helps stabilize the head of the humerus in the glenohumeral joint.

Teres minor

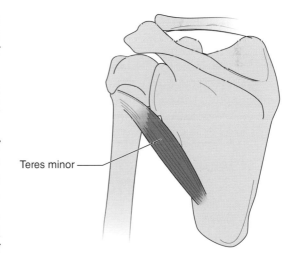

Real-life movement example: Works in a traditional sense in situations where the arm and hand are turned upward, like when carrying a tray of food. Acts like a bungee cord to help slow down the arm as it comes across and in front of the body—for example, in the follow-through part of a golf or baseball swing. It also helps stabilize the shoulder during movements like pull-ups.

Helpful tips: The teres minor and infraspinatus are called external rotator cuff muscles because, when they contract, they help stabilize the shoulder as the arm rotates outward. These two muscles can get overly lengthened, irritated, and sore from prolonged rounded shoulder postures.

Biceps Brachii

Muscle specifics: A dual-headed muscle on the front of the upper arm. It originates from the top of the scapula, runs down the arm, crosses the elbow, and attaches to the lower arm on the radius (Gray 1995).

Muscle action(s): Bends the elbow and supinates the forearm (i.e., turns the palm upward). Due to its origin on the shoulder blade, it also helps lift the arm at the shoulder (Gray 1995).

Real-life movements: The bungee cord action of the biceps brachii decelerates the elbow as it straightens and the forearm as it pronates (i.e., turns the palm down). The biceps brachii also helps stabilize the shoulder blade.

Real-life movement example: Acts like a bungee cord to help slow down the arm as it straightens and turns inward, which happens when the arms swing behind the body during gait or when a ball is thrown. Also helps stabilize the shoulder blade during these movements.

Helpful tips: People who sit with their elbows bent for prolonged periods, such as when typing or driving, can have chronically shortened biceps brachii muscles. When they try to extend their elbows while walking, the biceps brachii cannot lengthen effectively, and this can pull the shoulder blade out of alignment.

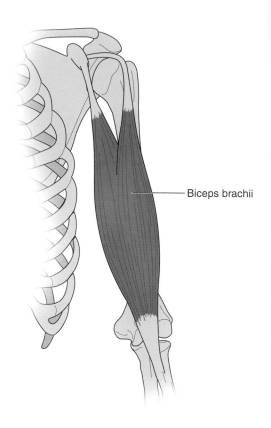

— Biceps brachii

 Go to the online video to watch video 11.1, where Justin talks about how the biceps brachii muscle works in real-life.

EFFECT OF THE THORACIC SPINE AND SHOULDER GIRDLE MUSCLES ON THE MOST COMMON MUSCULOSKELETAL DEVIATIONS

Today's high-tech environment can have adverse effects on the structures of the thoracic spine and shoulder girdle. People often spend hours with their shoulders and upper backs rounded forward and their arms internally rotated as they use computer devices (Plotnik and Kouyoumdjian 2014). When not at a computer, they are often either driving or sitting in front of a television. Many people spend most of their waking hours in a seated, rounded posture.

These prolonged positions can lead to chronic musculoskeletal imbalances that disrupt function in the thoracic spine and shoulder girdle, causing pain and affecting arm and torso movements (Sahrmann

2002). The neck, lower back, hips, knees, ankles, and feet then must compensate for immobility and dysfunction in the thoracic spine and shoulder girdle. The resulting overuse in these other areas can lead to more imbalances and pain. So the alignment of the thoracic spine and shoulder girdle is important to the entire body.

Here are three examples of how the bungee cord feature of specific groups of muscles can prevent the most common deviations of the thoracic spine and shoulder girdle.

EXAMPLE ONE: THE LATISSIMUS DORSI AND PECTORALS

The latissimus dorsi and pectoral muscles work together to control the movement of the arm and torso. The latissimus dorsi lengthens like a bungee cord to slow the arm as it swings forward during gait. During this forward movement of the arm, tension in the latissimus dorsi also helps keep the lower thoracic spine upright (see figure 11.4).

Conversely, the pectorals (minor and major) act like bungee cords to slow down the arm as it swings behind the body during gait. Tension in the pectorals as they lengthen also pulls on the upper part of the rib cage, keeping it upright and keeping the thoracic spine extended (see figure 11.5). Therefore, it is the combined working of these muscles during gait that helps control movement of the arms and shoulder girdle and keeps the thoracic spine upright, thereby reducing excessive thoracic kyphosis (Price and Bratcher 2010).

EXAMPLE TWO: THE RHOMBOIDS, TRAPEZIUS, SERRATUS ANTERIOR, AND BICEPS BRACHII

The rhomboids, trapezius, serratus anterior, and biceps brachii muscles work together to control movement of the scapula on the rib cage to ensure correct functioning of the shoulder girdle and arm. As the arm swings forward during gait, for example, the shoulder blade rotates up and away from the spine (i.e., it elevates and protracts). This lifting of the shoulder blade is initiated by momentum and contraction of the upper fibers of the trapezius. The rate at which the shoulder blade elevates is controlled by the lengthening of the lower fibers of the trapezius. The middle fibers of the trapezius and the rhomboids also lengthen during this movement to slow the protraction of the shoulder blade as it moves away from the spine (see figure 11.6).

The serratus anterior also helps to control movement of the shoulder blades as the arm swings forward by helping keep the vertebral border of the scapula flat so that it glides smoothly over the ribs as it protracts. Conversely, as the arm swings behind the body, the serratus anterior lengthens like a bungee cord to help control the position of the scapula on the ribcage, and the biceps brachii lengthens to control the extension of the arm and to stabilize the scapula (Hertling and Kessler 2006) (see figure 11.7).

The correct functioning of the trapezius, rhomboids, serratus anterior, and biceps brachii can

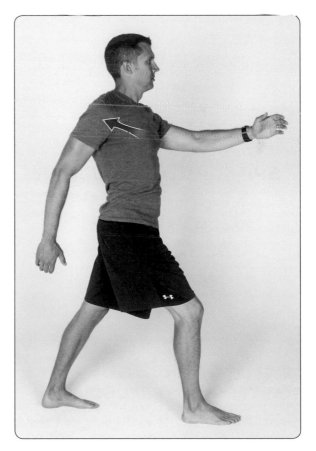

Figure 11.4   Example of bungee cord action of the latissimus dorsi decelerating the forward movement of the arm and promoting thoracic extension.

Figure 11.5   Example of the pectoral muscles lengthening to control extension of the arm and thoracic spine.

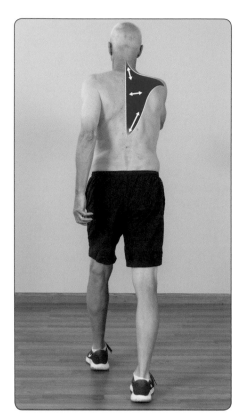

Figure 11.6 Example of the trapezius and rhomboids lengthening to control scapular elevation and protraction.

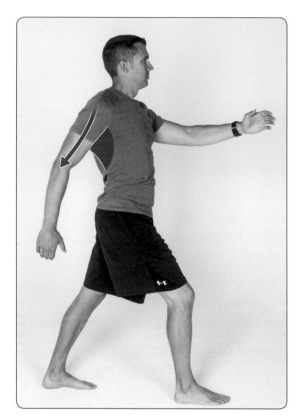

Figure 11.7 Example of bungee cord action of the biceps and serratus anterior controlling scapular retraction and arm extension.

minimize the potential for imbalances such as elevated scapulae and a protracted shoulder girdle. Moreover, because the function of the shoulder girdle directly affects the position of the thoracic spine, these muscles also influence the presence or absence of excessive thoracic kyphosis (Price and Bratcher 2010).

 Go to the online video to watch video 11.2, where Justin talks about how dysfunction of the biceps brachii muscle can affect the most common imbalances.

EXAMPLE THREE: THE ROTATOR CUFF MUSCLES

The rotator cuff muscles work together to control the movement of the humerus in the glenohumeral

joint. When the arm swings forward during gait, for example, it internally rotates and moves slightly toward the midline of the body. This turning inward of the arm is controlled and decelerated by the bungee cord action of the subscapularis, infraspinatus, and teres minor. If these rotator cuff muscles are chronically lengthened or dysfunctional, they cannot effectively control the extent to which the arm moves forward and across the body. Therefore, these muscles must work properly to minimize the effects of internally rotated arms.

When the weight of the arms is increased by holding a heavy object, or when they come in contact with a surface to perform a movement like a push-up, it is important that all the rotator cuff muscles effectively stabilize the humerus in the glenohumeral joint so that the rest of the shoulder girdle and thoracic spine can function properly (Hertling and Kessler 2006).

Review of Key Points

Optimal alignment of the thoracic spine and shoulder girdle is important to long-term health. Since the shoulder girdle articulates with the thoracic spine and rib cage, the shoulders and arms can be affected by imbalances in these areas.

- The diaphragm and intercostal muscles attach to the rib cage and are the key muscles used for breathing. Imbalances in the thoracic spine directly affect the rib cage and thus can affect a person's ability to breathe correctly.

- The rhomboids help retract the shoulder blades and help to correctly align the thoracic spine and shoulder girdle. Prolonged sitting can result in a protracted shoulder girdle, which can lead to chronic lengthening of the rhomboid muscles.

- The trapezius muscles form a large diamond shape that runs downward from the head, out to the shoulders, and then back inward toward the bottom of the thoracic spine. The upper, middle, and lower fibers of the trapezius help to elevate, depress, and retract the scapulae. The upper trapezius also helps extend the neck and head.

- There are four rotator cuff muscles of the shoulder. Working together, these rotator cuff muscles help move the arm and stabilize it in the glenohumeral joint.

Self-Check

The following exercise is designed to increase your awareness of daily activities that might exacerbate imbalances in the thoracic spine and shoulder girdle.

Think of three static positions you assume throughout the day. For each, write down how much time you spend in that position, and list what muscles of the thoracic spine and shoulder girdle (and the rest of the body, if you can) might be adversely affected and why. An example is provided.

Posture/position	Duration	Muscles affected and why
Sitting on the couch watching TV with arms crossed	2 hours	• Thoracic erectors lengthened • Pectorals shortened • Abdominals shortened • Rhomboids and middle traps lengthened • Infraspinatus and teres minor muscles lengthened
POSTURE 1		
POSTURE 2		
POSTURE 3		

CHAPTER 12

Functional Anatomy of the Neck and Head

Most of the human head is made up of several fused bones that create a dome-shaped cavity called the skull. The skull protects our brain and many of our sensory organs, such as the eyes, ears, nose, and tongue (Halim 2009). The head articulates with the neck, and together with the muscles, tendons, ligaments, and other soft tissues of this part of the body, it makes for a very mobile structure that helps us maintain balance, vision, posture, and musculoskeletal alignment (Clarkson 2000).

BONES AND JOINTS

The skull joins with either side of the mandible at the temporal bones (figure 12.1; see Temporomandibular Joint later in this chapter for more information) (Adds and Shahsavari 2012). The skull also connects to the cervical spine via the atlas bone, which is the topmost vertebra of the neck (i.e., C1) (Gray 1995). The rest of the neck is comprised of the remaining six vertebrae of the cervical spine. Positional changes of the head up and down, side to side, and in rotation are made possible by movements of the neck (Peterson and Richmond 1988).

SOFT TISSUE STRUCTURES

Here we discuss some key structures in the neck and head so that you can understand how they influence movement and participation in activities of daily living. These structures are intricately linked with the muscles of the neck and head, and therefore they can be negatively affected by musculoskeletal imbalances in these areas.

TEMPOROMANDIBULAR JOINT

The temporomandibular joint (TMJ) is one of the most important joints in the neck and head area. This joint is formed where the mandible articulates with the temporal bone of the skull (see figure 12.2). There is a small disc of fibrous cartilage positioned on either side of the jaw between the end of the mandible and the temporal bone that enables the jaw to move smoothly during activities like talking, chewing food, and taking in oxygen through the mouth (e.g., yawning) (Willard, Zhang, and

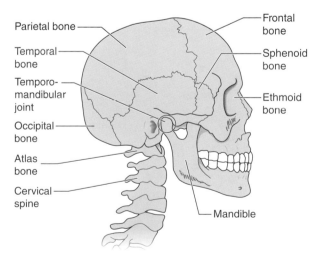

Figure 12.1 Anatomy of the head and neck.

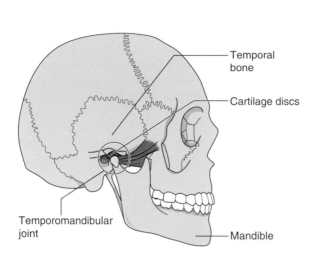

Figure 12.2 Temporomandibular joint.

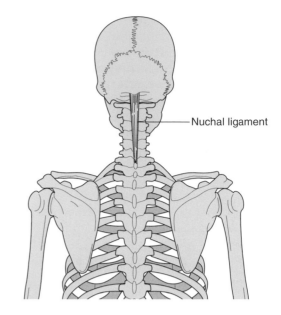

Figure 12.3 Nuchal ligament.

Athanasiou 2017). The tissues surrounding these discs are highly innervated, so when the TMJ is pulled out of alignment by a forward head position or excessive cervical lordosis, it often produces pain and discomfort (Salvo 2009).

NUCHAL LIGAMENT

The nuchal ligament extends from the base of the skull down to the body of the seventh cervical vertebra (see figure 12.3). This connective tissue acts like a guide rope to help hold up the head and prevent excessive neck flexion (such as when looking down at a book). The nuchal ligament also helps separate the muscles on either side of the neck (McGowan 1999). Since it also serves as an attachment site for some muscles of the neck, an irritated, painful nuchal ligament can disrupt neck and head movements.

MUSCLES

There are many muscles that flex, extend, side bend, and rotate the neck (Clarkson 2000). This chapter examines muscles that facilitate these movements and originate from or attach to the skull or cervical spine. They include the following:

- Longus colli
- Longus capitis
- Sternocleidomastoid
- Semispinalis capitis
- Semispinalis cervicis
- Splenius capitis
- Splenius cervicis

Longus Colli

Muscle specifics: A muscle on the front of the neck. It is divided into three portions (superior oblique, inferior oblique, and vertical) and originates from the top of the thoracic spine and the bottom of the cervical spine, travels up the neck, and inserts at the top of the cervical spine (Gray 1995).

Muscle action(s): Bends the neck and head down and forward toward the chest (i.e., neck and head flexion). Due to the position of the muscle on either side of the neck, when only one side of the muscle activates, it also helps with side flexion and rotation of the cervical spine (Palastanga, Field, and Soames 1994).

Real-life movements: The bungee cord action of the longus colli decelerates the neck and head as they arch or tilt backward (i.e., neck and head extension). They also help decelerate side bending and rotation of the neck and head when they are in extension.

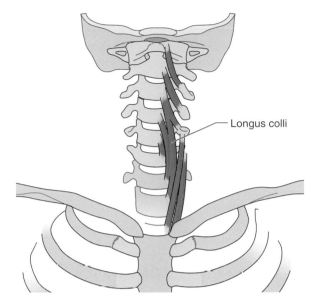
Longus colli

Real-life movement example: Works in a traditional sense to produce movement of the neck and head toward the chest during activities like sit-ups. Acts like a bungee cord to slow down the neck and head when you lean your head back or have to decelerate the head and neck, such as when going to lie down on the floor or a bed.

Helpful tips: The longus colli is most often damaged during activities where the head is violently thrown backward, such as the whiplash action that can occur during a car accident.

Longus Capitis

Muscle specifics: A muscle on the front of the neck. It originates from the middle of the cervical spine, travels up the neck, and inserts into the base of the occipital bone (Gray 1995).

Muscle action(s): Bends the upper cervical spine and head forward and down (i.e., neck and head flexion) (Palastanga, Field, and Soames 1994).

Real-life movements: The bungee cord action of the longus capitis decelerates the top of the neck as it arches backward (i.e., extends) and the head as it tilts back.

Real-life movement example: Works in a traditional sense to flex the top of the neck and head toward the chest during movements like looking down to see if you have spilled something on your shirt. Acts like a bungee cord to slow down the top of the neck and head when they are thrown backward, such as what would happen if a person were forcefully shoved forward from behind.

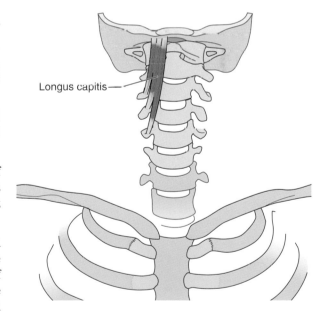
Longus capitis

Helpful tips: The literal translation of *longus capitis* from Latin means "long (muscle) of the head," and its position at the top of the neck places it in a useful anatomical position to control movements of the head.

Sternocleidomastoid

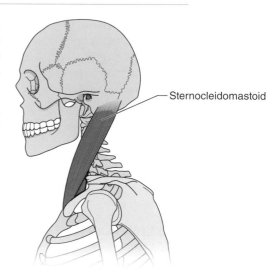

Sternocleidomastoid

Muscle specifics: A muscle on the front side of the neck. It originates on the uppermost part of the sternum and the medial portion of the clavicle, travels up and across the side of the neck, and inserts below the ear on the mastoid process of the temporal bone and on the occipital bone (Gray 1995).

Muscle action(s): When both sternocleidomastoid muscles contract together, they bend the neck forward (i.e., flex the neck) and tip the head backward (i.e., extend the head). If only one muscle contracts, the neck and head tip to the same side that is flexed and rotate to the opposite side (Palastanga, Field, and Soames 1994).

Real-life movements: The bungee cord action of the sternocleidomastoid decelerates the lower neck as it arches backward (extends) and slows the head and upper neck as they tilt down and forward. It also helps decelerate side bending and rotation of the neck when only one side is lengthened.

Real-life movement example: Works in a traditional sense to hold the head up, such as when performing sit-ups or oblique crunches. Acts like a bungee cord during movements that require tucking of the head and chin such as the lowering phase of a sit-up.

Helpful tips: The longus colli and sternocleidomastoid work together to slow down neck extension. This is especially important in situations where the body is hit and the neck arches backward, like when one is hit from behind in bumper cars.

Semispinalis Capitis

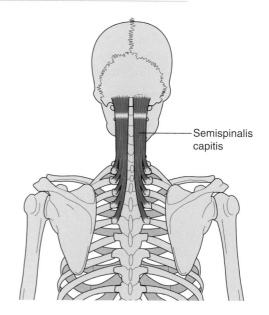

Semispinalis capitis

Muscle specifics: A muscle on the back of the neck. It originates on the upper thoracic spine and lower cervical spine, travels up the neck, and inserts at the back of the skull on the occipital bone (Gray 1995).

Muscle action(s): Extends the neck and head. If only one side of the semispinalis capitis contracts, then the head bends to the same side and rotates toward the opposite side (Chaitow and DeLany 2008).

Real-life movements: The bungee cord action of the semispinalis capitis helps decelerate forward bending (flexion) of the neck and head. It also decelerates side bending and rotation of the neck and head when they are in flexion.

Real-life movement example: Works in a traditional sense during all seated postures where the head and neck are tilted back and up to enable the eyes to look up like when sitting on the floor to watch TV. Acts like a bungee cord to slow down the weight of the head as it tips forward and from side to side, such as what might happen if you were to fall asleep in a chair.

Helpful tips: There are actually three semispinalis muscles: capitis, cervicis, and thoracis. As the name implies, semispinalis thoracis is primarily involved in extension and rotation of the thoracic spine, whereas capitis and cervicis affect movements of the head and neck, respectively.

Semispinalis Cervicis

Muscle specifics: A muscle on the back of the upper torso and neck. It originates from the vertebrae of the middle and upper thoracic spine, runs up along the spine, and inserts on the vertebrae of the middle and upper cervical spine (Gray 1995).

Muscle action(s): Extends the neck. If only one side of the muscle contracts, then the neck bends to the same side and rotates toward the opposite side (Chaitow and DeLany 2008).

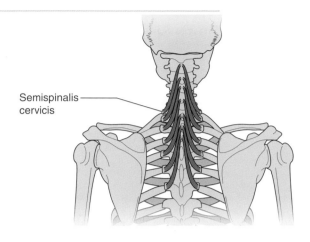
Semispinalis cervicis

Real-life movements: The bungee cord action of the semispinalis cervicis decelerates bending of the neck forward (flexion of the neck). It also helps decelerate side bending and rotation of the neck when it is in flexion.

Real-life movement example: Works in a traditional sense to lift the head up by extending the neck during activities such as bicycle riding, where you must lift your head up to look where you are going. Acts like a bungee cord to help slow down the head as it tips forward or from side to side by decelerating bending of the neck during activities like looking down at your feet.

Helpful tips: Neck muscles react to the many pain receptors in this area. This may explain why muscular tension in the neck is so common (Ferrari 2006).

Splenius Capitis

Muscle specifics: A muscle on the back of the neck. It originates from the upper thoracic spine, the last vertebrae of the cervical spine and the nuchal ligament, and travels up and outward along the neck before inserting behind the bottom of the ear on the skull (Gray 1995).

Muscle action(s): Helps extend the neck and head. If one side of the splenius capitis muscle contracts without the other, then the head bends and rotates to the same side (Lee 2017).

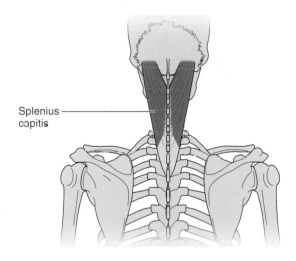
Splenius capitis

Real-life movements: The bungee cord action of the splenius capitis decelerates flexion of the neck and head (i.e., nodding downward). It also decelerates side bending and rotation of the neck and head when they are in flexion.

Real-life movement example: Works in a traditional sense during all movements that require the head to be lifted up to keep the eyes focused and level with the horizon, such as when walking. Acts like a bungee cord to slow the neck and the head as they tip forward, such as when looking down to pet a dog.

Helpful tips: The splenius capitis acts as a fastener of sorts that holds the head firmly to the neck. In fact, its name comes from the Latin words *splenium* meaning "plaster" and *capitis* meaning "of the head."

Splenius Cervicis

Muscle specifics: A muscle on the back of the upper torso and neck. It originates from the middle of the thoracic spine, travels up the neck, and inserts at the top of the neck (Gray 1995).

Muscle action(s): Helps with arching the neck backward (neck extension). If one side of the muscle contracts without the other, then the head bends and rotates to the same side (Lee 2017).

Real-life movements: The bungee cord action of the splenius cervicis decelerates flexion of the neck. It also helps decelerate side bending and rotation of the neck when it is in flexion.

Splenius cervicis

Real-life movement example: Works in a traditional sense to keep the neck extended so the head can sit correctly on top of the shoulders during all upright and weight-bearing movements, like walking and running. Acts like a bungee cord to slow down the neck as it rounds forward, such as when reading a book or looking at your lap when seated.

Helpful tips: The splenius cervicis originates on the thoracic spine and attaches on the neck. Therefore, imbalances in the thoracic spine can affect the function of this muscle and the resulting position of the cervical spine and head.

EFFECT OF THE NECK AND HEAD MUSCLES ON THE MOST COMMON MUSCULOSKELETAL DEVIATIONS

Musculoskeletal imbalances in the neck and head can affect the position of the entire body because the structures beneath must compensate to keep balance mechanisms like the eyes and inner ears working correctly (Lieberman 2011). Similarly, dysfunctions below the neck and head can place the neck and head muscles under stress as they try to compensate for problems elsewhere (Price and Bratcher 2010).

Here are three examples of how the bungee cord feature of specific muscles covered in this chapter factor into the most common deviations of the neck and head.

EXAMPLE ONE: LONGUS COLLI AND LONGUS CAPITIS

The longus colli and longus capitis muscles help flex the neck. However, excessive cervical lordosis

(extension of the neck) can cause chronic lengthening of these muscles, and this can affect their function. Specifically, dysfunctions in these muscles can inhibit the neck from flexing well and can prevent the head from achieving its optimal position. For example, imagine that during a consultation with a prospective client you slouch with your fist under your chin supporting your head as you sit listening. In this position, your neck must arch backward to keep your eyes on your customer. When you try to correct your posture at the end of the chat by sitting upright, pulling your head back, tucking your chin in, and flexing your neck, irritation in the longus colli and longus capitis muscles can make it difficult (Price and Bratcher 2010).

EXAMPLE TWO: STERNOCLEIDOMASTOID

The sternocleidomastoid muscles originate on the front of the rib cage and attach to the base of the skull just behind the ears. When the thoracic spine rounds forward, it causes the sternum and clavicle bones to drop down with the rib cage. This downward shift of the rib cage creates a pull via the sternocleidomastoid on the back of the skull, which in turn causes the head to tip backward and the top of the cervical spine to arch, causing excessive cervical lordosis (see figure 12.4).

Over time, this series of compensation patterns can affect the functioning of the sternocleidomastoid muscles, making it difficult to return the head and the cervical and thoracic spine to their optimal positions. However, if the sternocleidomastoid muscles are healthy and functional, they can be used to pull up the front of the rib cage and correct many of the musculoskeletal imbalances found in the thoracic and cervical spine. For example, when the head is pulled back and the chin is tucked in to achieve a neutral position for the head, the insertions of the sternocleidomastoids on the back of the skull pull away from their origins on the sternum and clavicles. This produces extension of the thoracic spine, flexion of the upper cervical spine, and a correct position for the head (see figure 12.5) (Price and Bratcher 2010).

EXAMPLE THREE: SEMISPINALIS CAPITIS, SEMISPINALIS CERVICIS, SPLENIUS CAPITIS, AND SPLENIUS CERVICIS

Musculoskeletal imbalances in the neck and head can cause the muscles that extend them to become chronically shortened. As a result, they cannot lengthen effectively when you try to perform such everyday movements as rounding your neck forward or tilting your head down. This can produce dysfunctional compensations like the thoracic spine rounding forward instead (see figure 12.6). When the extensor muscles of the neck and head are supple and healthy, they can work in a bungee cord fashion to help keep the neck and head (and consequently the thoracic spine) functioning as they should (Price and Bratcher 2010).

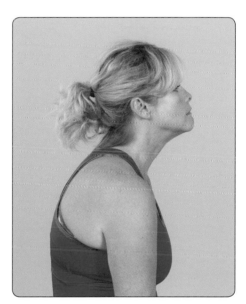

Figure 12.4 Example of excessive thoracic kyphosis causing excessive cervical lordosis via the sternocleidomastoid.

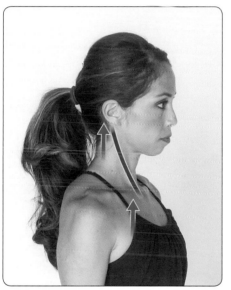

Figure 12.5 Healthy sternocleidomastoids can negate excessive cervical lordosis, excessive thoracic kyphosis, and a forward head position.

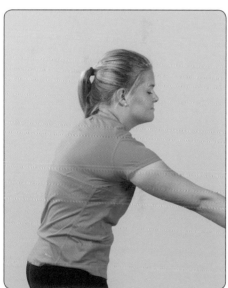

Figure 12.6 Excessive kyphosis as a compensation for restricted neck extensors.

Review of Key Points

The head contains our most vital organ, the brain, which enables us to perceive our environment through sensory organs and maintain balance through the vestibular system. To help keep this part of the body working well, the neck and head must be correctly aligned and functioning effectively.

- A forward head position shifts the body's center of gravity forward and effectively increases the weight of the head in relation to the body. For every inch that the head is forward of its optimal position, the effect of its weight on the body approximately doubles.

- The alignment and function of the temporomandibular joint are affected by musculoskeletal imbalances in the neck and head. Popping and grinding noises in the jaw, difficulty chewing, jaw ache, headaches, or any pain or dysfunction in this area may result from such imbalances.

- The sternocleidomastoids can be used to help align the head, neck and thoracic spine. Pulling the head back and the chin in will lift the rib cage upward and will promote neck and head flexion and thoracic extension.

- Excessive cervical lordosis can lead to irritation of the muscles on the back of the neck. This can prevent these muscles and soft tissues from lengthening correctly when the neck and head must flex.

- While neck flexor muscles such as the longus colli, longus capitis, and sternocleidomastoid help flex the neck toward the chest, they also lengthen like bungee cords to protect the neck from unnecessary stress as it arches backward.

- Musculoskeletal imbalances in the neck and head create compensation patterns throughout the rest of the body, and vice versa.

Self-Check

The following exercise is designed to help you become aware of how postural positions in different parts of the body affect the head and neck.

Stand in front of a full-length mirror and perform the movements listed in the following chart. Observe how your neck and head change position in response to these movements. Use your structural assessment knowledge and understanding of muscles and movement to identify what structures of the head and neck are affected as you change the alignment of different areas of the body. Record your findings in the chart. An example has been provided.

Movement	What happens to head and neck?	Why does movement affect head and neck?
Round your shoulders and look up.	Back of head moves downward, neck arches, chin tilts upward	Neck extensors shorten and get restricted, TM joint moves out of alignment
Lean forward so your weight is in your toes.		
Arch your lower back.		
Bend your knees and do a small squat.		

CHAPTER 13

Fascia

Fascia is a type of connective tissue that intertwines and binds every muscle, organ, and soft tissue structure throughout the body. It links the body together as an integrated system of functional parts. Therefore, when musculoskeletal imbalances occur anywhere in the body, the whole system is affected because of the interconnections created by this fascial network (Myers 2008; Rolf 1989).

There are two levels of fascia in the body. The first level is called the superficial fascia. It lies near the surface of the body and helps bind our skin to the muscles and other structures underneath. The second layer is called deep fascia. It helps bind together different layers of a muscle and also helps hold our nerves, blood vessels, and organs in place (Myers 2008; Rolf 1989).

To help you visualize fascia in the body, imagine a time when you tried to take the skin off a chicken or turkey leg. The skin was attached by a thin film to the muscle underneath. That tissue was the superficial fascia. When you tried to remove the meat from the drumstick, you would have noticed another thin membrane that wrapped around bunches of muscle fibers and then to the bone. That membrane was the deep fascia.

Fascia has elastic properties that help the body deal with gravity and ground reaction forces by absorbing and redistributing shock (Karageanes 2003). When the musculoskeletal system is functioning well, fascia is pliable and lengthens like a bungee cord during movement to help reduce stress. On the other hand, musculoskeletal imbalances, injuries, myofascial restrictions (e.g., trigger points, adhesions, scar tissue), pain, and inflammation can inhibit fascia's ability to moderate tension (Houglum 2016).

Fascia is arranged in a series of systems that follow the paths of muscles, bones, ligaments, and tendons as they travel up, down, and around the body, resulting in an inseparable link between the musculoskeletal system and the fascia. Fascial systems that specifically surround muscles are called myofascial networks. The purpose of these myofascial networks is to help the body to move forward and backward, side-to-side, and in rotation—that is, in all three planes of motion. However, musculoskeletal imbalances can disrupt these myofascial systems, causing more dysfunction and pain, both at the site of the imbalance and elsewhere in the body (Myers 2008; Rolf 1989; Price and Bratcher 2010).

Understanding fascia's influence on the entire body will help you to appreciate that, while individual parts can experience pain and dysfunction, the long-term remedy for musculoskeletal imbalances is to improve the functioning of the body as a whole (Price and Bratcher 2010).

FASCIAL SYSTEMS FOR FLEXION AND EXTENSION

Many movements made throughout the day require the body to flex and extend. For example, when you bend forward at the hips and round your spine to pick something up off the ground, you must then extend your hips and spine to stand up straight again. You learned in previous chapters that muscles and other soft tissue structures can both help initiate these movements and help decelerate the transfer of forces.

There are three systems, or chains, of fascia that link the muscles and their accompanying soft tissue structures on the front and back of the body: the superficial back line, the superficial front line, and the deep front line (see figure 13.1).

- Traveling down the body from top to bottom, the superficial front line includes the sterno-cleidomastoid, rectus abdominis, quadriceps, and tibialis anterior.

- The deep front line includes the longus colli and longus capitis, the diaphragm, the hip flexors, the adductors, and the tibialis posterior.

- The superficial back line includes the erector spinae, sacrotuberous ligament, hamstrings, gastrocnemius, and plantar fascia.

All of these systems of fascia help to synchronize the movement of these muscles, predominantly in the sagittal plane (i.e., movements that require the body to either bend forward or arch backward) (Myers 2008).

When these myofascial systems are functioning effectively, they ensure that all the musculoskeletal structures of these systems work together to integrate and coordinate movements. In doing so, they also protect individual parts of the body and the rest of the kinetic chain from unnecessary stress (Starlanyl and Sharkey 2013).

Many of the most common musculoskeletal imbalances affect the health and function of these myofascial systems responsible for flexion and extension. Excessive lumbar lordosis and excessive cervical lordosis, for example, can cause tension and restrict mobility of the fascia on both the lower back and the back of the neck and head (Hyde and Gengenbach 2007). Consequently, when the spine has to flex, other parts of the spine, such as the thoracic spine, must compensate for the lack of movement in the lower back and neck. Over time, these repeated compensation patterns can lead to the development of additional musculoskeletal imbalances, such as excessive thoracic kyphosis (DiGiovanna, Schiowitz, and Dowling 2005).

Go to the online video to watch video 13.1, where Justin gives an overview of fascia.

FASCIAL SYSTEMS FOR LATERAL MOVEMENT

In addition to sagittal plane movements, many daily activities and sports require side-to-side (frontal plane) movements. Walking, for example, involves transferring weight from side to side and requires

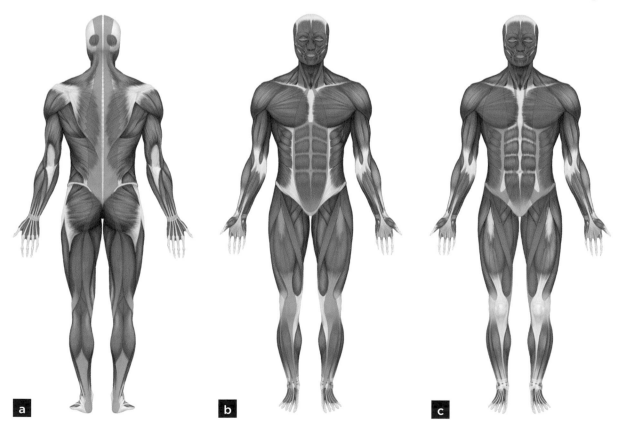

a   b   c

Figure 13.1   Flexion and extension fascial systems: *(a)* superficial back line, *(b)* superficial front line, and *(c)* deep front line.

that the pelvis shift from left to right, that the legs and hips abduct and adduct, and that the spine flex from one side to the other.

Many muscles and other soft tissue structures help produce sideways movement and slow the transfer of forces as our body moves laterally. The musculoskeletal elements involved in these movements are all part of the lateral line of fascia, a myofascial system that connects the structures that run along the sides of the body and facilitate movement in the frontal plane (Myers 2008). There is a left and a right lateral line; each line starts under the foot, and it connects with the peroneal muscles as it wraps around the outside of the ankle and up the side of the lower leg. It then integrates with the iliotibial band running up the outside of the thigh and into the tensor fasciae latae and gluteus maximus muscles. It then continues up the side of the torso by way of the obliques and the intercostals, where it terminates on the side of the neck (see figure 13.2) (Myers 2008).

Many of the most common musculoskeletal imbalances also affect the health and function of the myofascial systems that lie on sides of the body (Houglum 2016; Price and Bratcher 2010). For example, overpronation causes the foot and ankle to collapse inward. Over time, this imbalance can restrict foot and ankle movement, causing other areas of the body to compensate, like the knee deviating too far toward the midline into a valgus position (Hutson and Ward 2016).

FASCIAL SYSTEMS FOR ROTATIONAL MOVEMENT

In addition to forward, backward, and sideways motion, the body also performs movements that require rotation (i.e., movements in the transverse plane). Activities such as swinging the arms and turning the torso when walking, taking a backswing and following through in golf, and hitting a forehand in tennis all involve rotation. The musculoskeletal elements involved in transverse plane movements are part of myofascial networks called spiral lines that wrap around the body (Myers and Earls 2017).

There are two spiral lines running from head to toe that also wrap around the body from front to back (see figure 13.3). They begin under the foot and wrap around the inside or the outside of the ankle, travel up the front and side of the lower leg by way of the tibialis anterior and peroneals, connect with the side and back of the thigh via the iliotibial band and biceps femoris muscle, continue up the spine by way of the erector spinae muscles, and wrap around the torso and rib cage by means of the obliques and

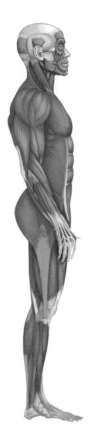

Lateral line

Figure 13.2 The lateral line of fascia.

serratus anterior muscles. The system then crosses over the back of the upper torso by way of the rhomboids and terminates at the base of the skull (Myers 2008). These spiral systems of fascia connect all of the soft tissue structures that help rotate the body as an integrated and coordinated chain.

A number of common musculoskeletal imbalances affect the health and function of the myofascial networks that wrap around the body (Houglum 2016; Price and Bratcher 2010). For example, when a person is walking, protraction and retraction of the shoulder blades helps the body to remain balanced as the arms swing in opposition to the legs. However, excessive protraction of the shoulder blade causes it to move too far forward on the rib cage (and the arm to internally rotate disproportionately). Over time, this can irritate the fascia surrounding the shoulder blades and affect the ability of the rhomboid muscles to contract and lengthen appropriately. This in turn affects the arm swing in relation to the opposite leg swing, causing that leg, knee, and ankle to compensate by moving too far toward the midline during gait (i.e., a valgus knee position and overpronation) (Giangarra and Manske 2011).

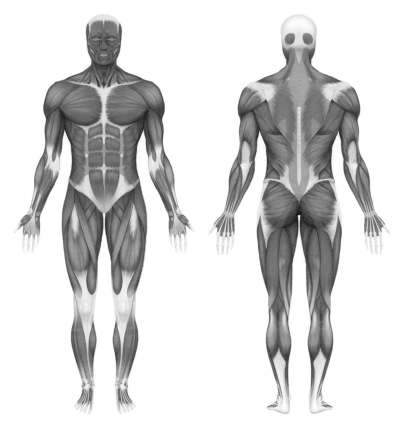

Spiral line

Figure 13.3   The spiral lines of fascia.

FASCIAL SYSTEMS AND COMPLEX MOVEMENT

Myofascial systems are not limited to helping people to move either forward, backward, sideways, or in rotation. Integrated real-life movements require the body to move in multiple directions at the same time (Myers 2008; Price and Bratcher 2010). When we run or walk, for example, we move forward, side-to-side, and in rotation simultaneously. The legs are swinging forward and backward (flexion and extension) as they roll inward and outward (internal and external rotation). The spine is moving from side to side as weight is transferred from left to right, and it is also rotating with the arm swing (Swinnen et al. 1994). These multiplanar movements are possible because, like the musculoskeletal system, the body's myofascial systems are interconnected. In fact, many of the muscles and soft tissue structures of one myofascial network are also contained in others. The obliques, for instance, are part of both the lateral and spiral lines, and the erector spinae group is part of both the superficial back line and the spiral line. The coordination of these complex myofascial networks facilitates sophisticated movement in multiple planes during weight-bearing activities (Myers 2008).

Having an understanding of fascia and how it can affect the movement of the whole body is important to your future success as you help people who have musculoskeletal imbalances. You must consider the myofascial systems as you begin to select corrective exercises and to design programs to address the causes of your clients' pain and movement dysfunction.

Review of Key Points

Fascia is a three-dimensional network of connective tissue that envelops every structure in the body, including muscles, tendons, ligaments, and internal organs. While the interconnectedness of fascia enables multiplanar and multidirectional movement, it also means that musculoskeletal imbalances in one part of the body have a direct impact on movement and function (or dysfunction) elsewhere.

- There are two levels of fascia: superficial and deep. The superficial level primarily binds muscles to skin, and the deep level binds muscles together.

- Restrictions, adhesions, and scar tissue can affect the ability of fascia to lengthen and be pliable. This can cause pain and can restrict movement.

- The term *myofascial* refers to fascia that is specifically associated with muscles.

- There are myofascial systems on the front, back, and sides of the body and others that also wrap around the body.

- The myofascial systems on the front and back of the body are called the front and back lines. Those on the sides are called the lateral lines, and those that wrap around the body are called the spiral lines.

- The myofascial systems intertwine so that movements in all three planes can occur in a coordinated fashion.

- Musculoskeletal imbalances can restrict movement in one area of the body or in a particular muscle or group. These restrictions can affect the functioning of the entire myofascial system, causing the body to compensate elsewhere and creating additional musculoskeletal imbalances.

Self-Check

The ability to explain to clients what fascia is and how myofascial systems affect the body as a whole is a vital part of successful corrective exercise programming. The following activity will enable you to help clients truly appreciate the interconnectedness of their bodies and to experience firsthand the amazing impact appropriate corrective exercise strategies can have on their musculoskeletal systems. Practicing this activity before introducing it to clients will help you to develop your coaching and communication strategies, and you will be more confident when you use it to explain the importance of restoring and maintaining a healthy myofascial system.

Perform the Activity

Gently bend forward from a standing position and reach down toward the ground while keeping your legs fairly straight. Do not force the movement. Note how far down you can reach (e.g., just past your knees, to the tops of your feet, fingertips touching the ground).

Return to a normal standing position and place a golf or tennis ball on the underside of your left foot. Roll it around under your foot, pausing on any sore spots to massage away tension before moving on to the next sore spot. Do this for one minute, and then transfer the ball to your right foot and massage the underside of that foot for one minute.

Once you have massaged both feet, put the ball to one side and repeat the forward bending stretch you performed initially. You will notice that you can now reach farther down.

Explain the Results to Your Client

This increased range of movement is a direct result of loosening up the plantar fascia on the underside of your foot. This fascia is part of the superficial back line of fascia that runs from under your foot, up the back of your leg, across the back of your pelvis, up your back and neck, and over your head to the top of your forehead. By increasing the flexibility of the fascia on the underside of your foot, you increased the movement potential of the myofascial system on the back of your body. That is why it is now easier to bend forward and lengthen your reach (Myers 2008).

Part III

Fundamentals of Corrective Exercise

In part III, you will learn about the elements of a successful corrective exercise program and how to select and adapt exercises that address the most common musculoskeletal imbalances you learned about in part I. The results of your structural assessments, and your enhanced knowledge of functional anatomy gleaned from part II, will enable you to evaluate the suitability of available options. Then you can make the appropriate recommendations for clients' corrective exercise programs.

Part III will teach you specifically about the three most effective types of corrective exercise: self-myofascial release techniques, stretching exercises, and strengthening exercises. You will learn about the history of these exercises, the unique benefits of each, and how these modalities have proved successful for addressing and correcting musculoskeletal imbalances. A variety of different myofascial release techniques, stretches, and strengthening exercises are introduced, and you will be taught when to use each one based on your client's needs. You will also learn ways to reduce your clients' anxiety surrounding the performance of corrective exercises and strategies to boost their confidence and commitment to their corrective exercise programs. Furthermore, you will learn when and how to progress a client's program and, conversely, when and how to regress it when necessary. You will also learn about specific contraindications for each exercise type to ensure safety and effectiveness.

In addition to choosing appropriate corrective exercises, you must be able to educate clients about nonexercise-related issues that may be contributing to their problems, such as footwear choices, the use of arch supports, or prolonged static standing, sitting, and sleeping postures. The last chapter in part III explains the negative effects of prolonged static postures, and it offers tips on helping clients to make better lifestyle choices and assume better body positions throughout the day.

CHAPTER 14

Elements of Corrective Exercise Programs

Chronic imbalances can affect the health and condition of all musculoskeletal structures, including the bones, joints, muscles, fascia, tendons, and ligaments. Therefore, the corrective exercises you recommend must first promote the rest, recovery, and rejuvenation of all structures you identified as problematic during the assessment process. You must then help these areas regain function, health, and suppleness by introducing corrective exercises to retrain, reinforce, and strengthen them in order to improve the overall health of the musculoskeletal system, and curtail future problems.

Many things factor into the selection of appropriate corrective exercises for your clients' programs. In addition to choosing safe and effective techniques, you must also address clients' practical and emotional needs and abilities, and the exercises you recommend should build their confidence (Price and Bratcher 2010). You must also know how to introduce corrective exercises in a logical sequence so that clients can achieve the greatest possible benefits in the least amount of time.

BUILDING CLIENT CONFIDENCE

When clients first come to you to discuss their goals or the musculoskeletal issues they are experiencing, understand that they have probably been concerned about it for some time. As a result, they may have lost confidence in their ability to perform certain activities, especially those that require the use of the affected or painful areas (Bandura 1986)

Bearing this in mind, it is important to build clients' confidence when you first introduce them to corrective exercise. This is best done by taking the time to listen to their concerns and answering their questions honestly, avoiding the use of technical jargon. Proceed slowly at first, and use different teaching approaches as you explain each technique and the corrective exercise process in general. If you notice that a client appears confused, is not asking questions, or is simply agreeing with everything you say—or if he seems overenthusiastic—do not assume that he understands (Fuller 2004) These types of responses often indicate just the opposite. Clients who lack confidence in their abilities are less likely to tell you when they do not understand. Learning to recognize when a client is feeling anxious or overwhelmed will allow you to address these issues as they arise, gain the client's trust, and build a positive, long-lasting relationship (Whitworth et al. 2007).

In addition to addressing clients' concerns about their physical condition, you can boost their confidence by choosing easy-to-perform exercises at the outset of the program. When they can try and successfully perform a new corrective exercise, their self-confidence increases. This will motivate them to repeat the action (i.e., it will increase their adherence), and it will make them more likely to try the next exercise you ask them to perform (Feltz 1992; Rejeski 1992).

Remember, the guiding principle of corrective exercise programming is the same as that of traditional fitness programs: gradual progression (Bryant and Green 2010). This strategy applies from both a mental and a physical standpoint. Introducing concepts and exercises at a manageable pace will improve the likelihood that your clients will adhere to their programs and reach their goals.

 Go to the online video to watch video 14.1, where Justin provides tips for building client confidence.

ORDER OF EXERCISES

Successful corrective exercise programs must address a client's imbalances and deviations in a logical and sequential format. Structures that have been damaged and stressed must first be allowed to rest and regenerate before any attempts at retraining through stretching or strengthening can be made (Price and Bratcher 2010). Therefore, when designing a corrective exercise program, use activities that achieve the following goals in the order listed:

1. Let inflamed joints rest while incorporating techniques for rejuvenating and regenerating the fascia, muscles, and tendons.

2. Increase blood flow and range of movement.

3. Strengthen the muscles and challenge the nervous system.

In other words, every corrective exercise program should begin with self-myofascial release techniques, then progress to stretching, and ultimately advance to strengthening exercises.

- *Self-myofascial release:* The term *myofascial* comes from "myo" meaning muscle and "fascial" referring to fascia. This technique of self-massage is used to restore and rejuvenate soft tissues that have become adversely affected by chronic musculoskeletal imbalances (Rolf 1989; Myers 2008; Travell and Simons 1992). Self-myofascial release also helps clients feel better by reducing aches and pains that accompany excessive soft tissue stress. Always start each exercise session and each program with some form of self-massage that clients can also do between sessions at home, at the office, or anywhere they feel completely comfortable.

- *Stretching:* As the soft tissue structures become more fluid and healthy with the regular performance of self-myofascial release exercises, the next step in the corrective exercise process is to increase flexibility of the muscles and fascia and to increase the range of motion of the joints. Many different types of stretching exercises can be used to increase safe ranges of motion and retrain movement in those parts of the body that have become dysfunctional because of chronic musculoskeletal imbalances (Walker 2011).

- *Strengthening:* Once a client has begun to improve the condition of specific soft tissue structures, add strengthening exercises to the program. These will fortify the soft tissue structures and will increase the client's confidence about movements that were previously difficult. Strengthening exercises are also used to reeducate the client's body so it can eliminate musculoskeletal imbalances (Price and Sharpe 2009).

The appropriate application and progression (or regression, when appropriate) of self-myofascial, stretching, and strengthening exercises is vital to the design of corrective exercise programs. Each of these modalities will be discussed in greater detail in later chapters.

Go to the online video to watch video 14.2, where Justin talks about The BioMechanics Method corrective exercise program design process.

EVALUATING EXERCISES

Selecting effective corrective exercises involves determining whether the techniques you recommend are both effective and practical. Clients are unlikely to adhere to exercises that call for equipment they cannot easily obtain. Therefore, you should always evaluate both the usefulness and the practicality of an exercise before choosing it.

The following SIMPLE exercise evaluation process can help you determine the suitability of an exercise by identifying the target structures, the imbalances being addressed, the clients' ability to do the exercise, practicality, and possible alternatives, regressions, and progressions.

- *Structure:* What structures (muscles, fascia, joints, bones) are targeted with this exercise?
- *Imbalance:* Which musculoskeletal imbalance(s) are you addressing with this exercise?
- *Mechanics:* What are the correct mechanics of the exercise (so the imbalance is addressed and not exacerbated), and can the client perform it correctly?
- *Practical:* Will the client perform this exercise effectively and regularly? (Are the constraints of the exercise reasonable, and are the equipment needs practical?)

- *Level:* Can this exercise be progressed or regressed for a greater or lesser challenge to meet the client's needs?
- *Exercise alternatives:* Is there a similar exercise that targets the same imbalance that is more likely to increase client adherence—that is, an exercise the client likes better or that can more easily be incorporated into his or her daily routine?

Use this SIMPLE procedure to evaluate every corrective exercise you recommend to ensure that you meet each client's needs.

Review of Key Points

Many factors must be considered when selecting effective corrective exercises.

- The three most important components of successful corrective exercise selection are:
  - the ability to assess clients' musculoskeletal imbalances and evaluate the condition of their soft tissue structures,
  - the ability to recognize client anxieties and build their confidence using appropriate communication strategies, and
  - knowing which corrective exercises to use for each client and the order in which they should be introduced.
- Corrective exercise programs will be most successful if the strategies you first recommend promote healing and regeneration of the affected structures and can also be easily adhered to.
- Clients with musculoskeletal imbalances, injuries, or pain will likely feel anxious about their condition. Look for indications that anxiety levels may be rising as you discuss exercises and other program variables with them. You can adapt your strategies as needed to help keep them comfortable, confident, and focused.
- The best strategies for building client confidence are:
  - Speak in a straightforward manner and avoid using complex, technical terms.
  - Begin a program with exercises you know they can perform successfully.
  - Apply the guiding principle of gradual progression to all aspects of a corrective exercise program.
- Every corrective exercise program should incorporate self-myofascial release techniques, stretches, and strengthening exercises, in that order.
- Evaluate every corrective exercise using the SIMPLE procedure so that those you choose are appropriate, effective, and practical.

Self-Check

Due to the anxiety that accompanies chronic musculoskeletal imbalances and pain, it is important to explain corrective exercise to your clients without using technical jargon. To help you hone this valuable skill, use the following spaces to explain the concepts and benefits of self-myofascial release, stretching, and strengthening exercises in simple, everyday language. An example for self-myofascial release has been provided.

Type of exercise	Jargon-free description
Self-myofascial release	Self-myofascial release is just a fancy name for self-massage. Self-massage is used to bring blood supply to tight muscles and other tissues that have been affected by the imbalances we found during your assessment. These techniques will rejuvenate and regenerate your body, which will alleviate some of your symptoms and prepare to you progress with your program when the time comes.
Stretching	
Strengthening	

CHAPTER 15

Self-Myofascial Release

In this chapter, you will learn about various self-myofascial release techniques and why they should be used at the outset of a client's program before stretching and strengthening exercises are introduced. (The terms *self-myofascial release* and *self-massage* are interchangeable. Many clients prefer the term *self-massage* because they are familiar with massage and are more enthusiastic about learning the techniques.) You will learn how these techniques rejuvenate and rehabilitate soft tissue structures, address musculoskeletal imbalances, and alleviate musculoskeletal dysfunctions and pain. You will also learn tips for teaching and cueing clients on these techniques and ways to progress and regress these techniques.

WHAT IS SELF-MYOFASCIAL RELEASE?

Self-myofascial release may sound complex and technical, but it is really a very simple concept. The term *myofascial* refers to muscles and the fascia that surrounds them; the prefix *myo-* simply means "muscle." Therefore, self-myofascial release is a massage technique of applying sustained pressure to an area of myofascial tissue that contains restrictions, tightness, inflexibility, adhesions, knots, or scar tissue, or lacks proper movement. The sustained pressure stimulates circulation to the area, reduces pressure buildup from sluggish blood flow and toxins, and improves tissue elasticity and suppleness (Travell and Simons 1992; Simons, Travell, and Simons 1998). It is important to understand the properties of muscles and fascia before using self-

myofascial release. This will enable you to appreciate how they can be helped by the appropriate application of these techniques.

MUSCLES

Skeletal muscle is the most common form of muscle tissue in the body. Apart from the tongue, all skeletal muscles are connected at both ends to bones by tendons. The origin point of a muscle is the end that is attached to a bone that is either fixed in position or has less movement capability (usually nearer the body's center of mass). The insertion point is the end that is attached to a bone with greater movement capability (Hyde 2002). Muscles are comprised of bands of tissue that typically run in the same direction as the force they apply to the bones and joints. For example, the tissues of the biceps brachii muscle originate from portions of the scapula and insert on the end of the radius and the fascia in the lower arm near the elbow (Scheumann 2007). The bands of fibers in this muscle run lengthwise down the upper arm because their function is to help pull the lower arm toward the shoulder when contracted. There are also muscles, such as the gluteus maximus, that have multiple functions and contain fibers that run in multiple directions. The origin and insertion points of muscles, and the direction the muscle fibers run, determine the actions of each muscle or muscle group (Hyde 2002). Adhesions, nodules, knots, scar tissue, and inflexibility in muscles can affect the muscle's ability to perform these actions correctly. The regular application of self-myofascial release techniques can help realign these muscle fibers so that the muscle can function effectively (Clark and Lucett 2011).

Skeletal muscle can lengthen and stretch, shorten and contract, and return to its normal shape. These properties are called elasticity, contractility, and extensibility, respectively (Hyde 2002). From a corrective exercise standpoint, all three are extremely important. The contraction function of muscles enables the skeleton to move. The ability of muscles to lengthen and stretch appropriately facilitates the "bungee cord action" that decelerates movement and reduces stress on joints. The ability of muscles to return to their usual shape enables all the parts of the body to return to normal, allowing rest and preventing the onset of negative musculoskeletal changes. The regular application of self-myofascial release techniques has been shown to help improve all three of these muscle functions by improving the sensitivity, repair and recovery, growth, and performance of muscle tissue (Beck 2010).

FASCIA

Fascia is connective tissue that wraps around and separates bundles of muscle fibers, entire muscles, and every other layer of tissue in the body. It runs throughout the body, connecting all the structures into one inseparable kinetic chain (see figure 13.3) (Myers 2008; Scheumann 2007).

The overall condition and health of the fascia should be addressed from the outset of any corrective exercise program. This is because restrictions or tightness in the fascia is generally manifested as musculoskeletal compensation patterns and imbalances, which often present as muscle tension and pain. The regular application of self-myofascial release helps to regulate myofascial tension throughout the body to decrease movement stress, improve blood flow, and increase range of motion (Rolf 1989).

Unhealthy fascia and muscle fibers are prone to develop very dysfunctional (and sometimes painful) characteristics such as excessive tightness, nodules, adhesions, and inflexibility (Scheumann 2007). Such symptoms can indicate where self-myofascial release might be applied to restore health and vitality to those tissues that need it most. Clients will appreciate the reduction and elimination of painful symptoms that self-myofascial release techniques can provide.

ORIGINS OF SELF-MYOFASCIAL RELEASE

The use of myofascial release techniques is not a new idea. Self-massage has been used in one form or another to promote health, relieve stress, and reduce pain for approximately 5,000 years. It is thought to have originated around 2500 to 3000 BC, and its use as a health tool was documented in early Chinese medical texts and depicted in ancient Egyptian tomb paintings (Calvert 2002). Massage also has documented roots in traditional Indian medicine dating as far back as 1500 BC. The ancient Greeks and Romans were among those who recognized the therapeutic qualities of massage, and they incorporated it into their daily health regimens. Even Julius Caesar (100 to 44 BC) used massage to help relieve pain (Sinha 2001). Practitioners in the Persian empire also believed in the benefits of exercise and massage, and they went about diagnosing and assessing conditions and prescribing massage techniques to help relieve pain. In the mid-1800s, the word *massage* was formally introduced in the Western medical community. Swedish massage became very popular, and many of the techniques developed during that time are still used today (Calvert 2002). Finnish and Russian influences further expanded the use of massage into sport massage and neuromuscular therapy.

Massage and myofascial release are now used in many settings around the world, from spas to hospitals, as a therapeutic and restorative strategy. Currently, the most popular forms of massage used for corrective purposes are applied to a general area of the body using a large tool like a foam roller or pinpointing a specific area of muscle or fascia using a small massage device like a tennis ball or Theracane (Price 2013; Price and Bratcher 2010; Simons, Travell, and Simons 1998; Travell and Simons 1992).

BENEFITS OF SELF-MYOFASCIAL RELEASE

There are many documented reasons why corrective exercise clients benefit from regularly performing self-myofascial release. Massaging the myofascial structures affected by the most common musculoskeletal imbalances has been shown to do the following (Abelson and Abelson 2003; Brummitt 2008; Calvert 2002; Inkster 2015; Price 2013; Simons, Travell, and Simons 1998; Travell and Simons 1992):

- Increases circulation, enabling oxygen and other nutrients to reach vital tissues, muscles, and organs
- Increases joint flexibility, preparing joints for the increased range of movement and load that accompanies stretching and strengthening exercises
- Reduces adhesions and scar tissue and improves the elasticity of muscles and other soft tissues

- Aids in the reduction of delayed onset muscle soreness (DOMS)
- Eliminates stored tension in muscles
- Releases endorphins to help reduce pain
- Relieves mental stress

TYPES OF SELF-MYOFASCIAL RELEASE

There are two kinds of self-myofascial release techniques: general and specific. Both are very effective for rejuvenating and regenerating muscles affected by musculoskeletal imbalances. They can be used to rehabilitate and restore the health of soft tissue structures, prepare them for movement at the beginning of a corrective exercise session, and also aid recovery after a bout of exercise or strenuous activity.

GENERAL TECHNIQUES

General self-myofascial release techniques are those that affect large areas of the body (Inkster 2015). Devices with a large surface area, such as foam rollers, are well suited for this type of massage (see figure 15.1).

These general techniques are typically applied at the beginning of a corrective exercise program to address wide-ranging muscle and soft tissue dysfunction (Myers 2008; Rolf 1989). For example, if your assessment reveals that a client has a valgus knee position, you know that his leg rotates in toward the midline of his body. From your understanding of muscles and movement, you also know that this imbalance affects many of the muscle groups that decelerate the inward rotation of the leg, such as the hip rotators, gluteals, adductors, and hip flexors. Each of these muscle groups consists of several

individual muscles. Expecting your client to massage each muscle in the group separately at the outset of his program would be overwhelming and perhaps unnecessary (the imbalance might affect some muscles in the group more than others). Therefore, general self-myofascial release techniques are very good for the introductory stage of a program.

Since general self-myofascial techniques take less time to affect a large area, they are also recommended if a client tells you that she lacks time to perform her corrective exercise homework. General techniques are also very useful for increasing blood supply and flexibility before exercise as part of a warm-up and for promoting rest and recovery as part of a cool-down (Clark and Lucett 2011).

SPECIFIC TECHNIQUES

Specific self-myofascial release techniques target individual muscles and precise "trigger" points in a muscle or area of fascia. These more exacting forms of self-massage usually require the use of sustained pressure on a specific part of the body to help restore movement and elasticity to individual muscles and their associated fascia (Abelson and Abelson 2003; Price 2013). Specific self-myofascial release techniques use massage tools with a smaller surface area (e.g., tennis balls, golf balls, lacrosse balls, baseballs, and trigger point therapy sticks such as Theracanes) that can pinpoint a precise area of muscle or fascia (see figure 15.2).

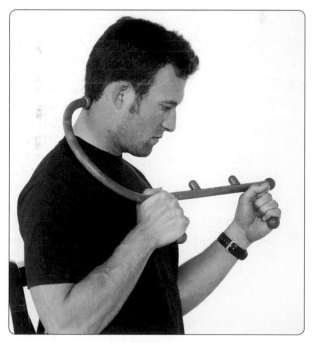

Figure 15.2 Specific self-myofascial release technique: Theracane on back of neck.

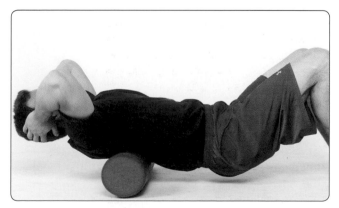

Figure 15.1 General self-myofascial release technique: Foam roller on thoracic spine.

Specific self-myofascial release techniques target smaller areas of the body like the foot or calf muscles. They also enable you to focus on individual muscles, or on a specific part of a muscle or fascia, as a corrective exercise program progresses and more precision is needed. For example, as you work with a client with excessive thoracic kyphosis and protracted shoulder blades, you might notice that his right shoulder blade is more protracted than his left. The use of a tennis ball on his right rhomboid (minor and major) muscle would be a great technique to address this specific imbalance.

Specific self-myofascial release techniques should also be used when general self-myofascial release techniques are not practical. This may include times when a client is traveling and cannot take a foam roller along, when buying a foam roller is impractical, or when a client cannot successfully perform a foam roller exercise you recommend (Price and Bratcher 2010).

TEACHING TIPS FOR SELF-MYOFASCIAL RELEASE TECHNIQUES

While self-myofascial release exercises are excellent for the outset of a corrective exercise program from a physiological standpoint, they offer the added benefit of enabling you to build a client's confidence by quickly alleviating symptoms of pain. Hence, it is crucial to choose exercises that are appropriate for a client's condition, will promptly help to reduce pain, and are presented in a way that will promote long-term adherence and program success.

Here are some suggestions for teaching self-myofascial release techniques so that your clients will implement them successfully:

1. When you first introduce clients to a self-myofascial release technique, they will often ask about performance variables such as sets, repetitions, duration, and frequency. It is important to remember that each client will have different needs, and the amount of time required will vary from person to person. Part IV of this text includes general guidelines for every exercise in the exercise library, but you should adjust the variables of any self-myofascial release exercise to accommodate each client's needs and abilities.

2. Once you have identified an area of myofascial restriction and chosen a self-myofascial release exercise, give the client ample time to explore the tight areas or sore spots for herself. A client's initial reaction to getting on a tennis ball or foam roller will often be to tense up in response to the discomfort or pressure she feels from the restricted tissue. However, if given time to adjust to these new sensations, she will begin to relax, and hormones will be released into her body to promote further relaxation. Furthermore, allowing clients to explore areas needing myofascial release allows them to find sore spots on their own. This self-discovery process will empower them to feel in control of this new exercise and of the program in general, increasing the likelihood that they will adhere to their programs (Price 2016).

3. The self-myofascial release techniques you suggest must be practical. Do not recommend pieces of equipment that are hard to buy or impractical to have on hand. For example, a full-sized foam roller is a very useful self-myofascial release tool. However, it will not fit in a carry-on-sized suitcase. If you have a client who flies often and prefers not to check bags, then an exercise requiring the use of a full-sized foam roller would not be appropriate.

4. Always tell clients *why* they are performing a particular self-myofascial release exercise and how it relates to their condition. Understanding the rationale behind your exercise recommendations gives them a good reason to perform the exercises regularly (Whitworth et al. 2007).

5. As clients perform self-myofascial release exercises, you will see their confidence level rise as their myofascial tension subsides. This growing confidence is usually accompanied by thoughts of what might be coming next in their corrective exercise program (Feltz 1992). You can harness this growing confidence to increase their adherence by explaining how the exercise being performed relates to the next stage of their program. This helps preserve their enthusiasm and prepares them mentally for what will be expected of them next (Pappaioannou and Hackfort 2014). For example, as a client becomes more confident with a particular exercise, prepare for the next one by saying something like, "Once we've warmed up your hips and lower back with the foam roller, we can start to teach the individual muscles around that area to move correctly by integrating some stretching exercises. This will help you get back to all those activities you enjoy, like hiking and gardening."

WHEN TO REGRESS SELF-MYOFASCIAL TECHNIQUES

Clients must always feel successful in performing the self-myofascial release techniques you recommend, both while under your supervision and when doing them on their own. Therefore, you need to know how and when to regress these exercises—that is, make them easier—if your client feels apprehensive, hesitant, or unable to perform the exercise correctly.

1. Self-myofascial techniques should be regressed any time a client feels uncomfortable or nervous in any way. For example, if a client performing a foam roller exercise keeps falling off or appears uneasy, regress him to a technique that he can perform more easily (see figure 15.3). Regressions that allow clients to remain in control of their bodies during an exercise are vital to increasing client confidence. They also help clients to enjoy the process and to ease into each exercise, allowing the myofascial structures they are addressing to relax and release.

2. Regress a self-myofascial release exercise if a client experiences any type of pain. Since self-myofascial release techniques are intended to rejuvenate unhealthy soft tissue structures, it is natural for clients to experience a little discomfort or soreness when first using a foam roller, tennis ball, or Theracane. However, if the sensation is intense or does not diminish once the exercise is underway, then the exercise should be stopped and regressed appropriately. Communicating with clients about what they feel while they perform the exercise, and watching their body language to monitor their level of discomfort, can help you determine whether a regression is needed.

3. If a client does not understand how to perform a self-myofascial release technique you have recommended, regress the technique. For example, if a client continues to place her body in the wrong position when performing a foam roller exercise, you must find a more appropriate exercise that she can perform successfully (such as a comparable tennis ball exercise).

4. Regress a self-myofascial technique if performing it causes pain or discomfort to another part of the client's body. For example, several foam roller exercises require clients to balance on one arm while rolling their legs or hips. Propping up their body weight with one arm may place excessive stress on the shoulder or cause pain. If this occurs, tell the client to stop performing the exercise and regress him to another exercise that does not require him to support himself on one arm.

5. If a client does not have a particular piece of equipment (and is not willing to purchase one), regress your self-myofascial exercise recommendation to a more accommodating option. For example, if a client does not have a Theracane and does not want to buy one, you will need to suggest an alternative exercise, such as one that uses a tennis ball instead.

WAYS TO REGRESS SELF-MYOFASCIAL TECHNIQUES

There are many ways to regress a self-myofascial release exercise:

1. Allow the client to use a softer tool for applying pressure, such as a less dense roller or a softer ball for any of the exercises.

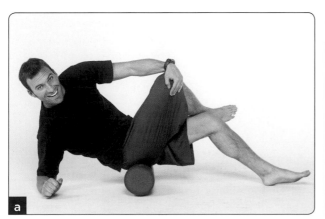
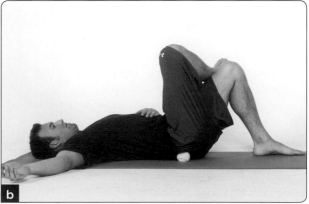

Figure 15.3   Regressing from (a) foam roller on glutes to (b) tennis ball on glutes.

2. Tell the client to perform an exercise while seated or lying down. For example, the Golf Ball Roll technique can be performed while seated using a tennis ball (see figure 15.4), thus reducing the amount of pressure on the client's foot.

3. Tell clients to use their fingers instead of a hard self-myofascial release tool to massage tender areas. You can further regress a self-myofascial exercise by instructing a client to apply heat to the affected area with a heating pad.

There are many different possibilities for regressing self-myofascial release exercises. A full library of exercises and suggestions for regressions can be found in chapter 19, Self-Myofascial Release Exercises.

WHEN TO PROGRESS SELF-MYOFASCIAL TECHNIQUES

Most clients would obviously like to improve their musculoskeletal health as quickly as possible so they can reduce their pain and improve their function. Progressing their programs as soon as they become proficient with an exercise is the most effective and efficient way to do this.

1. Progress a self-myofascial technique if a client no longer feels any tenderness when applying pressure to the target area. For example, if a client is rolling the quadriceps and no longer feels pressure or sensitivity in that area, a suitable progression would be to use a harder roller or to progress to an appropriate stretching exercise for that body part (see figure 15.5).

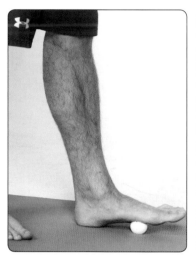
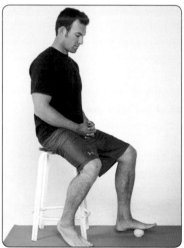

Figure 15.4 The Golf Ball Roll can be regressed by having the client sit while performing the exercise and using a tennis ball instead of a golf ball.

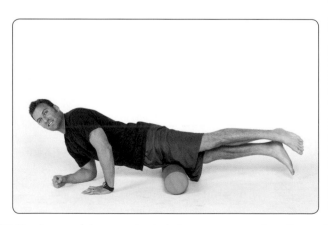
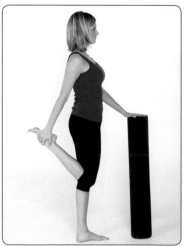

Figure 15.5 A quadriceps stretch is a progression from foam rolling this muscle group.

2. Progress or find alternative self-myofascial techniques if clients complain that their homework exercises take too long. For example, a tennis ball has a small surface area and takes considerable time to massage large areas of the body. A foam roller, on the other hand, is a more time-efficient tool due to its greater surface area.

3. Progress a self-myofascial release technique to a stretching exercise if the target tissues have released enough to perform the desired range of motion or movement with correct technique. For example, after a client has performed the Golf Ball Roll to loosen up the tissues on the underside of a foot, you can use a stretch (e.g., the Foot and Toe Stretch shown in chapter 20) to evaluate the flexibility and movement of the foot. If you find that the muscles are flexible enough to perform the stretch correctly, then progress and integrate it into the program. However, if you progress to a stretch and find that your client cannot perform the movement correctly, you will need to go back and spend more time releasing the area with the appropriate self-massage technique.

WAYS TO PROGRESS SELF-MYOFASCIAL TECHNIQUES

There are many ways you can progress a self-myofascial release exercise:

1. Direct a client to use a firmer roller or a harder ball for applying pressure to those areas that need releasing.

2. Integrate a stretch into the exercise. For example, while a client is releasing his gluteal muscles with the foam roller, you can coach him to pull his knee to his chest in order to stretch the gluteal muscles at the same time (see figure 15.6).

3. Coach the client to angle his body differently to apply more pressure to the area being massaged. For example, if a client is using the foam roller to massage his IT band, you can direct him to place his other leg on top of the leg that is in contact with the roller (see figure 15.7). This added weight will increase the pressure to the target area.

There are many different possibilities for progressing self-myofascial release exercises. A full library of exercises and suggestions for progression can be found in chapter 19, Self-Myofascial Release Exercises.

WHEN NOT TO USE SELF-MYOFASCIAL RELEASE TECHNIQUES

While SMR exercises are generally safe for most clients to perform, observe the following contraindications in a corrective exercise setting (Clark and Lucett 2011; Price and Bratcher 2010).

- Do not use SMR on areas of the body that are swollen or have edema (i.e., badly bruised or acutely inflamed areas).
- Do not use SMR on or near a blood clot.
- Do not use SMR with clients who have acute rheumatoid arthritis.
- Do not perform SMR on or near open wounds.
- Do not use SMR on clients who have had an aneurysm.

Figure 15.6 Integrated glute stretch.

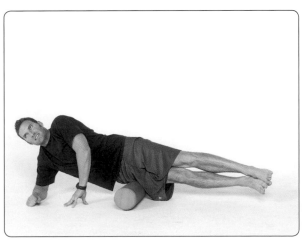

Figure 15.7 Foam roller on IT band with legs stacked.

- Do not use SMR on clients who have hypersensitive skin, hives, eczema, or rashes.
- Limit the use of SMR techniques with clients who have very high blood pressure. If you are ever in doubt about whether it is safe for clients to perform SMR exercises, contact their physicians to obtain clearance.
- Be conservative with the use of SMR on areas of the body that are excessively tight or currently in spasm.
- Pregnant women in their second and third trimesters should avoid sustained prone and supine positions. Do not recommend SMR techniques that require this population to assume prone or supine positions for prolonged periods.
- Clients should not perform SMR exercises when they have a high fever.
- Clients with a serious illness or an infectious disease like the flu should not perform SMR exercises while the condition is present.
- Do not use SMR techniques on the abdominal area if a client has hernias or has had recent abdominal surgery.
- Do not use SMR over broken bones.
- Be conservative using SMR on clients with osteoporosis. If you do recommend SMR for this population, choose exercises that do not place direct pressure on affected areas. For example, instead of instructing a client to lie on the ground over a tennis ball to massage her upper back, coach her to massage this area while standing by placing the tennis ball between her back and a wall. This will give her greater control over the amount of pressure she places on the ball and will reduce the risk that she will exacerbate her condition.
- Do not apply direct pressure on varicose veins when performing SMR exercises.
- People with certain types of cancer should avoid SMR. If a client you are working with has cancer, check with his physician first to obtain clearance.

- If you are ever in doubt about whether you should use SMR with a certain client, check with his physician first to obtain clearance.

ADDITIONAL CONSIDERATIONS

Here are a few more conditioning and safety tips to be aware of as you introduce self-myofascial exercises into clients' corrective exercise programs:

1. When clients perform self-myofascial release exercises, watch their body language for any hints of pain or problems. Watch their facial expressions for signs of discomfort or unease, listen to their voices or breathing for indications of distress, and watch their bodies for signals that they are not comfortable in the position you have suggested. If clients are uncomfortable for any reason, change the exercise to ensure that they can relax and will not harm themselves. Never encourage a client to try to push through the pain when performing any form of corrective exercise.

2. As clients experience pain relief from performing self-myofascial release, many will want to increase the pressure on the area they are massaging. While this is sometimes a good way to progress a program, it is also important to teach clients to be wary of applying too much pressure or staying on a sore spot for too long. Too much pressure may inadvertently damage the muscle tissue or the surrounding fascia (Fritz 2013).

3. Some self-myofascial release exercises may remain in a client's program for months, or even years. This is especially true for clients who are either very dysfunctional or who place their bodies under heavy physical stress. Long distance runners, for example, may need to use the foam roller on their IT bands and glutes almost daily to ensure that these structures recover from their high-intensity running programs.

Review of Key Points

Self-myofascial release techniques are used at the outset of a client's program to rejuvenate and regenerate unhealthy muscles and other soft tissues to prepare for later stretching and strengthening exercises. These self-massage techniques can be performed using minimal and low-cost equipment in the gym, at home, in the office, or on the road, and they should be done regularly to address the underlying causes of musculoskeletal issues.

- Two types of self-myofascial release techniques are described in this chapter, general and specific.

- Foam rollers or massage tools with a big surface area are ideal for performing general self-myofascial release techniques, which target large areas of the body at once.

- Tennis balls, baseballs, lacrosse balls, cricket balls, massage balls and sticks, and Thera-canes are massage tools with a smaller surface area that are used for targeting specific soft tissue knots and adhesions.

- Understanding a client's musculoskeletal imbalances and functional anatomy is essential to knowing what myofascial structures need addressing with self-massage.

- Although there are many documented benefits to the use of self-myofascial release techniques, there are also times when it is not appropriate to use them. Be aware of these important considerations so that the techniques you recommend will be beneficial.

- There are many ways to progress and regress self-myofascial release exercises. Watch clients' movements as they perform each technique to ensure that they will be able to perform it correctly at home. If you foresee any difficulties with an exercise, regress it or use an alternative.

Self-Check

Knowing how to regress or progress a self-myofascial release exercise is an important part of corrective exercise program design. To help you practice your exercise adjustment skills, list an appropriate regression and progression for each of the following exercises. (These exercises can be found in chapter 19, Self-Myofascial Release Exercises.)

Name of exercise	Possible regression	Possible progression
Foam Roller Gluteal Complex		
Tennis Ball Around Shoulder Blade		
Foam Roller Thoracic Spine		
Foam Roller IT Band		
Golf Ball Roll		
Calf Massage		

CHAPTER 16

Stretching

In this chapter you will learn how to progress a client's corrective exercise program from self-myofascial release by introducing stretching exercises. You will learn about various types of stretches and how they can be used to retrain, rehabilitate, and increase range of motion in those structures that have been hindered by musculoskeletal imbalances. You will also learn teaching and cueing tips to help you communicate these strategies to clients, and you will learn procedures for progressing and regressing these techniques as required.

WHAT IS STRETCHING?

Skeletal structures that have been chronically out of alignment can cause joints to become irritated and inflamed. In response to this inflammation, muscles and other soft tissue structures may tighten up or stiffen around a joint to prevent movement and to protect it from further injury or pain. Over time, these chronically tight muscles lose their ability to contract, stretch, and relax, which not only prevents movement locally, but also restricts motion in surrounding areas (Clark and Lucett 2011; Kovacs 2015). These chronically irritated or tight muscles limit function and can cause additional musculoskeletal imbalances as the body compensates for lack of movement. Chronically irritated muscles may also develop restrictions, nodules, or scar tissue that can cause additional pain (Rolf 1989).

Stretching is the process of elongating and lengthening muscle fibers (and their accompanying tendons and fascia) in order to restore blood flow, recondition or retrain deconditioned or injured tissues, and promote soft tissue elasticity (Karageanes 2005). The regular application of stretching can help break the cycle of protection created by irritated muscles by retraining them to contract, lengthen, and relax effectively. Stretching is also an ideal way to safely introduce range of movement to the body and to restore areas that have been adversely affected by musculoskeletal imbalances (Kovacs 2015).

Stretching involves moving parts of the body in directions that mimic the way those areas should move when they are working correctly. When performed properly, stretches not only improve the health and condition of the body, but they also reeducate the nervous system about the right way to move (Clark and Lucett 2011). In this regard, stretching (when combined with a program of self-myofascial release) helps set the stage for progressing the musculoskeletal, myofascial, and neuromuscular systems into the strengthening phase of a corrective exercise program (Price and Bratcher 2010).

ORIGINS OF STRETCHING

The use of stretching to increase range of motion, improve health, and alleviate pain has been around for centuries. The ancient Chinese are thought to have been the first civilization to have developed and used a regular program of exercise comprised mainly of stretching (known as kung fu) (Calvert 2002). The benefits of stretching were also touted throughout ancient India through the practices of yoga.

Today stretching is a standard practice used to improve athletic performance, increase range of motion, help the body recover and regenerate following an injury, prepare the body for exercise, help the body recuperate after strenuous activity, prevent injury, and decrease pain (Hyde 2002).

number of torso rotations while stabilizing the pelvis over the standing leg. This modification would result in an exercise that would stretch the hamstrings while strengthening the stabilizing muscles of the buttocks, hips, standing leg, and obliques (muscles that rotate the torso).

TEACHING TIPS FOR STRETCHING EXERCISES

It is important to thoroughly understand muscles and their functions so that you can identify which soft tissue structures you are stretching and what movements those muscles achieve. This will help you to teach clients how to perform the stretch correctly, where they should feel the stretch, and how to regress, progress, or adjust a stretch to make it more appropriate or effective.

When teaching stretching techniques, consider the following to ensure the successful implementation of these types of exercises into a client's program:

1. Some clients may believe that stretches must be held for long periods to be effective. However, that is not necessarily the case. Research shows that holding a stretch for more than 60 seconds generally produces no greater range of motion than holding a stretch for 30 to 60 seconds (Bandy, Irion, and Briggler 1997; Taylor et al. 2011). Additionally, injuries, adhesions, scars, tears, and muscle fatigue can affect a person's ability to perform or hold a stretch. Therefore, while general guidelines are provided in chapter 20 for each exercise, the physical capabilities of each client will ultimately determine how long and how often a stretch should be performed.

2. Always tell clients where they should feel a stretching sensation as they perform a stretching exercise. Knowing where they should feel a stretch serves several purposes. It enables clients to monitor their own stretching programs, reduces the potential for injury or harm when they are performing stretches on their own, increases their intrinsic motivation, and helps them to progress their stretching programs more quickly (Price and Bratcher 2010). For example, when stretching the piriformis muscle (see Piriformis Stretch in chapter 20), a client should feel the stretch across the back of the buttocks from the base of the spine to the outside of the hip (because the piriformis muscle originates at the sacrum, travels across the back of the hip, and attaches to the outside of the top of the upper leg) (Gray 1995).

However, if while doing this stretch the client experiences a weird sensation in his groin area (which is a common problem if this stretch is performed incorrectly), you would need to review his technique and adjust it accordingly. If you cannot adjust his form to target the piriformis muscle correctly, instruct the client to regress to a self-myofascial release exercise for that specific area. After the appropriate muscles have been massaged, when you return to the Piriformis Stretch, you will find that the area has released, and the client can now perform the stretch correctly, feeling it in the right area of his body. Communicating with clients about where they feel the stretch provides you with vital information about their progress, encourages greater client participation and feedback, improves their technique, and ensures program success.

3. As with any exercise recommendation, it is important to give clients a detailed rationale for *why* you are including specific stretching exercises in their programs. The sound reasoning behind your recommendations, linked to clients' assessment results, will increase their motivation to perform the exercises. Highlight how a given exercise will improve certain deviations and imbalances, or describe how performing a particular stretching exercise will release the muscles or tissues enough to enable them to progress to more challenging stretches or strengthening exercises. These communication strategies help involve clients in the exercise design process and motivate them to participate fully in their programs (Bandura 1986; Mason 2004).

4. Recommending appropriate and effective stretching exercises prepares clients for progression to the advanced challenges posed by strengthening exercises. The use of carefully selected stretching exercises also gives you an opportunity to build clients' confidence in moving and coordinating their bodies. This will help them feel optimistic about trying some of the more complex movements required in the strengthening portion of their programs.

WHEN TO REGRESS STRETCHES

It is important for clients to be successful at performing the stretching exercises you recommend, both when under your supervision and when completing them on their own. Therefore, you should know when it is appropriate to regress these types of exercises.

1. Always regress a stretching exercise if a client experiences pain or discomfort. If a muscle or group of tissues is not yet ready to be stretched, or has not been prepared adequately in advance, the joint associated with the muscles you are trying to stretch may experience strain or stress during the exercise. If a client indicates that a certain joint or area hurts when she performs the stretch, then either regress to a more subtle stretch or regress further to a self-myofascial release technique. Never persist with any stretch if a client indicates that it is painful (Clark and Lucett 2011).

2. Regress a stretching exercise if a client has difficulty performing the exercise correctly or remaining in control of the movement. For example, a client may struggle to remember all the key points of an exercise if there are too many components to it, or he may not be able to perform the movement properly. If this is the case, regress the stretch until the client can perform the movement completely and correctly.

3. Many standing or kneeling stretches require clients to stabilize their bodies during the exercise. However, if clients have trouble balancing during a stretch, regress the movement so they can maintain balance and concentrate on the key points of the exercise itself.

4. Regress a stretching exercise if a client indicates that the equipment needs for the exercise are not practical. A stretch that requires the use of a specialized piece of equipment (like a specific stretching band or strap), for example, may affect the client's ability to perform that exercise regularly at home if she does not have that piece of equipment.

WAYS TO REGRESS STRETCHES

There are many ways to regress a stretching exercise:

1. Allow clients to use a balance aid to assist with the movement (see figure 16.4).

2. Instruct a client to perform the exercise while sitting or lying down. For example, the Hamstring Stretch can be performed while lying down (see figure 16.5), and the Lower Back Stretch (both of these are described in chapter 20) can be regressed by coaching the client to lie on her back and hug her knees to her chest.

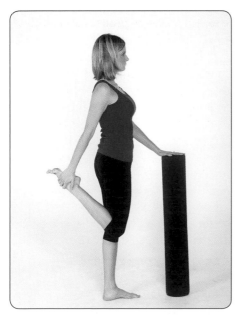

Figure 16.4 A foam roller provides assistance for the Quadriceps Stretch.

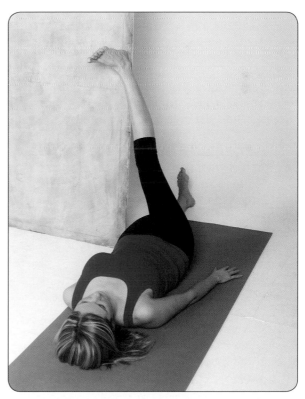

Figure 16.5 Performing a stretch while lying down is a way to regress it.

3. Regress a stretching exercise by revisiting a self-myofascial release exercise that will prepare the client to perform a stretching exercise more precisely. For example, if a client has pain in the front of the ankle or around the Achilles tendon during the Calf Stretch, regress to the Calf Massage (see figure 16.6). Then when you return to the Calf Stretch, the calf muscles will be better able to lengthen and will not place excessive stress on the ankle or on the Achilles tendon.

There are many different possibilities for regressing stretching exercises. Additional ideas and suggestions for regressions can be found in chapter 20, Stretching Exercises.

WHEN TO PROGRESS STRETCHES

Clients will want to make quick progress so they can move on to the strengthening portion of their programs. Knowing when and how to progress their stretching programs will help them to do this as soon as possible.

1. When clients have demonstrated that they can perform a stretch correctly (and regularly integrate that stretch into their daily routines) but are no longer seeing a benefit, progress to a more complex or dynamic stretch that integrates other parts of the body (Walker 2011).

2. Progress to a dynamic stretch that incorporates several areas of the body targeted with passive or active stretches as soon as a client has mastered those stretches, especially if the client says that the stretching program has become too time consuming (Price and Bratcher 2010).

3. If the desired range of motion and technique for a stretching exercise have been achieved, progress the exercise by introducing a strengthening component for the muscle or soft tissue structures being targeted.

4. When a client has demonstrated mastery of an exercise and is no longer experiencing progress, it is time to move on in the corrective exercise program.

WAYS TO PROGRESS STRETCHES

There are many ways to progress a stretching exercise:

1. Progress a stretch by telling the client to activate the opposite muscle (the antagonist) to the one being stretched (refer to the information on Active Stretching earlier in this chapter). For example, when a client is stretching her hamstrings, coach her to actively contract her quadriceps to produce a greater stretch in her hamstrings (Muscolino 2009).

2. Coach a client to move from a seated or kneeling stretch to a standing version of the same stretch. For example, progressing the seated Lower Back Stretch (see chapter 20) to a standing version (see figure 16.7) not only stretches

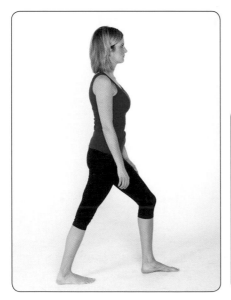
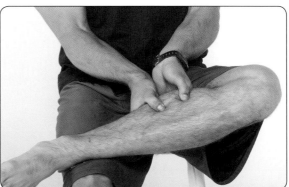

Figure 16.6 Regressing to a self-myofascial release technique from a stretching exercise.

the muscles and soft tissue structures of the lower back but integrates the hamstrings as well (Myers 2008).

3. Progress a stretch by removing a balance aid. For example, if a client places his hand on a foam roller for balance when performing the Quadriceps Stretch, remove the foam roller so he begins to strengthen the muscles of the leg that he is balancing on. However, you should never remove a balance aid if your client needs it to perform the exercise correctly or if the client does not feel confident performing the exercise without it.

4. Integrate additional areas of the body into a stretching exercise (refer to the information on Dynamic Stretching earlier in this chapter). For example, if a client has reached a suitable level of proficiency with the Calf Stretch, Hip Flexor Stretch, and Door Frame Stretch (see chapter 20), progress to a dynamic movement such as a Step Back with Arm Raise (see figure 16.8), which stretches the calf, hip flexors, and muscles of the trunk and torso to address the function of the entire lumbo-pelvic hip girdle (McGill 2002).

There are many different possibilities for progressing stretching exercises. Additional ideas and suggestions can be found in chapter 20, Stretching Exercises.

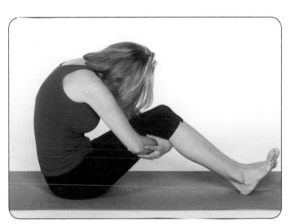
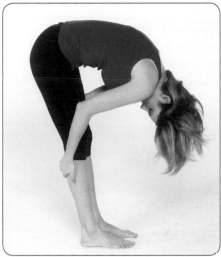

Figure 16.7   Moving from a seated to a standing stretch is a progression.

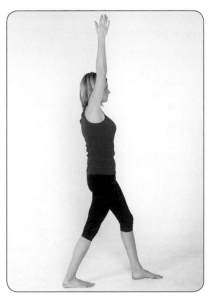

Figure 16.8   Progress to dynamic stretches that integrate several body parts as soon as a client is ready.

WHEN NOT TO USE STRETCHING EXERCISES

Stretching exercises are an incredibly beneficial and generally safe method for introducing movement to a client's program. However, following are some specific contraindications for the application of stretching exercises in a corrective exercise setting (Clark and Lucett 2011; Karageanes 2005; Kisner and Colby 2012; Price and Bratcher 2010).

- Discontinue stretching if a client complains of sharp pain in or around the target area.

- Do not stretch the soft tissue or muscles around a fracture site or broken bone that is still healing.

- Do not use stretching exercises around joints that are hypermobile or have sustained trauma (e.g., a dislocated shoulder, a labral tear).

- Do not stretch muscles or soft tissues that have recently sustained an acute injury like a tear or where bruising is present.

- Do not use stretching exercises around a joint that is acutely inflamed.

- Use stretching cautiously with clients who have rheumatoid arthritis or osteoporosis.

- Use stretching cautiously with clients who have a history of anticoagulant drug use.

- Use stretching cautiously with clients who currently use or have a history of steroid use.

- Do not recommend or use vigorous stretching exercises immediately following an injury or surgery.

- Obtain clearance from a physician before stretching clients with paralysis or chronic neuromuscular diseases.

ADDITIONAL CONSIDERATIONS

Here are a few more safety and conditioning tips to be aware of as you incorporate stretching exercises into clients' corrective exercise programs:

1. Stretching is used to facilitate the gradual lengthening of tissues, increase range of motion, and encourage the repositioning of the joints surrounded by those tissues being stretched. It is important to use gentle stretches. Ballistic stretching that involves bouncing or pulsing into a stretch may cause further injury to clients with chronic or extreme musculoskeletal issues (Walker 2011).

2. Muscles and tissues in areas of the body that are tight or restricted may not be willing (or able) to lengthen and stretch. These restricted muscles or soft tissue structures may need to be tight in order to protect an injured or dysfunctional part (Micheli 2011). If you persist with trying to stretch chronically restricted muscles or tissues, or if you try to mobilize a joint that is inflamed or injured, the muscles surrounding that area may tighten even further to protect the parts from moving, possibly risking further injury. You must understand the protective mechanisms of muscles and soft tissue structures, and this applies to all clients with chronic malalignment issues. When you recommend stretching exercises to a client with longstanding musculoskeletal issues, it is crucial to introduce stretching and movement *gradually*. This will reduce the risk that some areas will tighten up even further.

3. Passive stretches can bolster client confidence because they are relatively easy to perform, and they present a low injury risk. While this may seem ideal, this increased confidence can sometimes prompt clients to overdo passive stretches. Overstretching can damage muscle tissue and lead to excessive muscle soreness the following day, so teach clients not to overdo their passive stretching program, no matter how good they feel when performing the stretches (Alter 1998).

4. It is very important to thoroughly warm up the muscles and tissues to be stretched before instructing clients to begin their stretching programs (Bryant and Green 2010). The use of self-myofascial release techniques can help increase the core temperature of tissues prior to stretching. You can also suggest to clients that they take a warm bath or shower to help them warm up adequately before engaging in their stretching programs at home.

5. The body's soft tissues contain a lot of water, and their function and performance depend

on adequate hydration. Clients must be well hydrated before beginning any portion of their corrective exercise program, and they must remain hydrated during and after exercise (Hoffman 2014). Clients who are dehydrated (e.g., from drinking too much alcohol the night before or from having been in the heat for too long before exercising) may need to delay their exercise until they can adequately rehydrate.

Review of Key Points

Stretching exercises should be introduced into a client's program after the successful application of self-myofascial release techniques. Stretching exercises are designed to safely introduce range of motion to dysfunctional or previously injured parts of a client's body.

- Three types of stretches are described in this chapter: passive, active, and dynamic. Passive stretches are a safe and controlled way of introducing range of motion at the initial stages of a stretching program. Active stretches are a means of progressing a client's stretching program by integrating the contraction of an opposing muscle group as the target muscle is stretched. Dynamic stretches involve stretching (and coordinating) multiple areas of the body at once, and they represent the ultimate stage of a client's stretching program.

- A sound understanding of functional anatomy will help you to select appropriate stretching exercises and enable you to teach clients where they should feel each stretch.

- There are many documented benefits to integrating stretching exercises into a client's corrective exercise program. However, you should always be cautious. Chronic musculoskeletal dysfunction or imbalances may affect the manner in which your client can safely accept increases in range of motion to areas of their bodies that have been dysfunctional (or in pain) for some time.

- There are many ways to progress and regress the stretching components of a client's corrective exercise program. Pay careful attention to clients as they perform the exercises to make sure they will be able to do them correctly on their own. If you foresee any difficulties with an exercise, regress it or use another exercise.

Self-Check

In this chapter you learned how to progress and regress various stretching exercises. Take a few minutes to consider each stretch listed in column A and identify (in column C) whether the alternative exercise listed in column B is a progression or a regression for that exercise. *Note:* All the exercises identified in column A can be found in Chapter 20, Stretching Exercises.

Column A Stretch	Column B Alternative	Column C Progression or regression?
Calf Stretch (standing)	Standing Calf Stretch with activation of tibialis anterior	
Hamstring Stretch (standing)	Standing Hamstring Stretch with rotation	
Lower Back Stretch (seated)	Standing Lower Back stretch	
Quadriceps Stretch (standing)	Lying Quadriceps Stretch	
Chest Stretch (standing)	Chest Stretch with activation of rhomboids	
Palm on Wall Stretch	Self-massage of forearm muscles	
Why Stretch (seated)	Standing Why Stretch	
Biceps Stretch (standing)	Self-massage on biceps muscles	

CHAPTER 17

Strengthening

In this chapter you will learn how to progress from stretching exercises to introducing various techniques for strengthening muscles and other soft tissue structures that have been adversely affected by musculoskeletal imbalances. You will learn about several different types of strengthening exercises and how they can be used to recondition, retrain, and develop those parts of the body needed to address the underlying causes of a client's musculoskeletal imbalances. You will also learn teaching and cueing tips to help you communicate these strategies to clients as well as procedures for progressing and regressing these techniques.

WHAT IS STRENGTHENING?

Musculoskeletal imbalances have a dramatic effect on both the skeleton and the soft tissue structures. They cause myofascial restrictions that affect joint range of motion or function. Muscle length and tension are also affected, thus influencing the muscles' ability to contract, lengthen, and relax appropriately. As various muscles and other soft tissue structures lose their ability to function correctly, other musculoskeletal structures in the body take over for these dysfunctional areas, leading to further compensations and additional imbalances (Fritz 2013; Houglum 2016).

The appropriate and progressive application of self-myofascial release techniques and stretching exercises into a client's program helps to restore muscle function and range of motion. Once the soft tissue structures are reasonably healthy and pliable again, you can begin to introduce loads and resistance through the use of strengthening exercises

(Clark and Lucett 2011). Strengthening is the process of activating, coordinating, and continuing to reinforce correct motor and movement patterns by challenging the musculoskeletal and neuromuscular systems under load or tension (Clark and Lucett 2011; Price and Bratcher 2010). Strengthening exercises facilitate changes to these systems, resulting in physiological adaptations such as improvements in neural firing and increases in muscle size, endurance, power, and strength (Clark and Lucett 2011).

When performed correctly and consistently, resistance exercises help strengthen muscles to support the correct alignment and movement of the skeleton and to improve neuromuscular coordination. The successful performance of these exercises also increases clients' confidence in their ability to move a previously injured, painful, or dysfunctional body part. Strengthening exercises that address and correct musculoskeletal imbalances rather than exacerbate them will reduce unnecessary stress to other parts of the body. This allows overworked or inflamed areas to rest, recover, and recuperate. The introduction and regular use of corrective strengthening exercises is vital for helping clients to reach both their short- and long-term health and fitness goals (Price and Bratcher 2010).

ORIGINS OF STRENGTHENING EXERCISES

Resistance training programs have been used for over 3,500 years in different parts of the world to better prepare people for a task, such as sports or battle (Kraemer and Häkkinen 2002). The ancient Greeks, in particular, regularly integrated structured weight training into their daily routines to develop healthy, strong, and muscular physiques (Price 2008).

However, the development of precise and specialized exercise modalities to help people recover from injuries and to address musculoskeletal imbalances did not begin to develop until after the Industrial Revolution in the late 19th and early 20th centuries (Kraemer and Häkkinen 2002; Price 2008). After World War I, the modern practice of physical therapy was introduced to the medical community as a means of restoring movement and function to injured soldiers, primarily through the application of strengthening exercises (Price 2008).

Since that time, physical therapy has been used to treat incapacitated patients recovering from injuries. However, over the past several decades there has been an epidemic rise in the number of people suffering from common musculoskeletal imbalances that are not caused by an injury. These imbalances are caused by environmental factors, such as prolonged static postures, footwear choices, and sedentary lifestyles (Price and Bratcher 2010). Many people with common musculoskeletal imbalances do not need physical therapy, and so the field of corrective exercise is evolving to fill the gap in care for this population. As a result, the use of musculoskeletal assessments, self-myofascial release, restorative stretching, and corrective strengthening exercises in fitness settings is fast becoming commonplace.

BENEFITS OF STRENGTHENING EXERCISES

There are many documented benefits of strengthening exercises for corrective exercise clients. Specific benefits of corrective strengthening exercises include the following (Clark and Lucett 2011; McGill 2002; Miller 1995; Stone, Stone, and Sands 2007):

- Increases in muscular strength
- Increases in muscular endurance
- Promotion of growth and strength of connective tissue
- Improved joint stability
- Improved joint mobility
- Promotion of growth in joint cartilage

- Increased bone mineral density
- Increased muscular coordination
- Improved motor skill activity
- Improved motor unit and neuromuscular activation

TYPES OF STRENGTHENING EXERCISES

Six kinds of strengthening exercises are highlighted in this chapter:

1. Isometric
2. Concentric
3. Eccentric
4. Single joint
5. Multijoint and kinetic chain
6. Multiplanar and multidimensional coordinated movements

Each type of strengthening exercise offers a unique benefit to clients as they progress through their corrective exercise programs or exercise sessions.

ISOMETRIC

An isometric contraction occurs when a muscle becomes activated by neural input (i.e., movement information through nerves from the brain) but stays the same length during the contraction—that is, it neither shortens nor lengthens (Higgins 2011). This is the easiest type of movement for the nervous system to coordinate. Once the nervous system has generated an isometric muscle contraction, it can usually continue sending a strong signal to the muscles involved to maintain a state of activation. An example of an isometric exercise would be holding the Straight Arm Raise (see figure 17.1) in a static contracted state for an allocated amount of time.

When a muscle cannot activate correctly, or when it has disrupted neural input as a result of chronic musculoskeletal issues, it is important to get that muscle working again before progressing to more challenging types of strengthening exercises. You should never assume that a muscle that is not working correctly in isolation will work as part of a more complex multijoint or kinetic chain motion.

CONCENTRIC AND ECCENTRIC

A concentric muscle action involves shortening a muscle to bring the origin and insertion points of that muscle closer together, and it results in the movement of bones at a joint (see figure 17.2) (Fishman, Ballantyne, and Rathmell 2009). Concentric muscle contractions are usually easy for clients to see and feel because the muscle they are contracting will usually appear (or feel to the touch) larger as it contracts and shortens. An eccentric muscle action, on the other hand, involves the lengthening of a muscle and serves to slow down parts of the body as they move (Fishman, Ballantyne, and Rathmell 2009). For example, lowering a heavy weight from shoulder to waist height involves an eccentric muscle action of the biceps to counterbalance the weight of the dumbbell and the force of gravity as the elbow straightens.

Concentric strengthening exercises can involve a single joint (see Single Joint section that follows) or multiple joints (see Multijoint section later in this chapter). Concentric strengthening exercises are generally safer for clients to perform than eccentric exercises because a concentric action typically initiates movement at a joint. An eccentric action, on the other hand, involves slowing down forces on a joint. Clients who cannot perform an eccentric movement correctly may experience more stress on a joint or pain if they cannot perform it correctly. Therefore, strengthening exercises that involve concentric muscle actions are usually better initial choices to start the strengthening phase of a corrective exercise program. Bearing this in mind, always look to progress clients safely into incorporating eccentric movements that train their musculoskeletal system how to slow down movement and minimize stress to their body.

SINGLE JOINT

Single-joint strengthening exercises strengthen the muscles that move one joint at a time (Ackland, Elliott, and Bloomfield 2009). There is usually less risk for injury when you introduce single-joint strengthening exercises into a client's corrective exercise program because movement is controlled and is restricted to only one bony juncture. However, single-joint strengthening exercises should only be used once you are confident that a client is proficient at activating and controlling the muscle or group of muscles that must move the target joint. For example,

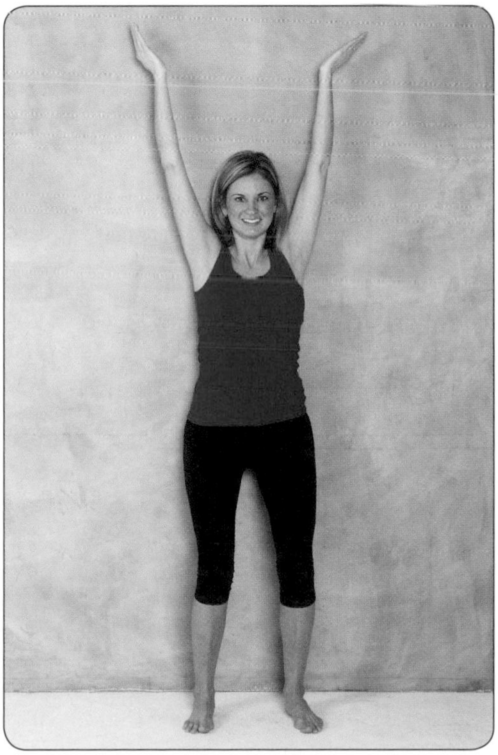

Figure 17.1 An isometric strengthening exercise.

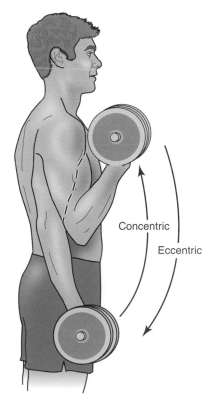

Figure 17.2 Example of a concentric contraction producing movement and an eccentric contraction decelerating movement.

a client must be able to activate her quadriceps muscles concentrically in order to extend the knee and eccentrically to slow down knee flexion. Isometric strengthening exercises (see Isometric section earlier in this chapter) can be used to evaluate the quality or strength of contraction for a muscle or group of muscles before you introduce either concentric or eccentric single-joint strengthening exercises.

If you recommend an exercise to a client and later find that a muscle or muscle group is not activating correctly, you may need to increase or decrease the input to those muscles by providing concentric or eccentric loading to stimulate the muscle to respond. For example, if you notice a client's abductors (e.g., gluteus medius and gluteus minimus) are not contracting—or she does not feel them contracting—when she performs a single-joint exercise like the Side Lying Leg Lift, you can help to activate those muscles by using your hand to place a gentle load on the movement. (Pushing down on the knee as she lowers the leg emphasizes the eccentric phase.) See figure 17.3. This extra pressure will help increase the neuromuscular demand on the muscles, stimulating them to activate in response (Reider, Provencher, and Davies 2015).

Adding a load in a controlled manner is a safe way to manipulate this particular exercise because the client is at little risk for injury when she moves a single joint while lying on the ground. However, when adding a load to any exercise, do not apply more pressure than a client can reasonably control. Otherwise, she will have to recruit other parts of her body to help with the movement if the force is too great (that is, she will have to "cheat").

Single-joint strengthening exercises are also recommended at the outset of a client strengthening program because they do not overload the nervous system with too much information, and they can be coordinated easily (Ackland, Elliott, and Bloomfield 2009). Clients can rapidly become proficient at single-joint strengthening exercises, thereby increasing their confidence in moving a previously painful or injured part.

MULTIJOINT

Multijoint strengthening exercises involve the movement of more than one joint (Ackland, Elliott, and Bloomfield 2009). Multijoint movements are designed to target one muscle that moves multiple joints, but they usually also involve the strengthening and integration of ancillary muscles that affect the joints being targeted. For example, the Gluteal Activation Over Ball exercise (see figure 17.4) is a multijoint exercise specifically designed to strengthen the gluteus maximus muscle. However, it also strengthens the hamstrings and quadriceps muscles isometrically because they are involved in stabilizing the knee and keeping the leg straight during this exercise. Multijoint exercises should be added to a client's program only when you are confident that the client has gained control over the muscle or muscle group involved in the movement.

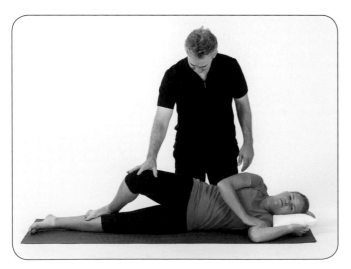

Figure 17.3 Example of a single-joint exercise with external load.

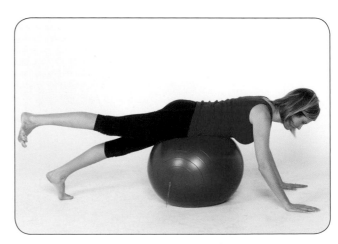

Figure 17.4 Example of a multijoint exercise.

KINETIC CHAIN

Kinetic chain exercises are comprised of a sequential series of motions or actions that rely on each other to produce a desired movement. This type of exercise is designed to teach a client how to use a number of muscles (or muscle groups) to create a chain of motion involving several areas of the body. Kinetic chain exercises are only appropriate for use when a client can control the muscles involved in the sequence both concentrically and eccentrically, and all of the joints those muscles cross. Kinetic chain movements can be open (i.e., the end of the "chain"—the hands or feet—can move freely) or closed (the end of the "chain"—the hands or feet—is restrained or fixed) (Ellenbecker and Davies 2001). For example, the Wave Goodbye (see figure 17.5a) is an open kinetic chain exercise because it involves coordination of the muscles that depress the scapula and bend the elbows while the rotator cuff muscles externally rotate the arms, which are not fixed (or closed) in any way.

On the other hand, The Pivot exercise (see figure 17.5b) is designed to strengthen many muscles that cross all of the joints in the lower body. However, one end of the chain (the foot) is in contact with the ground during the exercise. Therefore, this is considered a closed kinetic chain strengthening exercise.

Closed kinetic chain strengthening exercises typically require more neuromuscular coordination than open kinetic chain movements due to the increased demand of forces being exerted at the ends of the chain. Consequently, closed-chain exercises are potentially more stressful to the muscles and joints being targeted because any imbalances or restrictions can cause compensatory movements elsewhere (Ellenbecker and Davies 2001). Therefore, open-chain exercises should be introduced first when using kinetic chain exercises to reduce the likelihood of injury as you teach clients to coordinate multiple joints and multiple muscles working together as an integrated unit.

MULTIPLANAR AND MULTIDIMENSIONAL COORDINATED MOVEMENTS

Multiplanar exercises are those that move the body up and down, and in different directions, such as forward and backward, side-to-side, and in rotation (see figure 17.6). When groups of muscles work efficiently as part of a kinetic chain, you can progress to using whole-body, dynamic exercises that incorporate multiple planes and dimensions to ensure coordinated function of the entire body (Houglum 2016). Multidimensional exercises apply more scope to kinetic chain and multiplanar

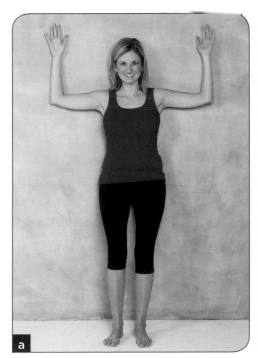
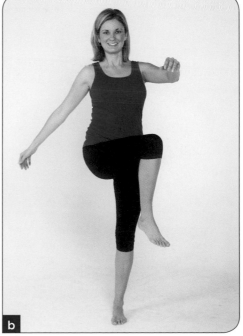

Figure 17.5 *(a)* Example of an open kinetic chain exercise and *(b)* a closed kinetic chain exercise.

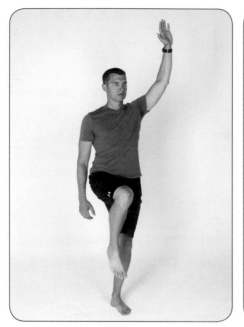
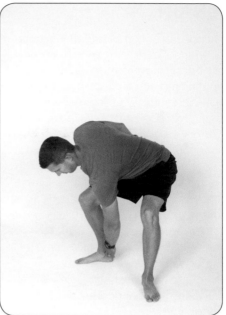

Figure 17.6 Example of a multiplanar exercise.

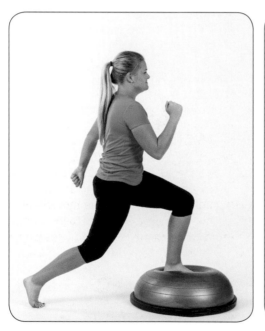
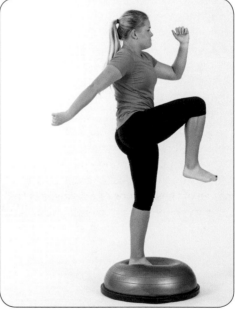

Figure 17.7 Example of a multidimensional exercise.

exercises by moving the body against resistance or on an unstable surface like a BOSU Balance Trainer, for example (see figure 17.7) (Shumway-Cook and Woollocott 2007).

Multidimensional and multiplanar exercises are designed to mimic real-life activities. They can be used to prepare a client for the performance of activities such as running or engaging in sports. Before introducing multiplanar and multidimensional strengthening exercises to a client's corrective exer-

cise program, however, you must evaluate whether she can correctly perform all of the movements required to execute the multifaceted movement you are proposing. Once you are confident she has the necessary skills, progress to using a multidimensional and multiplanar exercise that fosters improvement in those movements she needs to perform her chosen activity or sport. For example, if a client is an avid, right-handed tennis player, you can progress the Lunge With Knee Pull exercise (see figure 17.8)

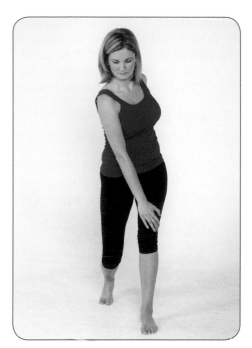

Figure 17.8 Lunge With Knee Pull can be progressed to mimic sporting moves.

when she is ready by coaching her to hold a medicine ball or tennis racket as she lunges forward onto her left leg. This will mimic setting up to hit a backhand in tennis.

You can progress any multiplanar and multidimensional kinetic chain exercise by adding external load, a variety of arm and leg movements, torso rotations, or multidirectional upper body movements to mimic real-life movements. The correct and efficient performance of these types of exercises is the ultimate goal for your corrective exercise program clients. When they have reached this level, they should be free from pain, highly functional, and able to perform coordinated, dynamic movements.

TEACHING TIPS FOR STRENGTHENING EXERCISES

There are a number of cueing, conditioning, and communication techniques to help you to implement strengthening exercises in clients' programs:

1. Clients will rarely perform strengthening exercises perfectly on their first try. Allowing clients to make mistakes as they try new movements and exercises gives them a wonderful learning opportunity that will help them to be more proficient in the long run. As they attempt an exercise, clients will begin to learn how to coordinate previously dysfunctional or injured parts, and their brains and neuromuscular systems will become stronger as they learn to correct mistakes and make improvements (Coyle 2009). It is very important, however, to watch them closely and offer detailed feedback when they try any type of new exercise in order to minimize mistakes that could result in pain or injury or exacerbate existing problems.

2. Strengthening exercises that are used to retrain the neuromuscular system use different variables than strengthening exercises that are used only to build muscle mass (Hoffman 2014). While general guidelines are provided in chapter 21, the variables of any corrective strengthening exercise—such as number of sets, repetitions, and frequency—should be tailored for clients' individual needs and abilities. When you establish these variables, bear in mind that the correct execution of the exercise is more important than achieving a specific number of sets or reps (Price and Bratcher 2010). As a client's abilities improve, the variables for each exercise should be adjusted accordingly.

3. As your teaching relationship with your clients builds, try to familiarize yourself with their learning styles. For example, you might find that one client learns more effectively by watching you demonstrate an exercise first, while another may need you to explain the exercise in words so he can process the information before attempting the movement. Yet another client may want to try to perform the exercise right away to get a feeling for what it is like. As you come to understand the learning styles of individual clients, you can teach subsequent exercises much more easily by using cues that match the way they learn (Wrisberg 2007). More information on learning styles can be found in chapter 23.

4. As clients progress into the strengthening phase of their corrective exercise programs, you can strengthen their motivation by reminding them of movements they are now doing that used to be difficult or impossible (Wrisberg 2007). For example, a client might have initially come to see you because she could not raise her arms very high without experiencing shoulder pain. However, as she performs strengthening exercises such as the Straight Arm Raise, you can remind her that she can now lift her arms

without pain. This will not only show her how far she has progressed, but it will also give her a reason to continue to perform these exercises at home.

5. As clients are introduced to various strengthening exercises, it is also important to link the reason why they are performing a particular exercise to the initial musculoskeletal imbalances you identified during the assessment process (Price and Bratcher 2010). For example, if you are at the stage of a program where you are teaching a client how to do a Pelvic Tilt, remind him that his assessment results revealed that he had an anterior pelvic tilt and that this exercise will help address this imbalance (with the goal of alleviating his back pain). Call attention to the fact that the muscles of his lumbar spine are now flexible enough to allow his lower back to round, permitting him to perform the Pelvic Tilt exercise correctly. This indicates that his lumbo-pelvic hip girdle is becoming more mobile and is releasing its "grip" on the structures of his lower back. Describing exercise selection in this way can help your clients to become more mindful of their habitual movement patterns and postures and give them a reason to adhere to their corrective exercise programs.

6. It is also helpful to link specific strengthening exercises you are recommending to those self-myofascial release and stretching exercises that helped prepare the client for such a progression. For example, if a client has progressed to the Butt Lift strengthening exercise (see chapter 21), point out how he can do this exercise correctly now because he first rejuvenated and regenerated the gluteal muscles with the Foam Roller Gluteal Complex exercise and then stretched the area with the Glute Stretch and Lower Back Stretch. Consequently, his lower back has released, and the glutes are now working effectively to lift the hips as they perform this strengthening exercise. This teaching technique not only helps your clients to see how they have progressed, but it also provides solutions (i.e., suitable regressions) for them if they are having trouble performing a strengthening exercise on their own.

WHEN TO REGRESS STRENGTHENING EXERCISES

It is important that clients be able to successfully perform the strengthening exercises you recommend, both under your supervision and when doing them on their own. Therefore, you will need to know when it is appropriate to regress any strengthening exercise.

1. If you are teaching an exercise and the client experiences pain of any kind, regress that exercise to one that she can perform without pain (Price and Bratcher 2010). For example, if you are trying to teach your client The Pivot exercise and she has knee pain, regress to an appropriate exercise such as the Duck Stand to help activate the gluteal muscles (see figure 17.9) or

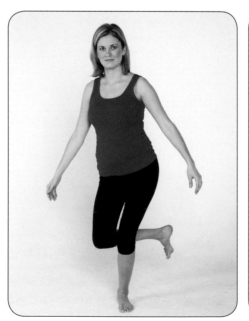
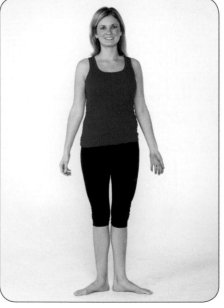

Figure 17.9 Regression of a strengthening exercise.

a self-myofascial release exercise, if necessary, such as Foam Roller on the Gluteal Complex or Foam Roller IT Band (see chapter 20) to loosen the structures that affect the knee first.

2. Regress a strengthening exercise if a client has difficulty performing or coordinating the movement correctly. You must watch your clients' body language when they perform any kind of strengthening exercise. If their breathing rate increases unnecessarily, or they bite their lips, stick out their tongue over their top lip, look uncomfortable, or exhibit other nonverbal signals of anxiety and discomfort, it could mean that they are overloaded with too much information. If you see indications of neuromuscular overload and confusion, it is wiser to regress than to have a client persist with the exercise (Chaitow and Delany 2005).

3. Regress a strengthening exercise if a client reports excessive soreness the next day or later the same day. Corrective exercises are designed to slowly retrain the way the body moves by gradually retraining the neuromuscular and musculoskeletal systems (Bryant and Green 2010). They are not designed to overtax the muscles, nervous system, joints, or connective tissues. If there is excessive muscle soreness or joint pain in one area after an exercise session, it can create additional musculoskeletal imbalances as they try to avoid the soreness in subsequent sessions.

WAYS TO REGRESS STRENGTHENING EXERCISES

There are many ways you can regress a strengthening exercise:

1. If clients have trouble maintaining balance when performing an exercise, have them use a balance aid (McGill 2002). For example, clients can tap their other foot on the ground for balance when performing The Pivot exercise (see figure 17.10), or they can perform the exercise beside a wall or chair in case they need something to grab onto during the exercise to feel more secure.

2. You can regress a strengthening exercise by having the client perform the exercise lying down (McGill 2002). The Straight Arm Raise (see figure 17.11) is an exercise that can be very easily regressed in this manner.

3. A strengthening exercise can also be regressed by revisiting or repeating a self-myofascial exercise or stretch that will help the client return to the strengthening exercise more adequately prepared (Price and Bratcher 2010).

There are many other possibilities for regressing strengthening exercises. Additional ideas and suggestions for regressions can be found in chapter 21, Strengthening Exercises.

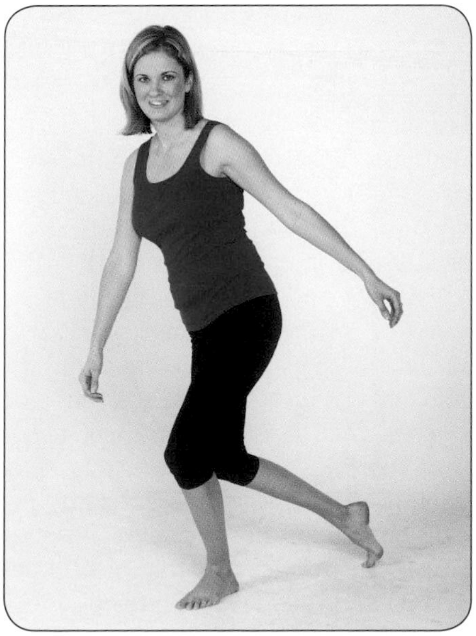

Figure 17.10 Adding a balance aid is a way to regress an exercise.

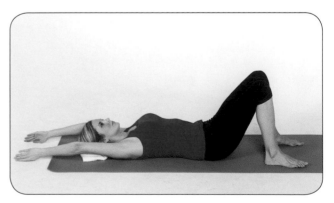

Figure 17.11 Lying down is a way to regress an exercise.

WHEN TO PROGRESS STRENGTHENING EXERCISES

Clients will enjoy progressing through the various stages of their strengthening programs as they improve their functional capabilities and experience less pain as they move. It is important to advance each exercise as soon as they become proficient with that movement or phase of the program.

1. Progress a strengthening exercise when a client has achieved a suitable level of competency and can perform the movement satisfactorily. If you find that clients can successfully do the desired number of repetitions with the correct technique, progress the exercise to keep challenging their musculoskeletal and neuromuscular systems.

2. Progress a strengthening exercise if a client has reached an acceptable level of proficiency and indicates that her program is taking too much time. For example, if when you are reviewing homework with a client, you learn that she regularly cannot complete the exercises because they take too long, progress her program (Price and Bratcher 2010). If the client has demonstrated proficiency at both the Gluteal Activation Over Ball exercise (which targets the gluteus maximus) and the Side Lying Leg Lift exercise (which targets the gluteus medius and minimus), replace both exercises with The Pivot (see chapter 21), which targets these muscles simultaneously as part of one kinetic chain movement.

3. As clients advance with their programs, they often quickly achieve many of their initial pain reduction goals (e.g., standing, sitting, and walking without pain). As a result, they will begin to feel more confident in their physical abilities and may indicate that they would also like to be able to play golf or tennis or engage in some other sport. If a client is physically and mentally ready to prepare to participate in an activity, progress his strengthening exercises so they start mimicking the movements required for the desired activity (Shumway-Cook and Woollocott 2007). For example, if a client says that she wants to resume playing tennis, you could combine Side Lunge With Rotation (see figure 17.12a) and the movement of the right arm in The Flasher exercise (see figure 17.12b) to create a full-body kinetic chain exercise that mimics the action of preparing to hit a forehand volley (assuming the client is right-handed) (see figure 17.12c).

WAYS TO PROGRESS STRENGTHENING EXERCISES

There are many ways you can progress a strengthening exercise:

1. You can progress any strengthening exercise by moving from one type of exercise to a more challenging movement. For example, progressions can be made from an isometric single-joint exercise to a concentric or eccentric multi-

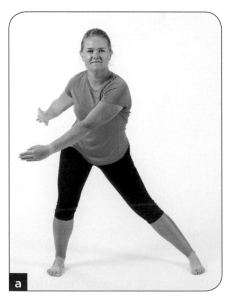
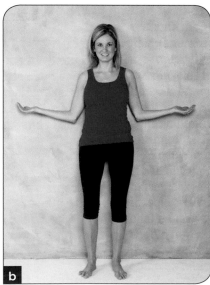
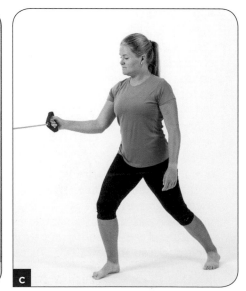

Figure 17.12 Progressing strengthening program by combining exercises to mimic athletic movements.

joint movement. Similarly, you can progress a strengthening exercise from a multijoint exercise to a kinetic chain or multiplanar and multidimensional exercise.

2. A strengthening exercise can be progressed by adding external load to the exercise (Clark and Lucett 2011). An example of this would be coaching a client to hold light weights when performing Back Step With Arm Raise (see figure 17.13) so that the muscles of the lumbo-pelvic hip girdle, trunk, and shoulder girdle all have to work harder to both accelerate and decelerate the extra weight.

3. Using fewer props, supports, or tactile feedback is another effective way to progress any strengthening exercise (Starkey and Johnson 2006). For example, once a client can maintain the correct spine position for the Straight Arm Raise against the wall, tell her to step away from the wall and perform the exercise (see figure 17.14). Without the wall to help guide her posture and movement, it will be necessary for her to tune into her body more to do the exercise correctly.

4. The ultimate goal of a strengthening exercise is to perform the movement at the speed at which it would happen in real life (Price and Sharpe 2009). Therefore, as clients improve their technique in executing a particular exercise, have them perform the movement more rapidly. For example, the Back Step With Arm Raise is similar to the manner in which a person might reach up to catch a ball. Having the client gradually progress the exercise, until they can perform the movement correctly at the same speed it would occur in real life, ensures that their neuromuscular and musculoskeletal systems learn to coordinate the right muscles and movements at speeds that mimic real-life activities.

There are many different possibilities for progressing strengthening exercises. Additional ideas and suggestions for regressions can be found in chapter 21, Strengthening Exercises.

WHEN NOT TO USE STRENGTHENING EXERCISES

When introduced gradually and monitored carefully, strengthening exercises are a safe and effective means for progressing a client's program. However, following are some specific contraindications for

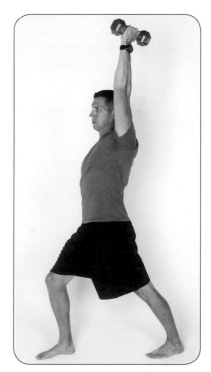

Figure 17.13 Progress a strengthening exercise by adding external load.

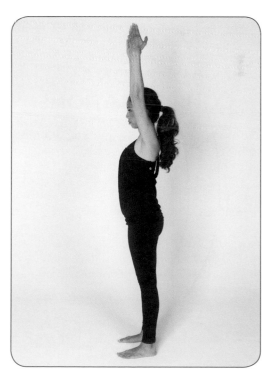

Figure 17.14 Progressing a strengthening exercise by removing tactile feedback, such as a wall.

strengthening exercises in a corrective exercise setting (Clark and Lucett 2011; Houglum 2016; Price and Bratcher 2010; Price and Sharpe 2009).

- Have clients stop a strengthening exercise if they complain of pain or discomfort.

- Do not try strengthening exercises for muscles that surround or cross a fracture site that is still healing.

- Do not try strengthening exercises with special populations such as clients with coronary heart disease, hypertension, or rheumatoid arthritis before clearance has been obtained from a licensed medical professional.

- Do not use strengthening exercises around joints that have sustained trauma (e.g., a dislocated shoulder or labral tear).

- Do not use strengthening exercises that involve muscles or soft tissues that have recently sustained an acute injury like a tear or have visible bruising.

- Do not use strengthening exercises that involve joints that are acutely inflamed.

- Use strengthening exercises cautiously and conservatively in those clients with osteoporosis.

- Obtain clearance from a physician before introducing strengthening exercises to a client's program immediately after an injury or surgery or after clients have been diagnosed with a chronic musculoskeletal or neuromuscular disease.

ADDITIONAL CONSIDERATIONS

Here are a few more safety and conditioning tips to be aware of as you incorporate strengthening exercises into clients' corrective exercise programs:

1. Corrective strengthening exercises are not just designed to build up muscles. Many of these techniques are also designed to retrain the way the body coordinates movement of the neuromuscular and musculoskeletal systems. This reeducation process requires patience and persistence. Allow clients enough time between their sessions with you to enable them to ade-

quately practice and hopefully improve their performance with each exercise. Scheduling strengthening sessions far enough apart will help ensure that clients are ready to progress to the next stage of their programs in subsequent appointments (Price and Bratcher 2010).

2. Do not overestimate either the number of repetitions or the number of sets you recommend. As clients tire during a session, their technique will deteriorate. If you see this happening, discourage them from performing additional repetitions or sets. It is always better to coach clients to do one less repetition or set than to do one extra and risk harm or injury (Bryant and Green 2010).

3. As you advance the strengthening elements of clients' programs, you should progress to incorporating the use of primarily closed kinetic chain movements that place particular focus on the eccentric portion of the movement (especially with exercises designed to strengthen the structures of the lumbo-pelvic hip girdle, knees, feet, and ankles). The ability to decelerate the body as it moves is an essential aspect of corrective exercise training to help strengthen the body to resist gravity and impact and reduce the likelihood of injury (Magee, Zachazewski, and Quillen 2007). However, since eccentric movements can tire the body easily and can potentially put clients at risk of injury, be conservative with the volume of eccentric work you recommend for clients' programs.

4. If a client has continued difficulty in performing a strengthening exercise or movement, it may be because that person's brain or nervous system is simply not ready to let go of an old movement pattern. In these cases, you must regress to either a self-myofascial release or a stretching exercise to help prepare the body to accept the new movement (Price and Bratcher 2010).

More information on strengthening techniques, and detailed information on how to construct the strengthening component of clients' programs, can be found in chapter 21, Strengthening Exercises.

Review of Key Points

Strengthening exercises are the ultimate progression for corrective exercise programming. They strengthen muscles and other soft tissues, retrain the nervous system, and teach the body how to coordinate dynamic, integrated movements to address the underlying causes of musculoskeletal imbalances.

■ Six types of strengthening exercises are described in this chapter: (1) isometric, (2) concentric, (3) eccentric, (4) single joint, (5) multijoint and kinetic chain, and (6) multiplanar and multidimensional coordinated movements.

■ There are many documented benefits of incorporating strengthening exercises into corrective exercise programs. However, it is important to progress carefully through the various types, introducing only those techniques that clients can successfully execute without compromising form or technique or causing discomfort.

■ As you introduce strengthening exercises to a client's corrective exercise program, do not recommend techniques that require a lot of equipment or are not practical for the client to perform at home or while traveling because this can hamper program adherence.

■ It is vital to know how and when to progress or regress the strengthening portion of a corrective exercise program. Incorporating or eliminating additional body parts, introducing or taking away unstable services, getting rid of or adding balance aids, and subtracting or adding weight are ways to control the level of effort (and subsequent success) the client experiences.

Self-Check

Take a few minutes to consider the unique aspects of each type of strengthening exercise you learned about in this chapter. In the lists that follow, you will find the strengthening exercise types listed on the left side of the page. Draw a line from each exercise type to the appropriate sample strengthening exercise (taken from chapter 21) that matches it on the right. There is one exercise match per exercise type.

Concentric single joint	Big Toe Pushdown (pushing toe down portion)
Eccentric single joint	The Wave Goodbye (with position held)
Multidimensional	Side Lying Leg Lift (lowering portion)
Isometric	Extension Crunch (lowering portion)
Kinetic chain	Lunge With Step Up (onto BOSU Balance Trainer)
Eccentric multijoint	Back Step With Arm Raise

CHAPTER 18

Static Postural Considerations

There are many common postures that people assume for extended periods of time each day, including sleeping postures, seated postures, and standing postures. They vary from person to person depending on occupation, lifestyle, and hobbies. However, the cumulative effect of spending time in certain static postural positions can be devastating from a musculoskeletal, movement, and myofascial perspective. Sustained postures have been found to negatively affect soft tissue structures, joint position, and movement, leading to musculoskeletal imbalances and pain (Sahrmann 2002). Nonexercise-based strategies to help clients both address and prevent prolonged postures must be considered in conjunction with a client's corrective exercise program.

The average person spends about six to nine hours per day sleeping (Plotnik, and Kouyoumdjian 2014). If we sleep in positions that stress certain body structures or exacerbate musculoskeletal imbalances, these sleeping postures can eventually cause pain or dysfunction (Sahrmann 2002). When we are awake, we may spend an additional seven to nine hours in a dysfunctional position slumped over a desk, driving a vehicle, or standing over a table, workstation, counter, or patient. The remaining six to ten hours of the day are then typically spent in positions that compound musculoskeletal issues, such as sitting on a couch in front of the television or playing on a computer.

STANDING POSTURES

Although the human body is designed to stand upright, the environments in which we stand today and the postures themselves are much different than our early ancestors experienced (Donatelli and Wooden 2010). With the advent of the Industrial Revolution, work speed became of paramount importance, particularly in the manufacturing, agriculture, and trade industries, and workplace environments were redesigned to enhance productivity. The lasting result of this innovative time in history is that unnecessary movements have been eliminated from most everyday jobs, and superfluous tasks have been eradicated with the goal of increasing production. Standing still for long periods of time, especially in a stressful environment that values speed, increases biomechanical stresses on muscles, tendons, joints, synovial fluid, and nerves (Hillstrom and Hillstrom 2007). Constrained standing environments designed to increase productivity have also helped create musculoskeletal imbalances. For example, an anterior pelvic tilt is a typical compensation pattern for continuously leaning forward over a workstation. Excessive rounding of the spine and shoulders, internally rotated arms, and a forward position of the head are also common postural adaptations that occur when confined in typical modern standing working environments (DeLisa, Gans, and Walsh 2005; Karwowski 2006; Price and Bratcher 2010).

The addition of technology and electronic devices to the modern environment compounds the problem of prolonged standing with poor posture. In today's high-tech society, people spend hours standing with shoulders rounded, heads forward, and arms crossed over their torsos using phones and other handheld devices to browse the Internet or communicate. This recent phenomenon has already reached epidemic proportions, with much research devoted to the problematic postural deviations and pain being caused by such activities (Atkins, Kerr, and Goodlad 2015).

Machines, electronic devices, and workstations are not the only things that have affected our standing postures and resulting musculoskeletal health. The pedestrian surface areas of the world until only 100 to 200 years ago were typically dirt floors, gravel trails, and uneven paths. Historically, this meant that standing and walking upright were always paired with a dynamic and ever-changing environment. This is vastly different from the smooth, concrete indoor surfaces, sidewalks, and roads of today. In the evolutionary scheme of things, smooth surface areas are a very drastic change for the body to have to contend with, both when standing still and when moving around. The musculoskeletal and neuromuscular systems are designed to instinctively interact far more gently with the ground when the foot comes in contact with or treads upon dynamic surfaces (Donatelli and Wooden 2010). This is because the foot must adapt to what it has encountered, and send signals back to the brain to be wary of the unpredictable terrain it might encounter next. Conversely, when interaction with the ground can be predicted consistently because the surface is smooth and flat, the feet (and brain and body) no longer have to anticipate what they will encounter. As a result, contact between the body and the ground becomes much less stimulating and more forceful.

In adapting to these predictable surfaces, the feet lose their ability to adjust to dynamic situations and undulating terrain. More accurately, they adapt so well to being on flat surfaces that they begin to habitually flatten out, or *overpronate*. As a result, the feet and ankles can no longer function optimally on the rare occasions when they must navigate unstable surfaces. You might even have observed this deterioration of foot and ankle function in yourself. For example, have you ever gone on vacation to a place such as the beach, kicked off your shoes, and headed straight for the sand, only to find that later that day or evening your feet and legs were cramping and sore? Or perhaps even your back hurt? This was probably due in part to the fact that your feet no longer can strongly support you on surfaces like sand that require the use of all of the muscles in your toes, feet, legs, hips, and back.

When the feet do not work properly or have pain and musculoskeletal imbalances, it is difficult and uncomfortable for them to support the full weight of the body. Consequently, people develop the habit of shifting their body weight more onto one leg in an effort to distribute their weight differently and alleviate the discomfort. However, propping the weight of the body on only one hip, leg, or foot can cause problematic changes in all the structures of the body as they adjust to keeping the body balanced in this perpetually unstable position. Not surprisingly, the cumulative stress of this fairly recent change in the pedestrian environment is showing up in the form of myriad musculoskeletal imbalances (Karwowski 2006).

TIPS TO HELP WITH STANDING POSTURES

There are many nonexercise-related suggestions that can help clients to alleviate some of the problems that can arise from standing with poor posture for long periods of time.

1. Help clients to become aware of any tendencies they have to chronically shift their weight from side to side or to prop their weight on one hip, leg, or foot when standing. For example, it is quite common for mothers to carry their young children predominantly on one hip. This can create heavily ingrained compensatory shifts in their bodies, especially on the side used to carry the child. These patterns can continue to exist long after their children are grown.

2. Educate clients about their footwear choices, and encourage them to select appropriate shoes. Radical changes in footwear or adding orthotics too quickly, however, will cause additional stress and will likely create other aches and pains due to tissues and structures not having sufficient time to adapt. Therefore, as with any element of an exercise program, remind clients to adopt the suggested footwear changes gradually. For more information on making appropriate footwear recommendations, see Footwear and the Role of Orthotics later in this chapter.

3. Make clients aware of the positions they assume with their hands and arms when they are standing. Prolonged positioning of these extremities can lead to myofascial and musculoskeletal changes and compensatory movement patterns.

For example, crossing the arms or resting the hands in pockets can round the shoulders forward; holding one's smartphone with one hand to text can shift the head, neck, and spine to one side; carrying a bag on one shoulder can tip the body to one side and shift the body's center of gravity; holding a cell phone to one ear while standing can tip the head to one side and cause side shifting. Over time, these habits can result in dysfunction and pain.

4. In cases where clients are forced by their work environment to stand for extended periods, encourage them to adjust their body position continually so that many parts can share the workload of maintaining an upright position. For example, you can suggest that clients switch hands throughout the day when performing repetitive tasks, vary the height of their workstations, raise or lower their computer monitors, take their shoes off or change shoes throughout the day, incorporate hands-free technology with their telephone, carry tools or bags on alternating sides of their bodies, and so on. These subtle changes will provide different stimuli and will ensure that undesirable long-term postural patterns do not become habitual.

5. Coach clients on the principles of standing with correct posture. When they stand upright looking ahead, instruct them to pull their heads back with their chins in (to minimize a forward head position and excessive cervical lordosis), keep the thoracic spine upright and the shoulders pulled back (to minimize excessive thoracic kyphosis and protracted shoulder blades), tuck the pelvis under (to minimize an anterior pelvic tilt and excessive lumbar lordosis), and be aware if they are collapsing their body weight into their feet (to avoid a valgus knee position and overpronation). These subtle adjustments will enable their center of gravity to shift back into the heels, permit the skeletal structures to support their weight more correctly, allow their soft tissue structures to rest, and help promote a better standing posture. For more detailed information on standing posture and a diagrammatic representation of ideal standing posture, see How the Head and Neck Relate to the Rest of the Body in chapter 6.

FOOTWEAR AND THE ROLE OF ORTHOTICS

The wrong footwear can contribute to the development of painful and dysfunctional standing postures.

Shoes with heels, such as pumps, high heels, running shoes, and boots, are designed to be higher in the back than they are in the front, and these types of shoes tip the body's center of mass forward (Greene and Roberts 2017). Hence, when feet are placed into shoes that have a standing surface not parallel to the floor, the entire body has to compensate in order to avoid tipping over forward. People who wear shoes with very high heels may even stand or walk with their knees constantly bent to stop themselves from falling forward. This continual, sustained flexion of the knees can, over time, lead to inflammation and pain and additional musculoskeletal imbalances. An elevated heel can also cause the back of the pelvis to tilt up at the back and down at the front (i.e., an anterior pelvic tilt), resulting in excessive lumbar lordosis and compensatory shifts all the way up the rest of the body to the head (see figure 18.1).

High-heeled shoes (and almost all footwear made for fashion-focused purposes) are also problematic for the musculoskeletal system for a different reason. These types of shoes are typically designed to be narrow toward the front of the shoe, which compresses the toes together. This squeezing together of the toes narrows the width of the foot and decreases the base of support for the entire body. As a result, balance is affected, and the rest of the body must compensate to maintain an upright and stable posture (Greene and Roberts 2017). Educating clients

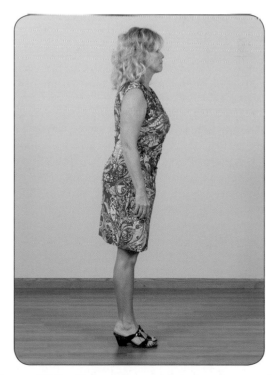

Figure 18.1 Example of high heels causing an anterior pelvic tilt.

about the effect of heeled shoes on the mechanics of the body, and encouraging them to wear more appropriate footwear like neutral-soled or flat-soled shoes with wide toe boxes, is an important supplement to their corrective exercise program.

 Go to the online video to watch video 18.1, where Justin talks about helping clients choose the right footwear.

In some cases, arch supports or orthotics, in addition to alternate footwear choices, may be advisable for clients to address their painful symptoms at the outset of a corrective exercise program. At the beginning of the program, their feet and ankles may benefit from the artificial support. However, as they progress with the corrective exercises, they should be able to phase out the use of artificial supports and begin to rely on their own bodies to support their feet and ankles naturally (Chinn and Hertel 2010; Price 2014). The use of arch supports, supportive footwear, and orthotics is usually only recommended as a long-term solution to specific and diagnosed conditions of the feet and ankles when a licensed medical professional has said that such devices are needed.

SEATED POSTURES

Prolonged seated postures can have a detrimental effect on various soft tissue structures and muscles (Sahrmann 2002). Similar to the changes in our pedestrian environment discussed previously, the everyday activities of humans have changed drastically over the past few hundred years. Daily life for most people in the Western world used to be full of various activities that required coordinated movements using the entire body. However, the standardization and automation of many tasks, coupled with huge technological advances in the past 50 years, has launched humans into a brand-new era where multiplanar and dynamic movements are greatly diminished. Instead of being weight-bearing to accomplish a variety of tasks throughout the day, people are spending more and more time in seated positions. Typical days spent sitting down to eat breakfast, driving to work, sitting at desks looking at computers all day, riding spinning bikes or performing seated exercises at the gym, driving back home, sitting down for dinner, and watching TV (or reading) are taking a toll on the human musculoskeletal system (Hertling and Kessler 2006).

The unique design of the human body enables people to assume practically any position they want. However, the body is distinctly designed to support essential weight-bearing functions that are performed in an upright position, such as walking. When a person is seated, the lumbo-pelvic hip girdle, thoracic spine, and shoulder girdle, legs, and feet no longer have to perform some of their major functions, like extending the hips to support the torso, keeping the spine erect on top of the hips, and bearing weight on the feet and ankles. Instead, the hips remain in flexion, and the body weight is supported by the chair on which the person is sitting. Since the glutes no longer have to extend the hips, they soon become dysfunctional and can no longer perform adequately. The hip flexors also become chronically shortened and dysfunctional as a result of sustained hip flexion (McGill 2016). Consequently, when we stand after a prolonged period of sitting, the glutes cannot extend the hips effectively, and the hip flexors are too tight to allow the hips and spine to extend as they should. Movement to an erect position is thus initiated incorrectly and by fewer muscles—for example, the lumbar erectors overworking to hyperextend the lumbar spine to pull the torso upright (Price and Bratcher 2010).

Several upper body problems can also develop as a result of constant and continual sitting. When a person is seated in front of a computer or in the driver's seat of a vehicle, for example, the tasks that must be performed in those situations require the arms and hands to be placed across and in front of the torso. This position of the arms requires the shoulders to round forward and the thoracic spine to flex, eventually leading to musculoskeletal imbalances such as excessive thoracic kyphosis, internally rotated arms, a protracted shoulder girdle, and elevated shoulder blades (Frontera, Silver, and Rizzo 2015; Price and Bratcher 2010). These changes in the thoracic spine and shoulder girdle affect the neck and head, causing the head to move forward of its optimal position and the neck to arch backward to keep the eyes aligned with the horizon or whatever they are focused on (see figure 18.2). Over time, these sustained postures can lead to imbalances in the head and neck (i.e., excessive cervical lordosis and a forward head posture) and resultant pain and dysfunction.

TIPS TO HELP WITH SEATED POSTURES

There are many nonexercise-related recommendations that can help clients to alleviate some of the musculoskeletal problems that can arise from sitting for long periods of time:

1. It may seem impossible in today's technologically advanced world, but coach clients to sit

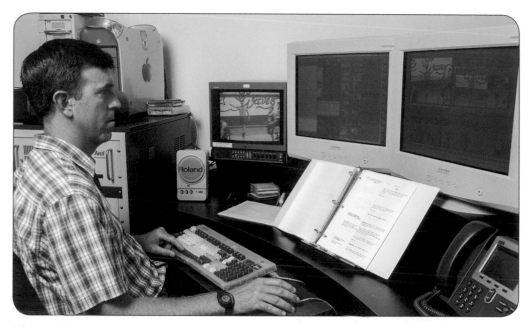

Figure 18.2 Example of forward head and rounded shoulders when seated.

down as little as possible. Reducing the overall amount of time spent in seated positions will complement the range of exercises you provide to address the detrimental musculoskeletal effects of continual sitting. Encourage clients to get out of their chairs several times a day to promote hip, leg, and spine extension.

2. Suggest proactive strategies to minimize the need for sitting, such as converting conventional desks and workspaces to standing desks or walking instead of driving when possible. In cases where clients have no choice but to remain seated, suggest that they use stretches or myofascial release techniques several times a day to target some of the undesired effects that prolonged sitting has on the musculoskeletal system (Higgins 2011; Price and Bratcher 2010).

3. Remind clients who must remain seated for prolonged periods to check the positioning and alignment of their computer monitors, telephones, steering wheels, chairs, televisions, computer accessories, and keyboards to ensure that these objects are situated in a manner that helps keep the spine upright, the head neutral, and the arms relaxed.

4. Remaining stationary in a fixed posture for any amount of time can have detrimental effects on the musculoskeletal system. Encouraging clients to fidget throughout the day when seated to encourage micromovements and lessen the negative effects of prolonged sitting may prove helpful (Weisberg and Shink 2015). Reminding clients to assume neutral positions of the thoracic spine, neck, and head whenever possible when seated will also prove beneficial.

SLEEPING POSTURES

Chronic muscular imbalances and myofascial restrictions that are exacerbated by prolonged standing and sitting can be made even worse by poor sleeping postures (Sahrmann 2002). For example, people with an anterior pelvic tilt and excessive lumbar lordosis will often have very tight hip flexors; as a result, they may find it difficult to sleep on their backs, especially with their legs straight. This is because the combination of an anterior pelvic tilt and tight hip flexors pulls the lumbar spine even further forward into extension, creating a greater arch in the lower back (see figure 18.3). When these people lie on their backs with their legs straight, the muscles and fascia in the lower back will compress and tighten. This can make it uncomfortable to bend forward and flex the lumbar spine after getting out of bed in the morning. Furthermore, an anterior pelvic tilt with excessive lumbar lordosis is also exacerbated by lying on the stomach (especially if the mattress is soft) because this places the spine into extension and tilts the pelvis anteriorly (Wilmink 2010). People with excessive lumbar lordosis and an anterior pelvic tilt will most likely feel most comfortable sleeping on their sides.

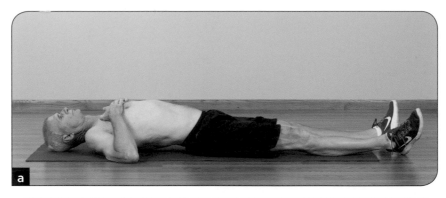

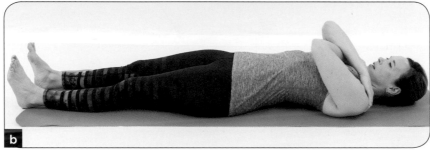

Figure 18.3   Example of (a) anterior pelvic tilt and (b) excessive lumbar lordosis when lying down.

Unfortunately, sleeping on the side of the body for prolonged periods can create musculoskeletal problems as well (Simons, Travell, and Simons 1999). Side sleeping promotes rounding of the shoulders throughout the night as the arms come across the front of the chest to meet on top of the mattress. This position protracts the shoulder blades, especially the shoulder blade not touching the mattress because it has to move farther across the torso in order for the top arm to rest on the bed. In addition, blood supply to the bottom arm and shoulder is restricted in a side sleeping posture because of the weight of the body on the arm (Scheumann 2007). These problematic sleeping positions can exacerbate musculoskeletal imbalances in the upper body, causing compensatory shifts of the pelvis, lower back, hips, and the rest of the lower kinetic chain upon waking and standing.

Occasionally, you will encounter clients who like to sleep on their stomachs. People who prefer this position may be younger clients with an anterior pelvic tilt and excessive lumbar lordosis who have not had these imbalances long enough to experience pain. However, it is very important to encourage clients who sleep on their stomachs to change this habit because it causes the lower back to arch excessively and the pelvis to tilt anteriorly, and it leads to habitually rotating the neck and head to

one side. These irregular spine and pelvis positions will exacerbate (or create) musculoskeletal problems that may eventually produce pain and dysfunction (Ombregt 2013; Simons, Travell, and Simons 1999).

TIPS TO HELP WITH SLEEPING POSTURES

There are many nonexercise recommendations that can help clients alleviate some of the problems that can arise from inappropriate sleeping postures:

1. Encourage clients to try to sleep predominantly on their backs on a firm mattress. The bed should be firm enough so that neither the lower back nor the thoracic spine sinks into the mattress. For those who can easily achieve a neutral lumbar spine, sleeping flat on their backs with their legs out straight is an ideal sleeping position. However, clients with excessive lumbar lordosis and an anterior pelvic tilt will find this position very uncomfortable to maintain. If this is the case, recommend that they place a wedge or pillow under their knees to help to posteriorly tilt their pelvises and flex their lumbar spines to help keep these structures closer to a neutral position (Sahrmann 2002). Coach clients to

start off in this position for just a few minutes a night, then to gradually increase their time in that posture. As the myofascial structures of the lumbar spine begin to adjust, the height of the pillows under the knees can be lessened. Eventually, they will be able to sleep on their backs with straight legs and no tightness or discomfort.

2. People with excessive lumbar lordosis also probably have excessive cervical lordosis. Therefore, a small pillow should be used to help keep the head and neck in a neutral position when sleeping on the back (Simons, Travell, and Simons 1999). Tell clients to choose a pillow thickness that puts their eyes in a position that is perpendicular to the ceiling to properly support the back head and align the neck. The pillow thickness should not be so great, however, that it pushes the head up into a forward head posture.

3. Encouraging clients to sleep on their backs with their arms at their sides will help promote thoracic extension and let the shoulder blades fall into a more neutral, retracted position. Moreover, sleeping on the back with the palms up will externally rotate the arms and help mitigate some of the negative effects of maintaining an internally rotated arm position throughout the day (Price and Bratcher 2010).

4. Although you should not coach clients to sleep on their sides, for some people it is inevitable. If you have a client who insists on sleeping on her side, have her place a pillow between her knees to help keep the upper and lower leg in line with the hip socket, and have her use a pillow thick enough to keep her neck in line with the rest of her spine. If the client is willing, encourage her to place a pillow under her top arm to prevent the arm and shoulder from rolling inward toward the chest. Finally, remind her to be aware of the placement of her head in relation to her neck on the pillow in order to avoid a forward head position as she sleeps (Simons, Travell, and Simons 1999).

Myriad structural and soft tissue changes can result from standing, sitting, and sleeping in malaligned postures. The impact of prolonged static positions can be far-reaching and can have a direct effect on the success of corrective exercise programs. While it is important to design at-home exercises to help undo myofascial restrictions caused by these postures, it is equally important to help clients to become aware of their posture throughout the day and to use the nonexercise strategies we have described to reduce their negative effects.

Review of Key Points

Posture refers to the way a person carries his body or assumes certain static positions.

- People assume different postures throughout the day that vary depending on their activities, occupations, and lifestyles. Muscular and fascial restrictions caused by prolonged static postures can lead to painful imbalances, and they should be addressed in a corrective exercise program.

- Technological advancements may make life easier, but they are harder on the musculoskeletal system when it must adapt to maintain rigid positions for extended periods. These problematic advancements include:
  - Smooth, paved, even surfaces for standing and walking
  - Standardization and automation in most trade industries
  - Comfortable office chairs, recliners, couches, and beds
  - Computers, TVs, automobiles, phones, and other handheld devices

- Standing and walking on dynamic surfaces requires coordinated use of all the muscles in the ankles, toes, and feet. Muscles and soft tissue structures that have become deconditioned by chronic exposure to flat surfaces and predictable terrain require attention throughout the course of a corrective exercise program. The recommendation of supportive shoes, arch supports, or orthotics may be helpful at the outset of a client's program to reduce their painful symptoms. However, these devices should rarely be considered a long-term and complete solution to addressing your client's musculoskeletal imbalances.

- Any type of footwear that is higher in the back than in the front is considered a high-heeled shoe. These types of shoes tip the body's center of mass forward, which can cause or exacerbate musculoskeletal imbalances.

- Sitting for prolonged periods of time can lead to a variety of musculoskeletal problems:

  - Excessive cervical lordosis

  - Excessive thoracic kyphosis

  - Internally rotated arms and a protracted shoulder girdle

  - Weak glutes and thoracic extensors, tight hip flexors

- Ideally, people should learn to sleep on their backs on a firm mattress. However, this position may not always be possible for clients to maintain. Provide recommendations to minimize the postural implications of side sleeping, and encourage clients not to sleep on their stomachs.

Self-Check 1

There are many postural habits that can contribute to musculoskeletal compensation patterns. To help you become aware of some of the most common ones, perform the following movements with your own body and make a note of the sensations you experience.

Movement	On which side of the body is it easier to perform the movement?	What areas on the difficult side do you feel are restricted?
Crossing your arms 1. First cross your right arm over your left. 2. Now cross your left arm over your right.		
Crossing your legs while seated 1. First cross your right leg over your left. 2. Now cross your left leg over your right.		
Propping weight on one leg 1. First shift your body weight onto your left leg. 2. Then shift your body weight onto your right leg.		
Reaching behind you to touch opposite glute while standing 1. First use your left arm to touch your right butt cheek (with palm down on butt). 2. Then use your right hand to touch your left butt cheek (with palm down on butt).		

Self-Check 2

Consider all the muscles, soft tissue structures, and fascia that can be adversely affected by prolonged static postures. Next to each activity in the following chart, list two possible musculoskeletal issues that could be caused or exacerbated by that activity, and identify one self-myofascial, one stretching, and one strengthening exercise that could be used to address the problems. (A complete library of corrective exercises is listed in chapters 19, 20, and 21).

Prolonged activity	Musculoskeletal issues caused	Exercises used to address problem
Driving long distance	1. 2.	Self-myofascial - Stretch - Strengthen -
Standing over an operating table	1. 2.	Self myofascial - Stretch - Strengthen -
Sleeping on one side of the body	1. 2.	Self-myofascial - Stretch - Strengthen -

(continued)

Prolonged activity	Musculoskeletal issues caused	Exercises used to address problem
Entering data on a desktop PC	1. 2.	Self-myofascial - Stretch - Strengthen -
Drawing plans at a drafting table	1.	Myofascial - Stretch - Strengthen -
Dancing in three-inch high heels	1. 2.	Myofascial - Stretch - Strengthen -

Part IV

Complete Corrective Exercise Library

In part IV, you will learn an array of the most effective self-myofascial release, stretching, and strengthening exercises for addressing the most common musculoskeletal imbalances. This comprehensive collection of techniques serves as an exercise guide to help you to create programs that are most appropriate for your clients. The information you have already gained about clients from the structural assessment, your insight into the condition of their soft tissue structures, and your knowledge about corrective exercise should make you feel confident and competent when selecting exercises from this library.

Part IV will highlight the fundamental principles of each corrective exercise category, underline the key teaching tips for each type of exercise, and describe effective ways to observe and monitor your client's progress as you introduce various corrective exercise techniques into their program.

Besides the discussion of general principles, you will find a variety of exercises and techniques for each category. Every exercise will include notations about the area of the body being addressed, the imbalances being targeted, the soft tissue structures involved, the benefits of performing the exercise, how to perform it correctly, progressions and regressions, recommended durations and repetitions, and tips and precautions to make sure you and your clients get the most out of each exercise.

> Go to the online video and watch video IV.1, where Justin provides an overview of the corrective exercise library.

CHAPTER 19

Self-Myofascial Release Exercises

Self-myofascial release (SMR) techniques are used at the outset of a client's corrective exercise program to rejuvenate and restore soft tissues that have been adversely affected by musculoskeletal imbalances (Rolf 1989; Myers 2008; Travell and Simons 1992; Price 2013). They are extremely useful for immediately reducing painful symptoms or movement restrictions while simultaneously allowing inflamed joints to rest and recover (Price and Bratcher 2010).

Generally speaking, the symptoms of unhealthy fascia and soft tissues are experienced as pain or discomfort in those target areas where the self-myofascial techniques are being performed. You and your client can use these sensations to help you gauge whether the SMR techniques you recommend are reducing the discomfort or, in rare cases, are exacerbating the symptoms. When a client performs SMR exercises under your supervision, watch his body language and his facial expressions for signs of discomfort or unease. Listen to his voice and breathing for indications of distress, and watch his body for signs that he is not comfortable in the position you have suggested for the exercise. If a client is stressed or uncomfortable for any reason, you have to change the exercise to make sure that he can relax and not hurt himself. Never encourage a client to try to "push through the pain" when performing any type of self-myofascial release exercise (Price and Bratcher 2010).

SELF-MYOFASCIAL RELEASE QUICK TIPS

There are a number of tips and cueing strategies for introducing clients to self-myofascial release techniques. Following is a brief recap of tactics to use when familiarizing clients with the SMR component of their corrective exercise programs (Barnes 1999; Price and Bratcher 2010).

- Always explain why they are performing a particular self-myofascial release exercise and how it applies to their musculoskeletal imbalances.

- When teaching these techniques, give your clients time to explore any tight areas or sore spots for themselves.

- Do not recommend SMR techniques that are not practical for clients to perform on their own. For instance, the equipment requirements must be reasonable for them.

- Regress an SMR technique if the client feels uncomfortable in any way or experiences pain. SMR techniques can be regressed by using a softer massage tool, by applying heat to the affected area, or by changing body position, such as lying down.

- If a client does not understand or cannot perform an SMR technique correctly, regress the exercise or suggest an alternative.
- Progress the SMR program when the client no longer feels tenderness in an affected area. SMR techniques can be progressed by using a harder massage ball or a firmer roller or by integrating movement into the technique.
- Progress a client's SMR program when the affected area has reached the range of motion needed to advance to stretching exercises.

- SMR may remain a part of your clients' ongoing daily corrective exercise homework.

Reminder

Review the comprehensive information in Chapter 15 on teaching tips, progressions and regressions, and when *not* to use self-myofascial release techniques before you introduce clients to any of the exercises in this chapter.

SELF-MYOFASCIAL RELEASE EXERCISE LIBRARY

The self-myofascial release techniques highlighted in this chapter can be used to benefit a wide variety of corrective exercise clients. They are easy to perform in a gym setting, at home, at the office, or when traveling because they require minimal equipment that is easily accessible to most people. As a rule, SMR exercises using foam rollers will enable clients to massage larger areas of muscle and tissues, while those that use small massage balls or tools are useful for targeting smaller trigger points in specific areas.

Golf Ball Roll

Area(s) of body: Feet and ankles

Imbalance(s): Overpronation, lack of dorsiflexion

Structures addressed: Plantar fascia and muscles of the lower leg that terminate on the underside of the foot

Exercise benefits: This exercise helps regenerate and rejuvenate the plantar fascia and muscles that terminate on the bottom of the foot, which can become irritated as a result of overpronation. Increasing the flexibility of these tissues will also help promote increased dorsiflexion.

How to perform

1. Place a golf ball on the underside of the foot.
2. Roll it back and forth until you feel sore or tender spots.
3. Pause on each sore spot and apply pressure to help each sore spot release.

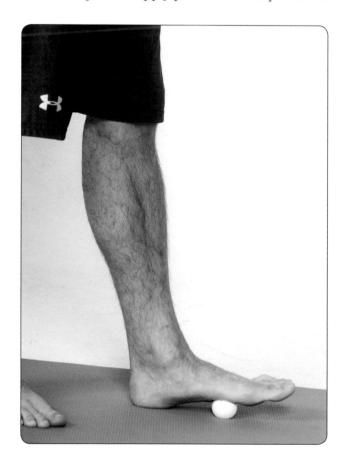

Duration and repetitions: Roll for 30 seconds to 1 minute under each foot at least once per day, spending more time under the side that has more sore spots.

Tip: To increase adherence encourage clients to keep a golf ball by the bed or couch so they can perform this exercise when they get up in the morning and at night before bed or while watching TV.

Precaution: Avoid using excessive pressure because it can irritate the structures of the feet.

Progress: Add an active stretch by pulling the toes up while rolling.

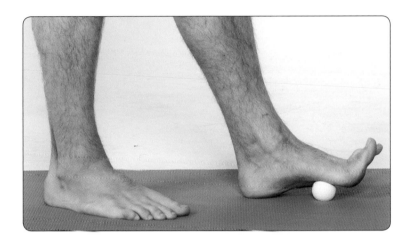

Regress: If a golf ball is too painful, use a tennis ball instead, or perform the exercise while seated.

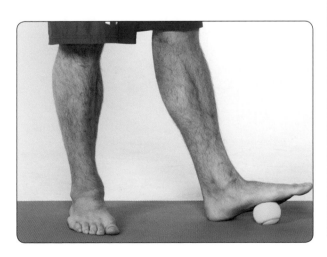

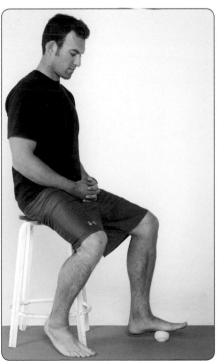

Calf Massage

Area(s) of body: Feet and ankles, knees

Imbalance(s): Lack of dorsiflexion, ovepronation, tracking problems of the knee

Structures addressed: Gastrocnemius and soleus

Exercise benefits: Massaging the muscles on the back of the calf can help realign and rejuvenate the soft tissue structures of the lower leg. Because the gastrocnemius and soleus muscles attach to the heel, this exercise will help improve dorsiflexion and consequently decrease overpronation. It will also help the knee bend more effectively (due to the fact that the ankle and knee bend together during many weight-bearing activities such as squatting, walking, and lunging).

How to perform

1. Sit down, place the ankle of the side being massaged on the knee of the opposite leg and grasp the belly of the calf with your hands.
2. Massage across the muscle or up and down.
3. Target knots or adhesions during the massage.

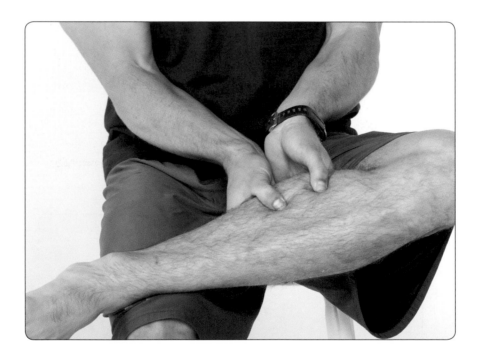

Duration and repetitions: Massage 1 to 2 minutes at least once per day.

Tip: To increase adherence encourage clients to use this massage technique while they are sitting at home watching TV or at work.

Progress: Use a massage device on the calf or perform the Calf Stretch.

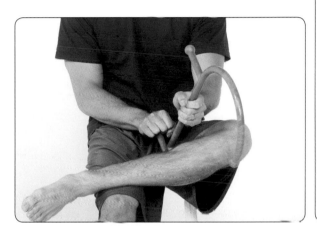

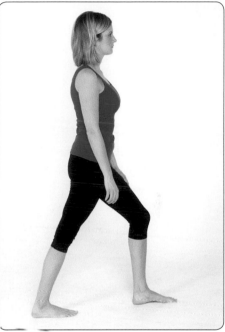

Regress: Use a hard ball (such as a baseball or lacrosse ball) placed on a book with the calf muscle placed on top of the ball.

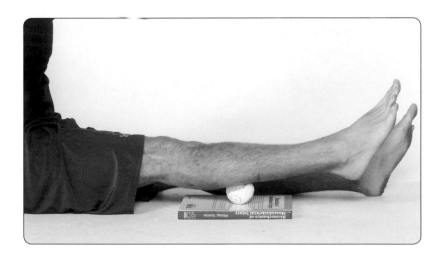

Foam Roller Quadriceps

Area(s) of body: Knees, lumbo-pelvic hip girdle

Imbalance(s): Tracking problems of the knee, anterior pelvic tilt

Structures addressed: Quadriceps muscles

Exercise benefits: This exercise helps rejuvenate and regenerate the quadriceps muscles to enable the knee and pelvis to function correctly. *Note:* Releasing all of the quadriceps muscles will help with tracking of the patella. However, releasing the rectus femoris will also help with an anterior pelvic tilt due to its origin on the front of pelvis.

How to perform

1. Place the roller perpendicular to the leg and lie over it; pressure should be on the thigh.
2. Find a sore spot and hold body weight on it for several seconds to help the tissues release.
3. Use the upper body to roll the roller to different sore spots on the upper leg; keep the abdominals engaged to ensure that the lower back does not arch too much.

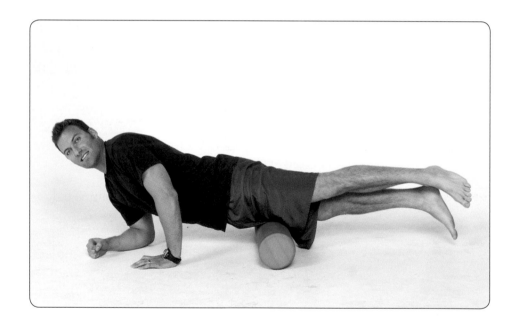

Duration and repetitions: Roll for 1 to 2 minutes on each leg at least once per day.

Tip: Moving toward the outside of the leg (about 6 inches [15 cm] below the hip) focuses on the rectus femoris. Centering releases all quadriceps muscles.

Progress: Bend the knee when rolling, or perform a Quadriceps Stretch.

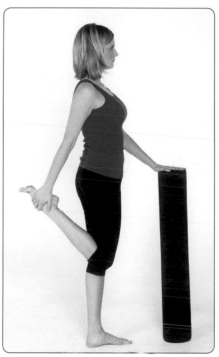

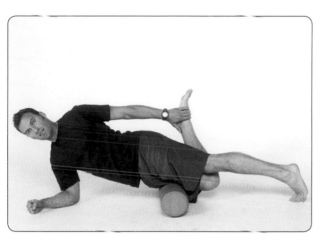

Regress: Lie on your stomach or side and use a half roller or tennis ball.

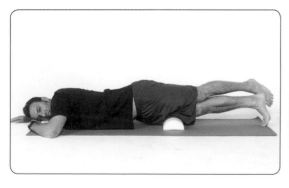

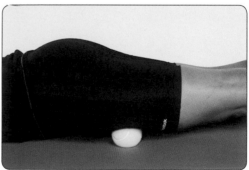

Foam Roller IT Band

Area(s) of body: Knees, lumbo-pelvic hip girdle

Imbalance(s): Valgus knee position, anterior pelvic tilt

Structures addressed: Iliotibial band (IT band)

Exercise benefits: The IT band attaches the gluteus maximus and tensor fasciae latae muscles to the lower leg. When the foot overpronates, the IT band gets stressed and can pull the leg, knee, and pelvis out of alignment. Foam rolling the IT band will help align these structures and allow them to function correctly.

How to perform

1. Lie on your side with hips stacked and forearm resting on the floor; the bottom leg rests on top of the foam roller so the pressure is on the outside of the leg.

2. To decrease pressure on the IT band, place the top leg in front of the body and rest the foot on the floor.

3. Roll from the hip to the knee without crossing the knee; move about 1 to 2 inches (3 to 5 cm) at a time, concentrating on the sore spots.

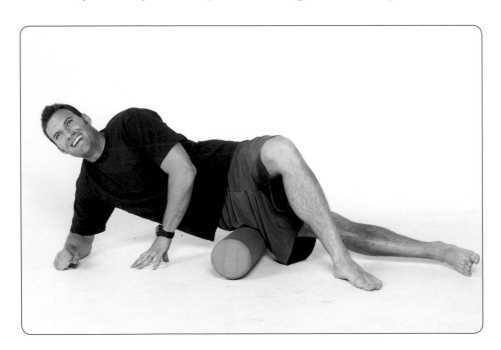

Duration and repetitions: Roll for 30 seconds to 2 minutes on both legs at least once per day.

Tip: A foam roller can be purchased for about $20 to $50.

Precaution: Do not roll over the knee joint when using the foam roller.

Progress: Use a harder (more dense) roller, or stack the legs so they are on top of each other.

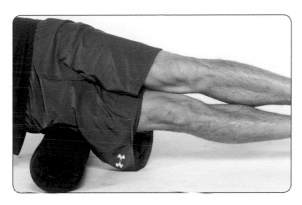
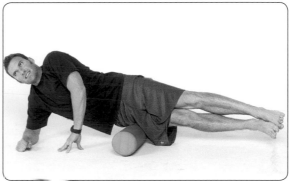

Regress: Lie on your side on a half roller or a tennis ball to massage the IT band; move the half roller or ball from each sore spot along the length of the IT band as tension decreases.

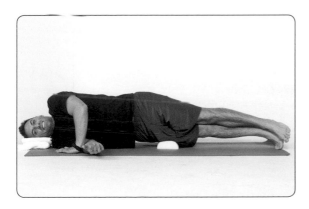
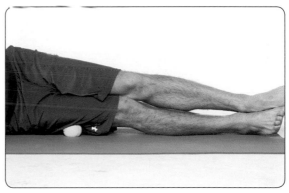

Foam Roller on Inner Thigh

Area(s) of body: Lumbo-pelvic hip girdle, knees

Imbalance(s): Valgus knee position, overpronation, anterior pelvic tilt, excessive lumbar lordosis

Structures addressed: Adductor group of muscles

Exercise benefits: The adductor muscles lengthen under tension during weight-bearing activities to slow down rotation, abduction, flexion, and extension of the leg. Rejuvenating and regenerating these tissues will help these muscles to function better to lessen the effects of excessive lumbar lordosis, an anterior pelvic tilt, a valgus knee position, and overpronation.

How to perform

1. Lie face down, bend the knee and hip of the leg being targeted, and place the roller perpendicular to the inner thigh.
2. Find a sore spot on the inner thigh, and hold body weight on it for a few seconds to help the tissues release.
3. Move the upper body to roll to different sore spots on the inner thigh.

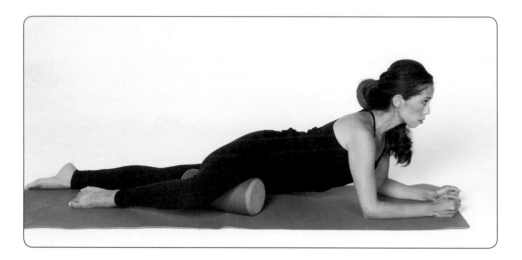

Duration and repetitions: Roll for 1 to 2 minutes on each side at least once per day.

Tip: Balance the body weight on the opposite side or hip, and use your arms to control the amount of pressure felt on the roller.

Precaution: Do not let the lower back over-arch when performing this exercise.

Progress: Perform the Adductor Stretch.

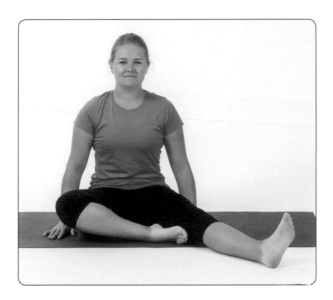

Regress: Use a heating pad on the adductors.

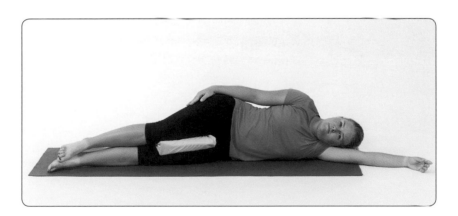

Foam Roller Hip Flexors

Area(s) of body: Lumbo-pelvic hip girdle

Imbalance(s): Anterior pelvic tilt, excessive lumbar lordosis, valgus knee position, lack of dorsiflexion, overpronation

Structures addressed: Hip flexor group of muscles

Exercise benefits: Rejuvenating and regenerating the hip flexor muscles will help the lumbar spine flex, enabling the pelvis to posteriorly rotate more effectively. The hip flexors also work eccentrically to slow down internal rotation and extension of the leg. Therefore, flexibility in these tissues will also help promote better movement of the hip, leg, knee, and ankle.

How to perform

1. Place the roller perpendicular to the front of the body, and lie over it at hip level.

2. Find a sore spot on the front of the hips, and hold body weight on it for a few seconds to help the tissues release.

3. Move the upper body to roll to different sore spots on the upper leg; keep the abdominals engaged to ensure that the lower back does not arch too much.

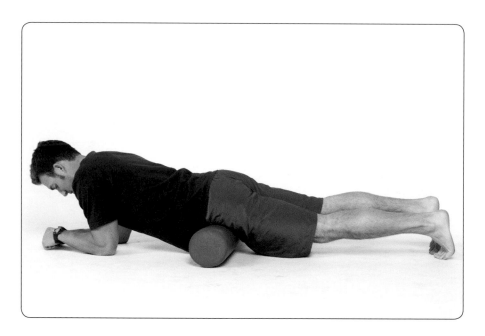

Duration and repetitions: Roll for 30 seconds to 1 minute on each side at least once per day.

Tip: Angle the roller so that it is in line with the crease of the groin (i.e., at 45 degrees to the hip and leg) to increase the pressure of the massage.

Progress: Perform the Hip Flexor Stretch (Sagittal).

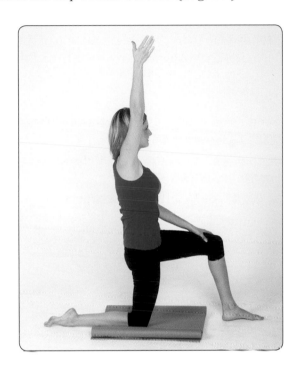

Regress: Use a tennis ball to massage the hip flexors (see detailed information in next exercise).

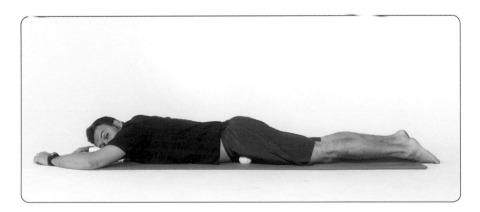

Tennis Ball on Hip Flexors

Area(s) of body: Lumbo-pelvic hip girdle, knees

Imbalance(s): Excessive lumbar lordosis, anterior pelvic tilt, valgus knee position, overpronation, lack of dorsiflexion

Structures addressed: Hip flexor group of muscles

Exercise benefits: Using a tennis ball to target the origin of the psoas major muscle (on the sides of the lumbar spine) and iliacus (from the front and inside of the pelvis) will directly help to improve the function of the lumbar spine and pelvis. Releasing these tissues will also improve the function of the legs, knees, feet, and ankles.

How to perform

1. Lie face down, and place a tennis ball on the abdominals beside the belly button to target the psoas major muscle (which lies under the abdominals).

2. Scoot your body to move the ball to any sore spots all the way down from beside the belly button to the top of the hip.

Note: Massaging just inside the ASIS (the bony protuberance on the front of the pelvis) will release the iliacus.

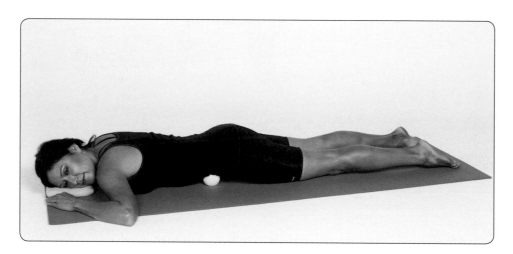

Duration and repetitions: Hold on each sore spot for 20 to 30 seconds. Perform at least once a day for a total of 2 to 3 minutes on both sides of the body.

Tip: Internally rotate the leg (i.e., turn the foot in) to help stretch the hip flexors while performing this exercise.

Precaution: If you feel a pulse under the tennis ball, simply move the ball slightly to reduce pressure on the femoral artery.

Progress: Use a larger and firmer ball, such as a softball, to help increase pressure through the abdominals to the hip flexor muscles. Perform the Hip Flexor Stretch (Transverse).

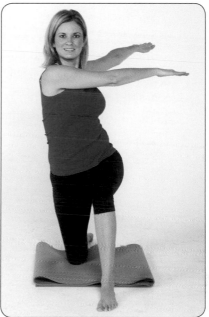

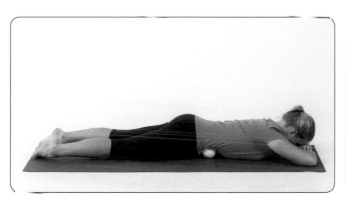

Regress: Apply heat to the area while you lie on your back with the leg straight.

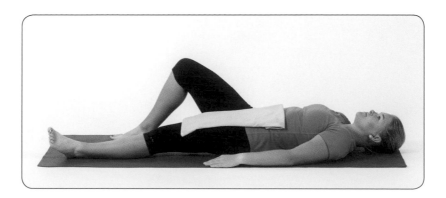

Foam Roller Gluteal Complex

Area(s) of body: Lumbo-pelvic hip girdle, knees

Imbalance(s): Anterior pelvic tilt, valgus knee position

Structures addressed: Gluteus maximus and hip rotators (e.g., piriformis). Also targets gluteus medius and gluteus minimus when roller is angled toward the side of the hip and buttocks.

Exercise benefits: An anterior pelvic tilt can adversely affect the muscles on the back of the hips. Foam rolling this area will help regenerate these tissues and enable the pelvis, hips, and legs to move into better alignment.

How to perform

1. Sit down on a foam roller, and lean your body to one side to place weight on the gluteal complex on that side.

2. Lift the foot of the side being targeted, and place the outside of that ankle on the opposite knee.

3. Pull your knee to your chest on the side being massaged, and roll back and forth to release and stretch the muscles of that area.

4. Increase stretch by pulling the knee in more toward the chest.

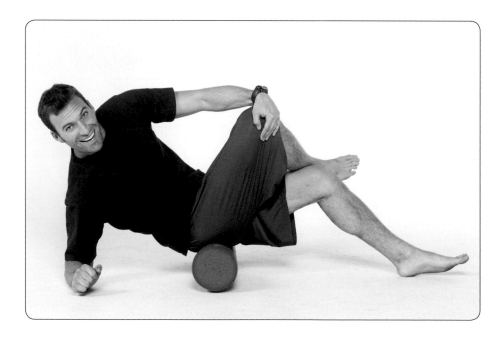

Duration and repetitions: Roll for 30 seconds to 2 minutes on both sides at least once per day.

Tip: The hip rotator muscles run transversely across the middle of the butt. This area will most likely be irritated and sore on those with an anterior pelvic tilt and valgus knee position.

Precaution: If numbing or tingling is felt, decrease pressure to the area or stop the exercise.

Progress: Use a harder foam roller or perform the Glute Stretch.

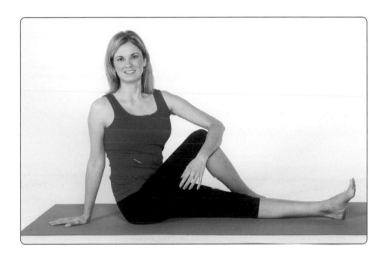

Regress: Massage the glutes using a tennis ball or baseball.

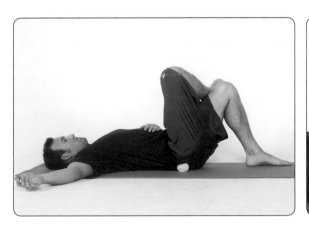
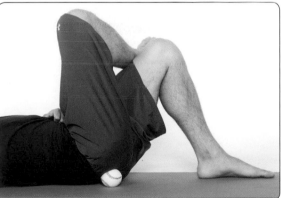

Tennis Ball Side of Hip

Area(s) of body: Lumbo-pelvic hip girdle, knees

Imbalance(s): Valgus knee position, anterior pelvic tilt

Structures addressed: Abductor group of muscles

Exercise benefits: This exercise helps the hip and leg complex and the knee to function correctly by rejuvenating and regenerating the abductor muscles on the lateral side of the hip and leg.

How to perform

1. Lie on your side with your head resting on a pillow to help keep the head and neck aligned.
2. Place a tennis ball under the lateral side of the hip just above the top of the leg on the side in contact with the ground.
3. Find a sore spot and hold there to release.
4. Move the ball gently to another sore spot and hold to release.

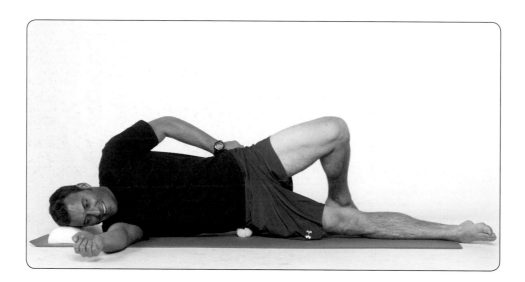

Duration and repetitions: Hold for 20 to 30 seconds on each sore spot. Perform at least once per day for a total of 2 to 3 minutes.

Tip: If the pressure felt in the area is too much, simply roll the body slightly off the ball to decrease the pressure.

Progress: Perform the Abductor Stretch or the Door Frame Stretch.

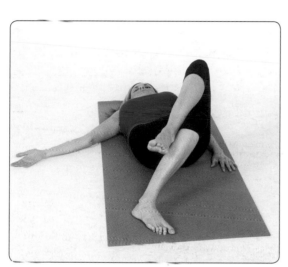

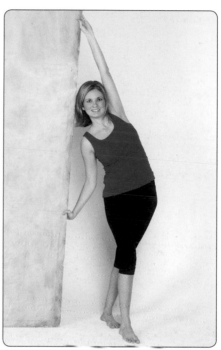

Regress: Use a foam roller to massage the side of the hip instead of a tennis ball.

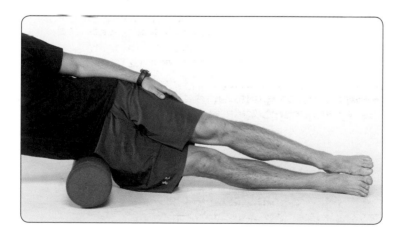

One Tennis Ball on Lower Back

Area(s) of body: Lumbo-pelvic hip girdle

Imbalance(s): Anterior pelvic tilt, excessive lumbar lordosis

Structures addressed: Lumbar erector spinae muscles and thoracolumbar fascia

Exercise benefits: An anterior pelvic tilt and excessive lumbar lordosis can cause the muscles and fascia of the lower back to become overworked and tight. This exercise helps rejuvenate and regenerate the muscles and fascia of the lower back to release tension in this area to enable the lumbar spine to flex and the pelvis to posteriorly rotate.

How to perform

1. Lie on your back; use a pillow under your neck if needed to make sure your eyes stay perpendicular to the ceiling.
2. Bend your knees to keep the pelvis posteriorly tilted, and place one tennis ball on one side of the spine in the lower back area; adjust the ball until a sore spot is found, and hold to release tension.
3. Move your body up or down to move the ball either up or down to find additional sore spots; hold to release tension.

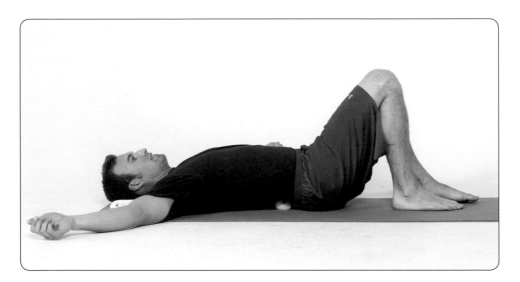

Duration and repetitions: Hold for 20 to 30 seconds on each sore spot. Perform at least once per day for a total of 2 to 3 minutes.

Precaution: Do not place the ball too close to the spine. Also, when traveling up the spine to the bottom of the rib cage, be careful not to place too much pressure on this area because this may cause discomfort.

Progress: Bend the knees and place the ankle of the side being massaged on the knee of the opposite leg. Perform the Lower Back Stretch.

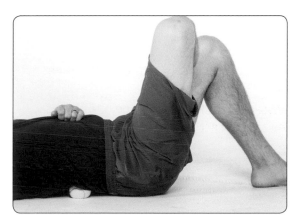 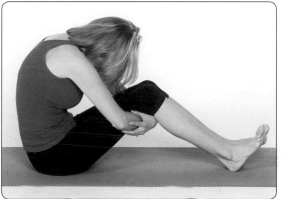

Regress: Support the opposite hip with a hand to help keep the pelvis level.

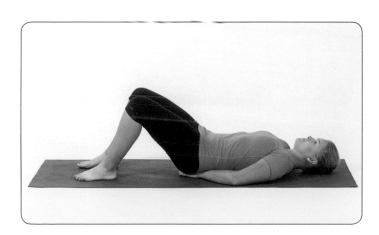

Foam Roller Quadratus Lumborum

Area(s) of body: Lumbo-pelvic hip girdle

Imbalance(s): Anterior pelvic tilt, excessive lumbar lordosis

Structures addressed: Quadratus lumborum

Exercise benefits: The quadratus lumborum (QL) is responsible for hiking the hip up toward the bottom of the rib cage, extending and side-flexing the lumbar spine. Releasing this muscle will enable the pelvis and lumbar spine to function more effectively.

How to perform

1. Sit down on a foam roller with knees bent and pelvis posteriorly tilted.
2. Gently slide down the roller until it is positioned just above the back of the hip.
3. Use the roller to release the area between the bottom of the ribs and the top of the pelvis, focusing on one side at a time.

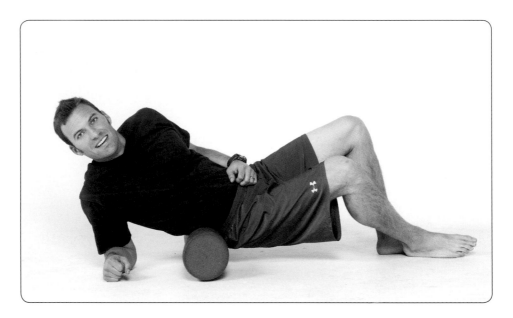

Duration and repetitions: Roll for 30 seconds to 1 minute on both sides at least once per day.

Precaution: Use caution when performing this exercise to avoid rolling over the bottom two ribs with too much pressure. They are floating ribs that do not attach to the sternum, and they can displace or become injured easily.

Progress: Perform the Door Frame Stretch.

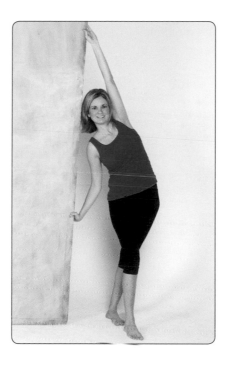

Regress: Place the ankle on the knee and use a tennis ball to massage the QL.

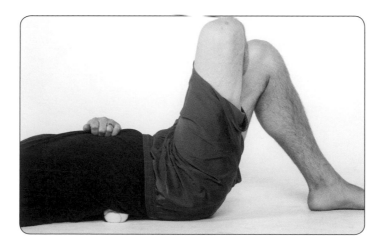

Two Tennis Balls on Upper Back

Area(s) of body: Thoracic spine

Imbalance(s): Excessive thoracic kyphosis, protracted shoulder girdle

Structures addressed: Thoracic erector spinae muscles, rhomboids, and middle fibers of trapezius muscle

Exercise benefits: Excessive thoracic kyphosis causes the erector muscles of the upper back and the retractors of the scapula to become chronically lengthened. Rejuvenating and regenerating these muscles will help release tension in this area and prepare the muscles of the thoracic spine and shoulder blades to be fortified with subsequent strengthening exercises.

How to perform

1. Lie on your back with your knees bent; place two tennis balls on either side of the spine under the upper back at approximately bra height or just below the shoulder blades.
2. Use a pillow to support your head and to keep your eyes perpendicular to the ceiling; the use of a pillow will also help control the amount of pressure felt on the back from the balls (i.e., a larger pillow will decrease the pressure felt).
3. Find a sore spot and hold to release tension.
4. Move your body up or down to move the balls either up or down to find additional sore spots; hold to release tension.

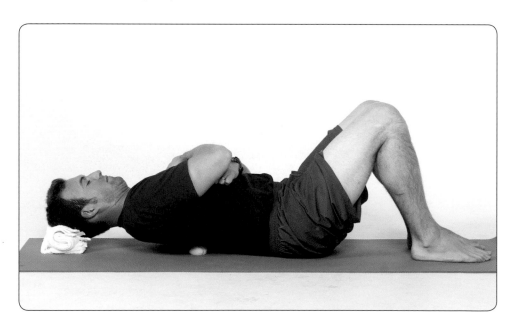

Duration and repetitions: Hold for 20 to 30 seconds on each sore spot. Perform at least once per day for a total of 2 to 3 minutes.

Precaution: Regress this exercise immediately if breathing feels restricted or if tension is experienced in the chest.

Progress: Tilt the pelvis to increase pressure from the balls, or perform the Shoulder Retraction on Floor exercise.

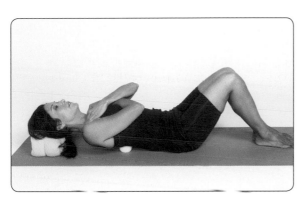 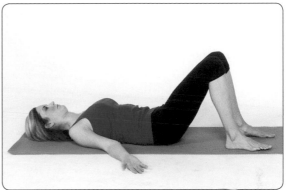

Regress: Use a higher pillow to support your head, or use one only ball at a time.

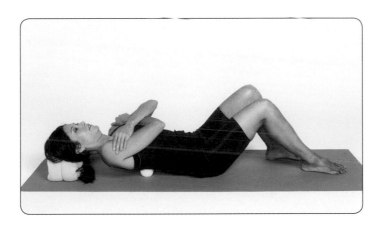

Foam Roller Thoracic Spine

Area(s) of body: Thoracic spine and shoulder girdle

Imbalance(s): Excessive thoracic kyphosis, protracted shoulder girdle

Structures addressed: Thoracic erectors, rhomboids, and trapezius

Exercise benefits: This exercise rejuvenates the muscles of the thoracic spine and shoulders by releasing excessive tension in this area to help correct excessive thoracic kyphosis and a protracted shoulder girdle.

How to perform

1. Lie on your back over the foam roller with your hands behind your head and your chin tucked in (the roller should be perpendicular to the torso).

2. Bend your knees, tuck your hips under, and lift your pelvis off the floor.

3. Roll back and forth along the thoracic spine, massaging sore or tender spots.

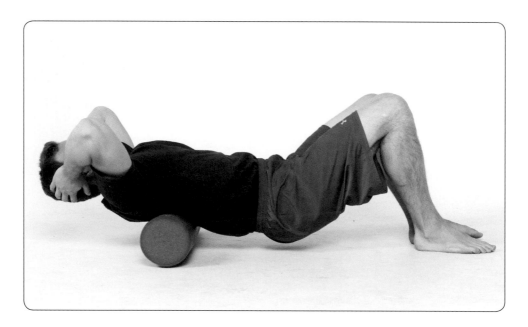

Duration and repetitions: Roll for 30 seconds to 2 minutes at least once per day.

Tip: Support your head while rolling to protect your neck from stress.

Precaution: Keep your pelvis posteriorly tilted to avoid excessive arching of the lower back.

Progress: Drop your hips to the ground and tilt your pelvis, or perform the Straight Arm Raise.

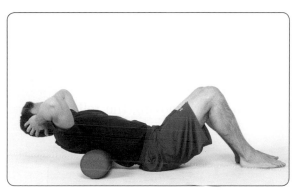
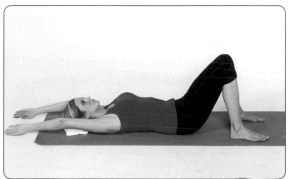

Regress: Two Tennis Balls on Upper Back.

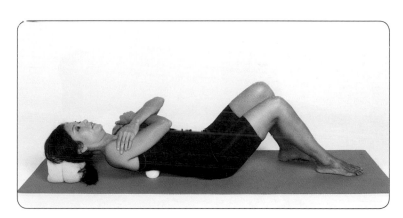

Tennis Ball Around Shoulder Blade

Area(s) of body: Thoracic spine and shoulder girdle

Imbalance(s): Protracted shoulder girdle, elevated scapula

Structures addressed: Rhomboids and trapezius muscles

Exercise benefits: Massaging the shoulder retractors will help you address imbalances throughout the thoracic spine and shoulder girdle and will prepare these tissues for subsequent strengthening exercises.

How to perform

1. Lie on the floor with your knees bent and your head resting on a pillow.
2. Pull one arm across your chest and place a tennis ball under your upper back beside the shoulder blade of that arm between the shoulder blade and the spine.
3. Find a sore spot and hold to release tension.
4. Move the ball gently to another spot and hold to release tension.

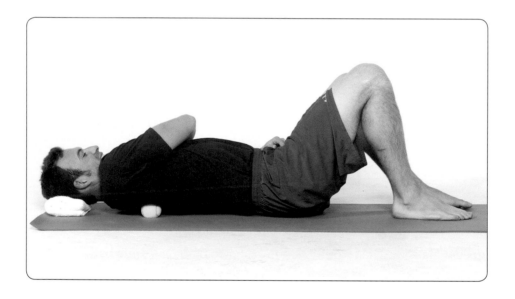

Duration and repetitions: Hold for 20 to 30 seconds on each sore spot. Perform at least once per day.

Precaution: Do not roll around dynamically when performing this exercise; this is to avoid damaging nerves of the shoulder complex. Hold pressure on each sore spot until it releases.

Progress: Perform the Seated Row.

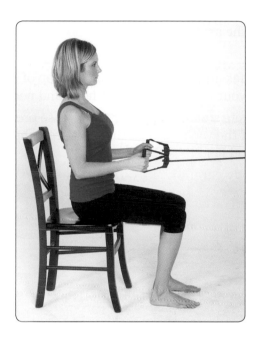

Regress: Use a softer ball (like a racquetball) or perform the exercise standing against a wall.

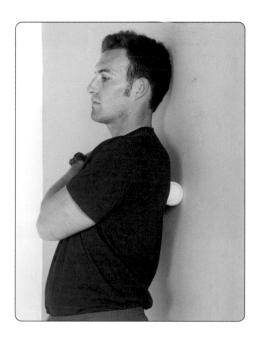

Abdominal Massage

Area(s) of body: Lumbo-pelvic hip girdle, thoracic spine, and shoulder girdle

Imbalance(s): Excessive thoracic kyphosis, protracted shoulder girdle

Structures addressed: Anterior abdominal muscles and abdominal fascia

Exercise benefits: Excessive thoracic kyphosis results in a chronic shortening of the abdominals. In this case, the muscles and fascia of the abdomen become restricted and tight, thereby affecting movement of the torso and spine. Releasing and regenerating the abdominal muscles and fascia will enable the thoracic spine to extend more effectively and the shoulders to retract, and this will allow greater movement throughout the torso, spine, and shoulder complex.

How to perform

1. Lie on your back with your knees bent and your head supported by a pillow to keep the head and neck neutral.

2. Use your hands to massage the abdomen from the bottom of the rib cage down to the pelvis, concentrating on any sore spots.

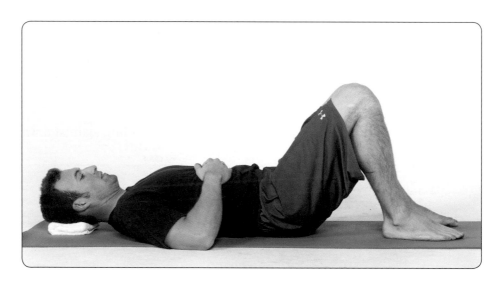

Duration and repetitions: Perform at least once per day for a total of 1 to 2 minutes.

Precaution: Some people may find initially that massaging their abdominal area makes them feel nauseous. If this is the case, regress or reduce the amount of pressure applied.

Progress: Use a handheld massage device to massage the abdominals, or lie face down on top of a massage ball like a tennis ball or baseball.

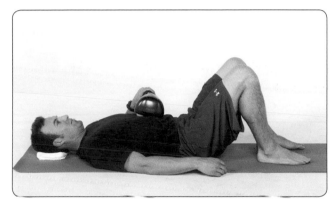

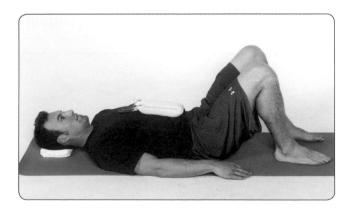

Regress: Use a heating pad.

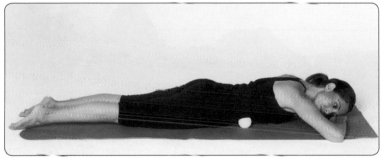

Front of Shoulder Massage

Area(s) of body: Shoulder girdle

Imbalance(s): Internally rotated arms, protracted shoulder girdle

Structures addressed: Supraspinatus, anterior deltoid, and origin of the biceps muscles

Exercise benefits: Internally rotated arms affect the function of the shoulder, arm, and shoulder girdle. Releasing tension in the muscles at the front of the shoulder will enable the arms to externally rotate and the scapula to retract. It will also prepare these muscles for subsequent stretching and strengthening exercises.

How to perform

1. Lie on your back with knees bent and head supported on a pillow to keep your head and neck neutral.
2. Using the fingers of one hand, gently massage the muscles of the front of the shoulder on the opposite side.

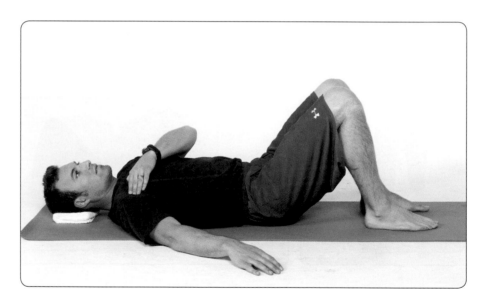

Duration and repetitions: Massage each sore spot for 20 to 30 seconds. Perform at least once per day for a total of 2 to 3 minutes.

Tip: Perform this exercise in conjunction with the Chest Massage to loosen up the entire anterior shoulder and chest region.

Progress: Perform the exercise lying on your stomach with a tennis ball on the front of your shoulder. Perform the Front of Shoulder Stretch (massage front of shoulder with opposite hand for maximum benefit).

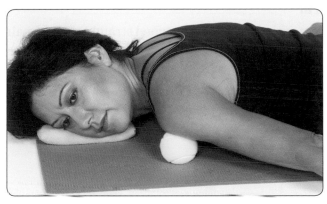

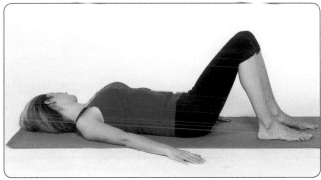

Regress: Use a heating pad.

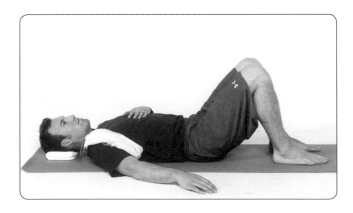

Forearm Massage

Area(s) of body: Thoracic spine and shoulder girdle

Imbalance(s): Internally rotated arms

Structures addressed: Forearm muscles and insertion of the biceps brachii

Exercise benefits: Restrictions in the upper or lower arm can affect the function of the glenohumeral joint and the shoulder complex. This exercise releases and rejuvenates the muscles and fascia in the forearm to enable the whole arm and shoulder to move more effectively.

How to perform

1. Sit in a chair and bring one arm across your abdomen; use the thumb and fingers of the other hand to massage the inside and outside of the forearm.

2. Apply steady pressure to each sore spot until it releases, and then move to the next spot.

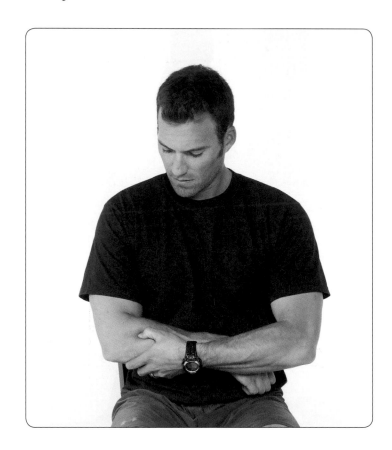

Duration and repetitions: Massage each sore spot for 20 to 30 seconds. Perform at least once per day for a total of 2 to 3 minutes.

Tip: This is a great exercise for everyone who uses a computer or their forearms regularly (e.g., tennis players, golfers, or people who work out a lot gripping heavy weights).

Progress: Perform the exercise using a tennis or a baseball placed on a desk with your forearm balanced on top of the ball. Perform the Palm on Wall Stretch.

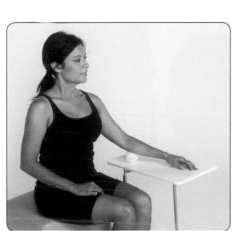

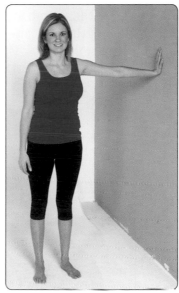

Regress: Use a heating pad or a handheld massager to massage the forearm.

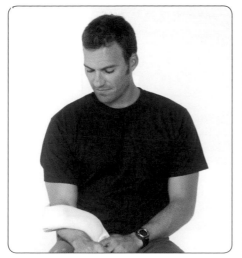

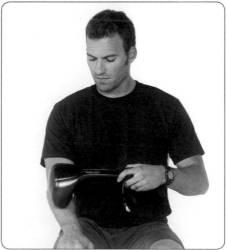

Theracane on Trapezius

Area(s) of body: Thoracic spine and shoulder girdle, neck, and head

Imbalance(s): Elevated scapula, excessive cervical lordosis

Structures addressed: Upper fibers of the trapezius and the extensors of the neck and head

Exercise benefits: The muscles that elevate the scapula and extend the neck and head can become restricted and tight as a result of excessive cervical lordosis and an elevated scapula. This exercise helps release tension in the upper traps and neck extensors to enable the shoulder blades to depress and the head and neck to flex more easily.

How to perform

1. Sit in a chair, and place the hook end of the Theracane on the top of the shoulder (i.e., on the upper trapezius).
2. Apply pressure to the upper traps by pulling the handle of the Theracane down and out to apply pressure to any sore spots on the trapezius and neck extensors; hold to release tension.
3. Move the hook end of the Theracane to other sore spots and apply pressure; hold to release tension.

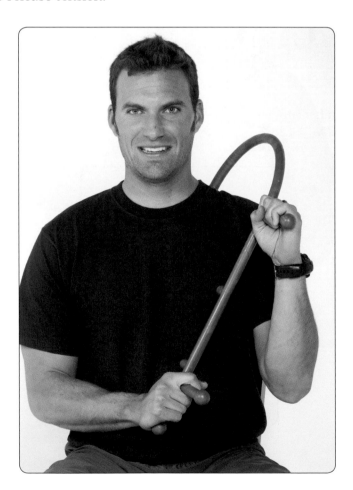

Duration and repetitions: Apply pressure for 20 to 30 seconds to each sore spot. Perform at least once per day for a total of 2 to 3 minutes.

Precaution: Apply steady pressure, and do not move the Theracane around vigorously; otherwise the device may slip or hurt the nerves in the neck.

Progress: Bend your neck to the side to add a stretch or perform the Straight Arm Pulldown.

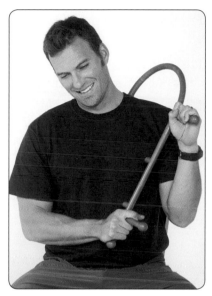
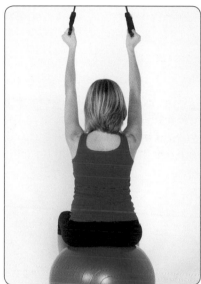

Regress: Use a heating pad.

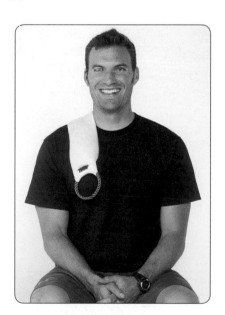

Theracane Back of Neck

Area(s) of body: Thoracic spine and shoulder girdle, neck, and head

Imbalance(s): Excessive cervical lordosis, forward head

Structures addressed: Neck extensors, upper trapezius, and fascia of the neck

Exercise benefits: A forward head position and excessive cervical lordosis can cause the muscles and fascia on the back of the neck to become irritated. This exercise helps rejuvenate and regenerate these tissues so that the neck can flex more easily and the head can move back into better alignment. It also helps prepare these muscles for subsequent strengthening exercises.

How to perform

1. Sit in a chair, and place the hook end of the Theracane on the back of your neck.

2. Apply pressure by pulling the Theracane down and out to apply pressure to any sore spot in the area; hold to release tension.

3. Move the hook end of the Theracane to other sore spots and apply pressure; hold to release tension.

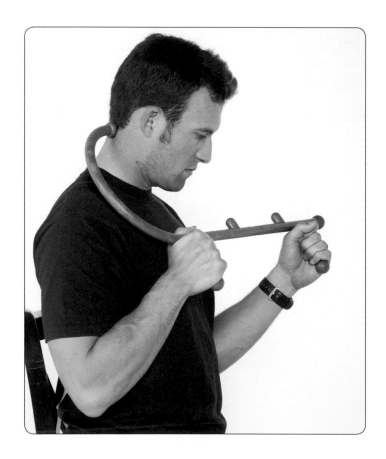

Duration and repetitions: Apply pressure for 20 to 30 seconds to each sore spot. Perform at least once per day for a total of 2 to 3 minutes.

Tip: This is a great exercise for people who look at a computer screen or watch television a lot throughout the day.

Progress: Perform this exercise lying on your back, cupping a ball in your hand, and pressing the neck down into the ball. Perform the Neck Extensors Stretch.

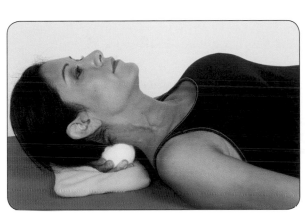

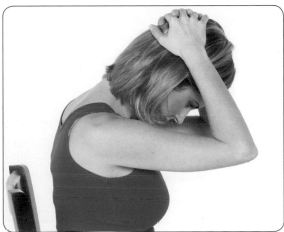

Regress: Use a heating pad.

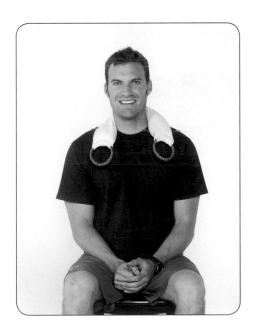

Review of Key Points

Self-myofascial release techniques are used at the outset of a client's program to rejuvenate and regenerate unhealthy muscles and fascia before moving on to stretching and strengthening exercises.

- When introducing your client to a specific self-myofascial release technique, it is important to explain why they are performing that exercise and to give them time to explore the tight areas on their own.

- Do not recommend SMR techniques that are impractical or require expensive equipment.

- Regress an SMR technique if your client experiences pain or cannot perform the exercise correctly.

- Progress an SMR technique if your client no longer feels any tenderness on the target area or if they have achieved the range of motion they need to progress to stretching and strengthening.

- There are a number of important contraindications to the application of self-myofascial release techniques. These are listed in chapter 15, and you should review them carefully before introducing these techniques into a client's corrective exercise program.

Self-Check

It is important to select self-myofascial release exercises based on the specific needs of each client. In this Self-Check, consider the client imbalance or situation described and identify three appropriate self-myofascial release techniques that could be incorporated into each client's program. Provide a brief rationale to support your selections. An example is provided.

Client imbalance or situation	SMR exercise selection
Your assessment results reveal a client with an over-pronated right foot, a valgus right knee, and right knee pain.	Golf Ball Roll to rejuvenate and regenerate the structures on the underside of the foot to help prepare the client for strengthening exercises later in the program. Calf Massage to increase dorsiflexion (effectively reducing overpronation and helping align the knee). Foam Roller on IT Band to release the structures on the lateral side of the leg and knee in preparation for strengthening the appropriate muscles to help decelerate the knee as it moves toward the midline of the body during activities like walking and running.
Your assessment results reveal a client with an anterior pelvic tilt, excessive lumbar lordosis, and lower back pain.	
Your assessment results reveal a client with internally rotated arms, excessive thoracic kyphosis, and pain between the shoulder blades.	

CHAPTER 20

Stretching Exercises

Stretching exercises are introduced into a corrective exercise program after the consistent application of self-myofascial release techniques (Clark and Lucett 2011; Price 2013; Price and Bratcher 2010). Once the overall condition of dysfunctional soft tissue structures has been addressed with self-myofascial release techniques, stretching exercises are used to introduce movement in order to increase range of motion in those areas that have been adversely affected by a client's musculoskeletal imbalances (Kovacs 2015; Price and Bratcher 2010).

Muscle tension, guarding, and movement restrictions are common in people with chronic musculoskeletal imbalances. While stretching exercises are designed to overcome these dysfunctional patterns, it is also important to remember that sensations of pain, joint inflammation, and current injuries can affect the success of any stretching program. In some cases, stretching can actually do more harm than good. Therefore, it is important to introduce isolated and gentle stretching exercises gradually. You must continually monitor your clients' sensations and body language, and you should progress to more advanced stretching exercises only when they are ready (Price and Bratcher 2010).

STRETCHING EXERCISE QUICK TIPS

There are a number of tips and cueing tactics that can facilitate the process of introducing clients to stretching techniques. Following is a brief recap of strategies for progressing your clients to the stretching portion of their corrective exercise programs.

- Use your knowledge of muscles and movement to teach clients to perform a stretch correctly, telling them where they should feel the stretch and how to adjust their technique if needed.

- Explain to the client why she is performing a specific stretch, and link the benefits of that exercise to the musculoskeletal imbalances that need correcting.

- Regress a stretching exercise if it causes discomfort or if clients have difficulty performing the exercise properly.

- Regress a stretching exercise if the equipment requirements make it impractical for the client to perform it on a regular basis.

- Regress a stretching exercise by allowing the client to use a balance aid or to perform the stretch lying down or seated, or return to a suitable SMR technique for the area being targeted.
- Progress a stretch by removing a balance aid, performing the exercise standing, or integrating other body parts into the movement.
- Progress a client's stretching program if she has demonstrated mastery and is ready for strengthening exercises.

Reminder

Review the comprehensive information on teaching tips, progressions and regressions, and when *not* to use stretching exercises in chapter 16 before you introduce any of the exercises in this chapter into a client's corrective exercise program.

STRETCHING EXERCISE LIBRARY

The stretching exercises highlighted in this chapter should be used as part of a complete corrective exercise program that involves both self-myofascial release and strengthening techniques. These stretching techniques are designed to be easy to perform in a gym or personal training setting, at home, at the office, or when traveling. The required equipment is minimal and is readily accessible to most people.

Foot and Toe Stretch

Area(s) of body: Feet and ankles

Imbalance(s): Overpronation and lack of dorsiflexion

Structures addressed: Plantar fascia and muscles of the lower leg that terminate on the underside of the foot

Exercise benefits: Overpronation and lack of dorsiflexion constantly stress the muscles that wrap around the ankle and terminate on the underside of the foot, causing them to become tight or restricted. Stretching the toes and underside of the foot can make the foot (and ankle) more flexible, allowing these areas to function more effectively.

How to perform

1. Stand barefoot with one foot forward and toes pushed up against a wall or half foam roller; keep the ball of the foot and the base of the toes in contact with the floor.
2. Slowly roll foot and ankle forward and inward (i.e., into pronation).
3. Slowly bend the knee and ankle forward toward the wall to stretch the underside of the foot.

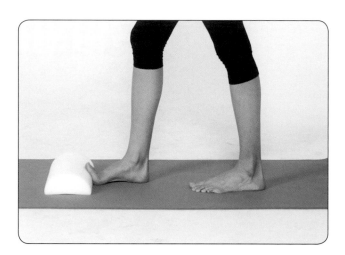

Duration and repetitions: Hold the stretch for about 10 to 15 seconds, release, and then repeat. Perform the cycle 1 to 3 times at least once a day on both feet.

Tip: When performing this stretch using a wall, place your hands on the wall to help keep your hips and torso straight and square.

Precaution: If a cramping sensation or discomfort is felt on the bottom of the foot or on the front of the ankle, ease off, regress, or stop performing this stretch.

Progress: Pronate the foot more by letting the knee fall toward the midline of the body to increase the stretch. When performing this progression, try to keep the hips level.

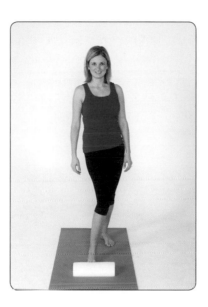

Regress: Perform the Golf Ball Roll or the Calf Massage.

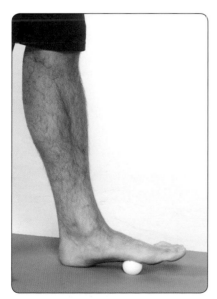

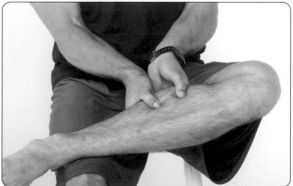

Calf Stretch

Area(s) of body: Feet and ankles, knees

Imbalance(s): Lack of dorsiflexion and overpronation

Structures addressed: Gastrocnemius and soleus; also activates and strengthens tibialis anterior when contracted to progress exercise

Exercise benefits: When the feet overpronate, the calf muscles and Achilles tendon can get irritated and may not be able to function effectively. This stretch helps release and realign the calf muscles to allow better dorsiflexion of the foot and ankle and prevent overpronation.

How to perform

1. Stand with feet in a staggered stance (one foot forward and one foot back).
2. Place your hands on a balance aid if needed (e.g., a wall in front).
3. Align your pelvis left to right and tuck it under (i.e., posteriorly rotate it).
4. Keep the arches of your feet raised, and gently lean forward, keeping both feet in contact with the ground.

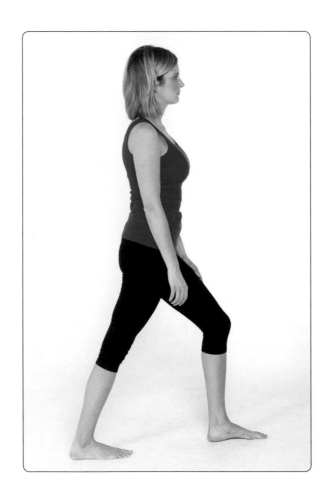

Duration and repetitions: Hold the stretch for about 20 to 30 seconds, release, and repeat. Perform this cycle on each side 1 to 2 times at least once a day.

Tip: You can vary this stretch by adding a slight bend to the back knee. This will stretch the soleus muscle (which will help increase dorsiflexion of the ankle when the knee is bent).

Progress: Actively pull up on the toes using the tibialis anterior muscle of the leg that is back, or add movement by bending and straightening the back leg while performing this stretch on a dynamic surface like a BOSU Balance Trainer.

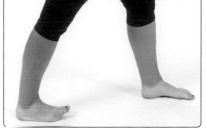
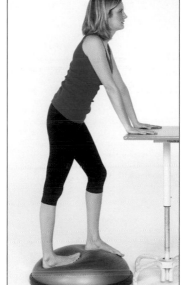
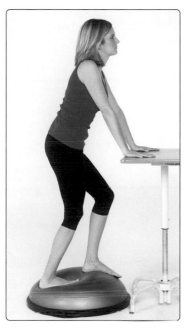

Regress: Perform the Calf Massage.

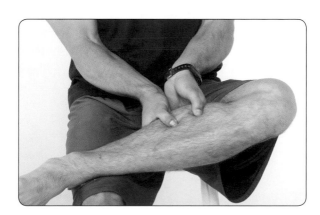

Quadriceps Stretch

Area(s) of body: Knees, lumbo-pelvic hip girdle

Imbalance(s): Anterior pelvic tilt and tracking problems of the knee

Structures addressed: Quadriceps muscles

Exercise benefits: Increasing the flexibility of the quadriceps muscles has many benefits. If the quadriceps are flexible (specifically the rectus femoris muscle, which originates on the front of the pelvis), the pelvis can posteriorly rotate and the hips can extend well. Also, since all of the quadriceps muscles attach at the knee, they are directly responsible for helping the kneecap to track correctly.

How to perform

1. Stand facing a tall object, such as a table or counter; place one hand on the object to stabilize your body.

2. Grab your foot with the other hand, and pull your heel up toward your buttocks.

3. Bring your knee back while gently rotating your pelvis under (i.e., posteriorly rotating) and straightening your upper back.

4. Do not excessively arch the lower back while performing this exercise.

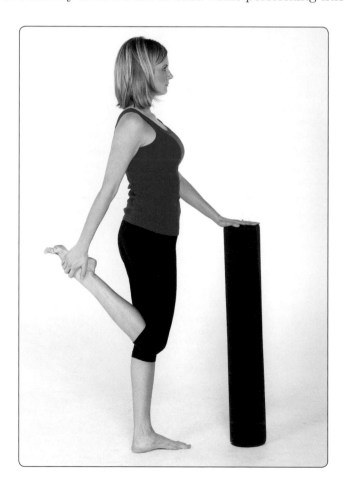

Duration and repetition: Stretch each side for 20 to 30 seconds at least once per day.

Tip: If the foot cannot be reached, simply wrap a towel under the foot of the leg being stretched and pull the towel toward the buttocks to feel the stretch in the thigh.

Progress: Place the ankle or foot of the stretching leg on a counter or bench. Use a balance aid, if needed.

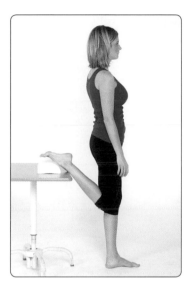
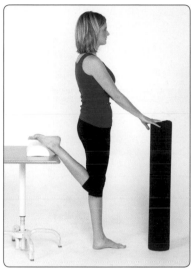

Regress: Use a towel to help with the stretch, and perform the exercise while lying down on your stomach or side.

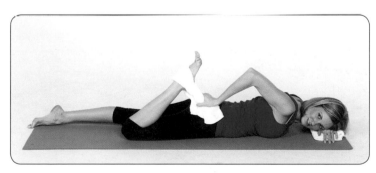

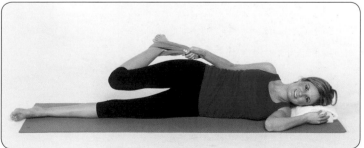

Hamstring Stretch

Area(s) of body: Feet and ankles, knees, lumbo pelvic-hip girdle

Imbalance(s): Overpronation, valgus knee position, anterior pelvic tilt, and excessive lumbar lordosis

Structures addressed: Hamstrings, gastrocnemius, and hip flexors; activates and strengthens tibialis anterior and quadriceps when exercise is progressed.

Exercise benefits: When the foot overpronates, the lower leg and knee rotate inward and the front of the pelvis tilts down. This can cause the hamstrings to become irritated because they must overwork to stabilize the pelvis and control the excessive rotation of the lower leg. Stretching the hamstrings can recondition these muscles and help the feet, knees, and lumbo-pelvic hip girdle function more effectively.

How to perform

1. Place your right leg up on a bench or chair, with your leg straight and both feet aligned forward.
2. Pull the right side of your pelvis back and away from the right foot as you dorsiflex the right foot.
3. Switch legs and repeat on the left leg.

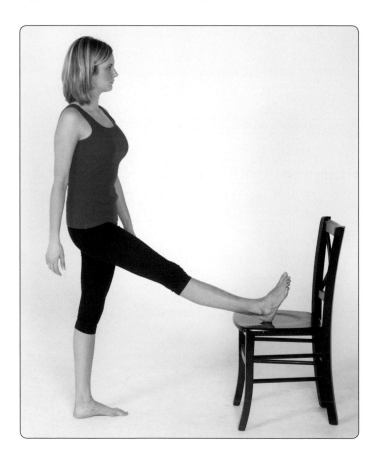

Duration and repetitions: Hold the stretch for 20 to 30 seconds, and repeat 2 to 3 cycles on each leg at least once a day.

Tip: The quadriceps muscles are antagonists of the hamstrings. Isometrically contracting the quadriceps during this stretch will help the hamstrings to release.

Precaution: Do not hyperextend the knee when activating the quadriceps.

Progress: Rotate the torso to the right by reaching the left hand over the right knee, and vice versa when stretching the other leg.

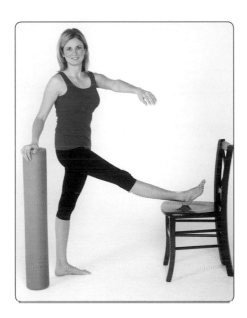

Regress: Perform this stretch lying down by placing the foot up on the corner of a wall or on a door frame. Rotate your torso for maximum benefit.

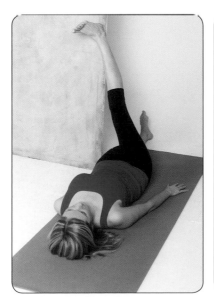 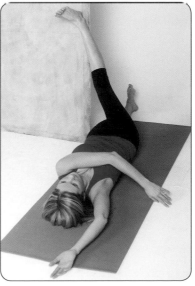

Glute Stretch

Area(s) of body: Lumbo-pelvic hip girdle

Imbalance(s): Anterior pelvic tilt, excessive lumbar lordosis, valgus knee position, and overpronation

Structures addressed: Gluteus maximus muscle and, to a lesser extent, other abductor muscles and hip rotators (e.g., piriformis).

Exercise benefits: Improving the flexibility of the gluteal muscles will enable them to work better eccentrically to assist with slowing down hip flexion during movements like squatting. This can prevent the pelvis from rotating too far down at the front and can prevent the lower back from arching too much. Healthy gluteal muscles also help to slow down the internal rotation of the leg, thereby controlling movement of the knee toward the midline and helping prevent a valgus knee position and overpronation.

How to perform

1. Sit on the floor with one leg straight out in front; bend the other leg at the knee and cross it over the straight leg.
2. Place the crossed foot flat on the floor and gently pull the bent knee toward the chest.
3. Be sure to keep the glute being stretched flat on the floor and do not let it rise up.

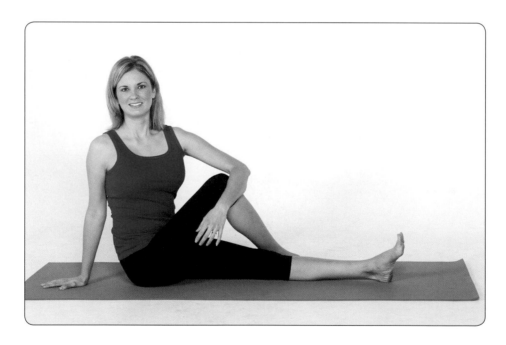

Duration and repetitions: Stretch each side for 20 to 30 seconds at least once per day.

Tip: Keep your torso upright and shoulders level while performing this stretch to maximize effectiveness.

Progress: Perform the Lunge With Knee Pull.

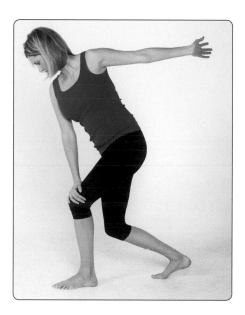

Regress: Use a countertop or bench to support the stretching leg.

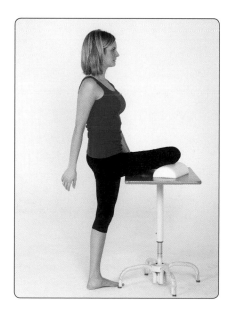

Piriformis Stretch

Area(s) of body: Lumbo-pelvic hip girdle

Imbalance(s): Anterior pelvic tilt and valgus knee position

Structures addressed: Piriformis muscle and hip rotator muscles

Exercise benefits: People who have overpronated feet usually have weak glutes. Consequently, the much smaller piriformis muscle (and other hip rotators) may try to take over the function of the glutes, and it can become irritated as a result. Releasing the piriformis (and other deep hip rotator muscles) and then strengthening the glutes can help improve the function of the entire hip and leg complex.

How to perform

1. Sit down on the floor and place your right ankle on your left knee.
2. Let the right side of the pelvis drop away from the right shoulder.
3. Hold the stretch to help release the piriformis and other hip rotator muscles.
4. Repeat with your other leg.

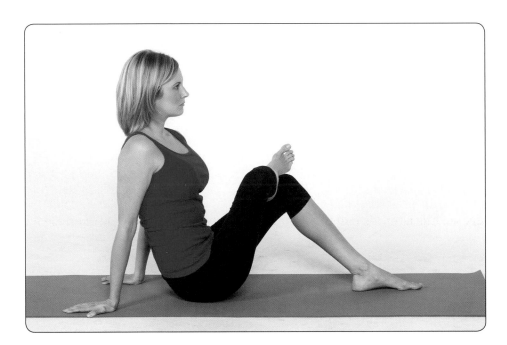

Duration and repetitions: Hold the stretch for 20 to 30 seconds at least once a day.

Tip: The sciatic nerve runs over, under, or through the piriformis muscle (depending on the individual). An irritated piriformis muscle is often responsible for the pain and symptoms of sciatica.

Precaution: If discomfort is felt in the groin area, ease off or stop performing this stretch.

Progress: Perform The Pivot.

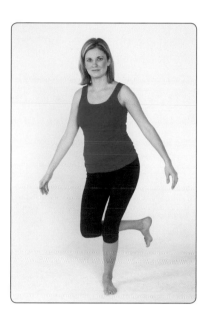

Regress: Use a tennis ball to massage the glutes, or perform the exercise lying down.

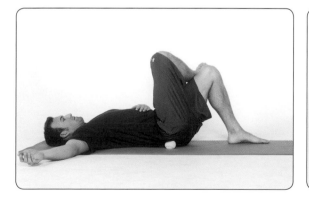
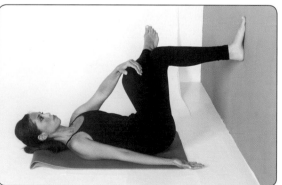

Abductor Stretch

Area(s) of body: Lumbo-pelvic hip girdle

Imbalance(s): Overpronation and valgus knee position

Structures addressed: Abductor muscles

Exercise benefits: This exercise helps increase the flexibility of the abductor muscles so that they can work more effectively to control the movement of the femur toward the midline of the body during weight-bearing activities like lunging and walking.

How to perform

1. Lie on your back with your knees bent and a pillow under your head.
2. Let one knee drop toward the midline of the body while ensuring that the pelvis on that side does not move excessively.
3. Place the ankle of the other leg over the knee that is toward the midline, and gently push down on the knee to increase the stretch.
4. Keep the pelvis level and flat on the ground during the stretch.
5. Repeat on the opposite side.

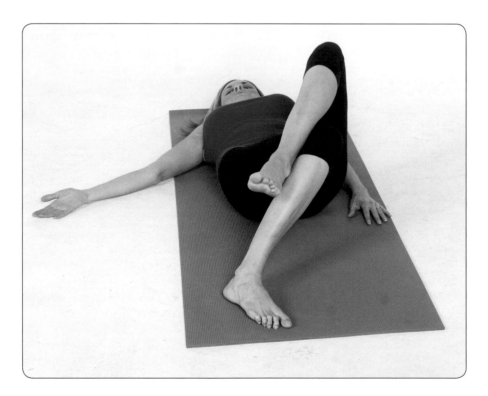

Duration and repetitions: Stretch each side for 20 to 30 seconds at least once per day.

Tip: Be sure to keep the back of the hips pressed into the floor while shifting the knee toward the midline. This stretch should be felt on the outside of the leg and hip.

Precaution: If pain is felt in the groin or lower back, regress or discontinue the stretch.

Progress: Raise the arm on the side that is being stretched over your head or perform the Lunge With Side Reach.

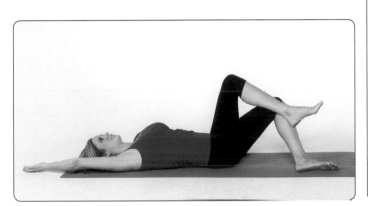

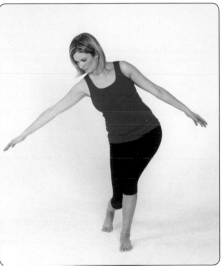

Regress: Perform the Tennis Ball Side of Hip or the Foam Roller IT Band.

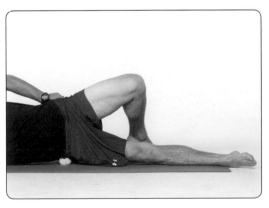

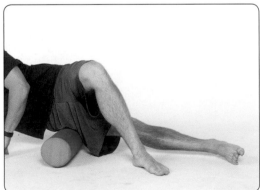

Adductor Stretch

Area(s) of body: Lumbo-pelvic hip girdle

Imbalance(s): Valgus knee position and excessive lumbar lordosis

Structures addressed: Adductor muscles

Exercise benefits: This exercise helps increase the flexibility of the adductor muscles so they can work more effectively during weight-bearing activities to control the movement of the leg and hip as they go into extension (to help prevent excessive lumbar lordosis) and the movement of the leg as it internally rotates when the foot is in contact with the ground (to help prevent a valgus knee position).

How to perform

1. Sit on the floor with your left leg straight and placed away from the midline of the body (abducted) and your left foot dorsiflexed.
2. Bend the right knee and place the sole of your right foot next to the inside of the left knee.
3. Sit upright, and do not bend the spine to the side.
4. Repeat on opposite side.

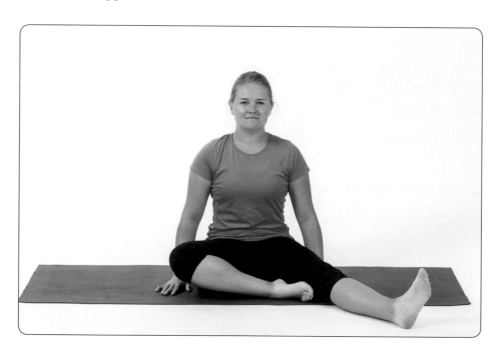

Duration and repetitions: Stretch each side for 20 to 30 seconds at least once per day.

Tip: Try to feel your "sit bones" (ischial tuberosities) in contact with the floor, and keep the pressure even as you perform the stretch. This will help keep the pelvis in the right place.

Precaution: If pain is felt in the knee, bend the leg that is straight slightly until you can progress to the point that the knee can be kept straight.

Progress: Bend forward at the hips, reaching the opposite hand toward the outstretched leg, or perform the Side Lunge With Rotation.

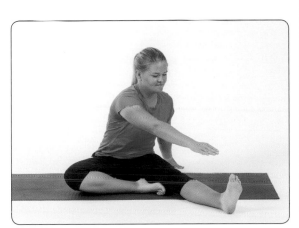 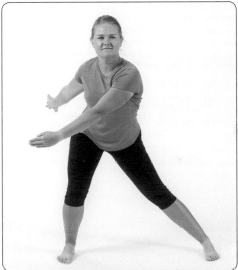

Regress: Foam Roller on Inner Thigh.

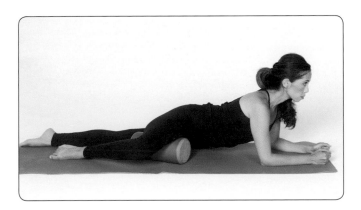

Lower Back Stretch

Area(s) of body: Lumbo-pelvic hip girdle

Imbalance(s): Excessive lumbar lordosis and anterior pelvic tilt

Structures addressed: Lumbar erector spinae muscles; also activates abdominals when contracted to assist with stretch

Exercise benefits: Releasing the lumbar erectors will enable the pelvis to posteriorly rotate and the lumbar spine to flex effectively.

How to perform

1. Sit on the floor with knees bent and feet forward.
2. Grab the backs of the knees, posteriorly tilt the pelvis, and lean forward to round the lower back.
3. The stretch should be felt in the muscles of the lower back.

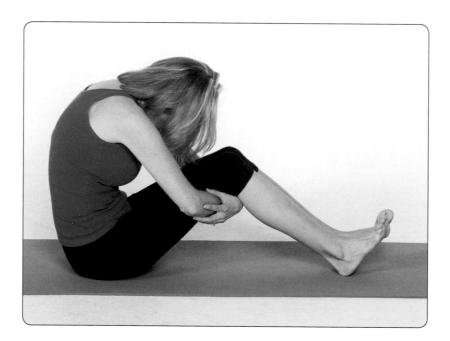

Duration and repetitions: Hold the stretch for 15 to 20 seconds. Repeat 2 to 3 cycles at least once a day.

Tip: Activate the abdominals to posteriorly tilt the pelvis and help flex the lumbar spine.

Precaution: People who have lower back pain should perform this stretch very gently and only once they are warmed up sufficiently. Discontinue immediately if any pain is felt.

Progress: Perform this exercise standing by bending forward toward the toes.

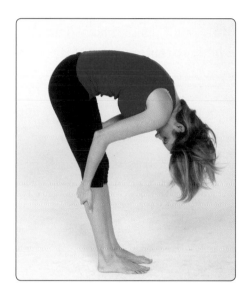

Regress: Perform the exercise lying supine by hugging the knees to the chest.

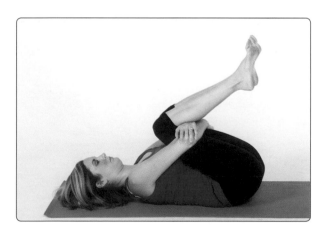

Lying Rotation Stretch

Area(s) of body: Lumbo-pelvic hip girdle

Imbalance(s): Excessive lumbar lordosis and excessive thoracic kyphosis

Structures addressed: Internal and external obliques, biceps, and pectorals

Exercise benefits: This exercise helps increase the flexibility of the oblique muscles to improve trunk and spine rotation. Sufficient trunk rotation helps prevent excessive lumbar lordosis and excessive thoracic kyphosis by encouraging the spine to rotate correctly during movements such as walking, hitting a golf ball, running, or throwing a Frisbee.

How to perform

1. Lie on your back, with knees bent and lifted up over your stomach.
2. Place a foam roller or pillow between the knees to minimize any potential for lower back discomfort.
3. Drop the knees to the left side of the body while keeping the shoulder blades, arms, and the palm of the right hand flat on the floor.
4. Turn your head in the direction of your legs.
5. Keep your hips bent to 90 degrees, and do not let the lower back arch.
6. Repeat the stretch on the opposite side.

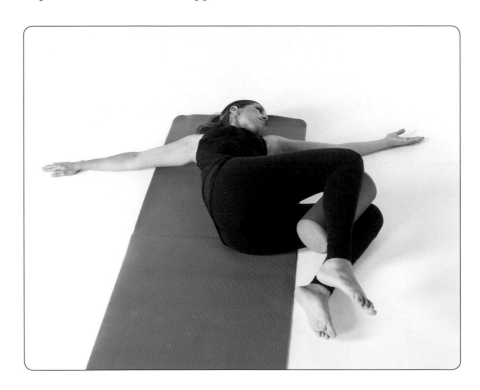

Duration and repetitions: Hold the stretch for 15 to 20 seconds. Repeat 2 to 3 cycles at least once a day.

Tip: Keep the pelvis tilted, and encourage clients to relax their breathing during this stretch.

Precaution: If pain is felt in the lower back, increase the thickness of the support prop between the legs. If pain is felt in the shoulder or chest, turn both palms up.

Progress: Remove the foam roller or pillow from between the legs, or perform the Wall Rotation Stretch.

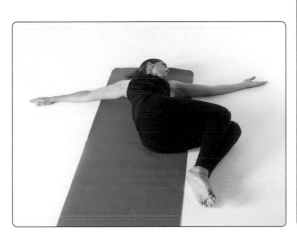
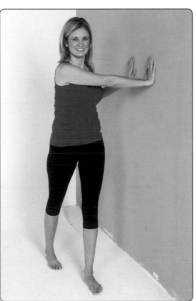

Regress: Perform the Foam Roller Thoracic Spine or Abdominal Massage.

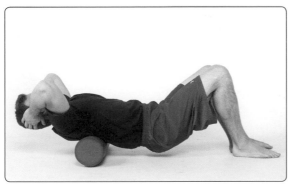
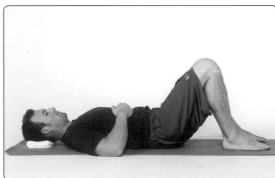

Hip Flexor Stretch (Sagittal)

Area(s) of body: Lumbo-pelvic hip girdle

Imbalance(s): Anterior pelvic tilt, excessive lumbar lordosis

Structures addressed: Hip flexor muscle group; also activates and strengthens the gluteus maximus and abdominals when isometrically contracted during stretch

Exercise benefits: Stretching tight or restricted hip flexors enables the lumbar spine to flex more easily, thereby reducing excessive lumbar lordosis. This in turn helps the pelvis to rotate posteriorly and addresses an anterior pelvic tilt.

How to perform

1. Kneel down on your right knee with your left foot forward; tuck the pelvis under using the glutes and abdominals to assist with this motion.

2. Align the hips straight from front to back, and then tuck the right hip in from the side (to keep the pelvis and hips in correct alignment); this stretch should be felt in the front of the hip (on top of the right leg).

3. Repeat on the opposite side.

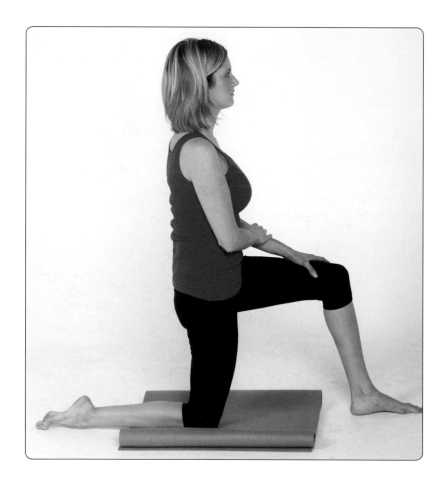

Duration and repetitions: Hold this stretch for 15 to 20 seconds, and repeat 2 to 3 cycles on each side at least once per day.

Tip: Make sure the hip stays tucked in and under by activating the glutes to keep the lumbo-pelvic hip girdle in good alignment.

Precaution: Avoid arching the lower back when you lift your arm overhead to progress the stretch.

Progress: Extend your right arm over your head (if your left foot is forward) and vice versa, or perform the Door Frame Stretch.

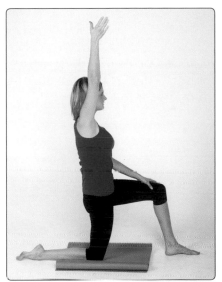 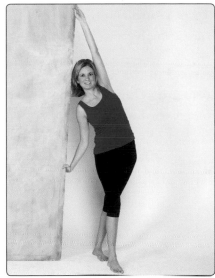

Regress: Round your lower back during the stretch, and use the rectus abdominis muscle to help tilt the pelvis under.

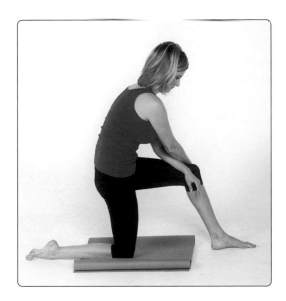

Hip Flexor Stretch (Frontal)

Area(s) of body: Lumbo-pelvic hip girdle

Imbalance(s): Anterior pelvic tilt, excessive lumbar lordosis, and valgus knee position

Structures addressed: Hip flexor muscles, quadratus lumborum, obliques; also activates and strengthens gluteus maximus and abdominals

Exercise benefits: Stretching the hip flexors in the frontal plane (i.e., from side to side) helps the pelvis, hips, and legs to move laterally more easily to take stress off the lower back and knees as weight is transferred from left to right during activities like walking and running.

How to perform

1. Kneel down on one knee; tuck the pelvis under using the glutes and abdominals to assist with this motion.
2. Raise your arm over your head on the same side as the kneeling leg, and reach over the head toward the opposite side of the body.
3. Repeat on opposite side.

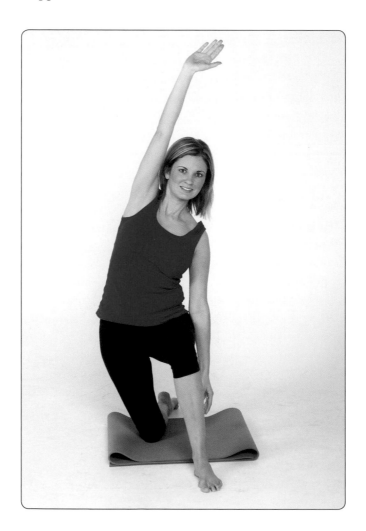

Duration and repetitions: Hold the stretch for 15 to 20 seconds, and repeat 2 to 3 cycles on each side at least once per day.

Tip: If there is difficulty activating the glute, try rounding the lower back to help activate this muscle.

Progress: Perform the Door Frame Stretch or the Gluteal Activation Over Ball.

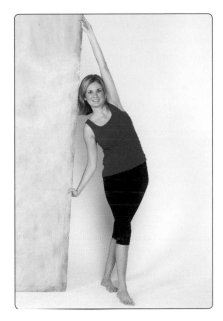

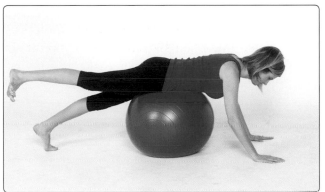

Regress: Do not raise the arm over the head.

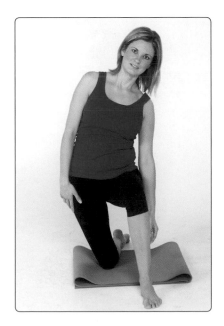

Hip Flexor Stretch (Transverse)

Area(s) of body: Lumbo-pelvic hip girdle

Imbalance(s): Valgus knee position, anterior pelvic tilt, excessive lumbar lordosis, and excessive thoracic kyphosis

Structures addressed: Hip flexor muscles and obliques; also activates and strengthens gluteus maximus and abdominals

Exercise benefits: As the hip and leg go into extension during activities like walking and running, the torso rotates over the front leg. The flexibility of the hip flexors in the transverse plane (i.e., in rotation) helps displace stress correctly through the legs, the lumbo-pelvic hip girdle, and the thoracic spine.

How to perform

1. Kneel down on one knee; tuck the pelvis under using the glutes and abdominals to assist with this motion.
2. Rotate your arms across your chest; make sure your body does not shift to the right or left.
3. Rotate the upper torso across the front leg; keep your head facing straight ahead; extend your arms to achieve a greater stretch.
4. Keep your shoulders level during the stretch.
5. Repeat on the opposite side.

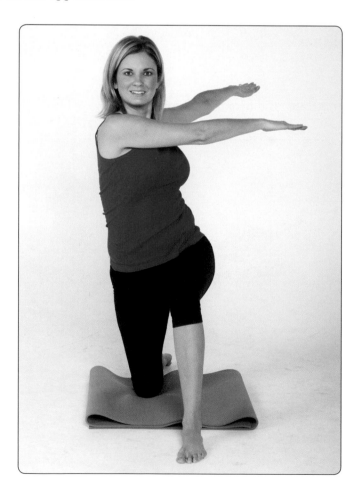

Duration and repetitions: Hold the stretch for 15 to 20 seconds, and repeat 2 to 3 cycles on each side at least once per day.

Tip: If you feel pressure on the kneecap during this exercise, place a pad or mat under the knee.

Progress: Perform the Wall Rotation Stretch.

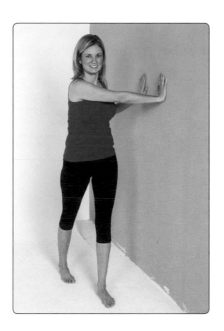

Regress: Perform the Foam Roller Hip Flexors.

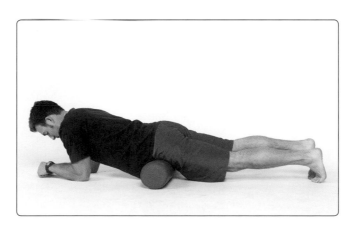

Door Frame Stretch

Area(s) of body: Lumbo-pelvic hip girdle and thoracic spine

Imbalance(s): Tracking problems of the knee, excessive lumbar lordosis, and excessive thoracic kyphosis

Structures addressed: Iliotibial band, abductors, obliques, latissimus dorsi, and quadratus lumborum

Exercise benefits: This exercise helps increase the flexibility of many of the muscles that help facilitate side-to-side movement of the legs, hips, and spine (and rotation of the trunk) to improve the function of the entire kinetic chain.

How to perform

1. Stand in a door frame; reach one arm over your head and grasp the side of the frame above head level; place the other hand lower on the frame at thigh level.
2. Tuck the foot farthest from the hands behind the other foot; push the hips away from the hands to stretch the side of your body that is away from the door frame.
3. To increase the stretch, gently rotate the sternum under the arm that is overhead while preventing the hips from rotating.
4. Repeat on the opposite side.

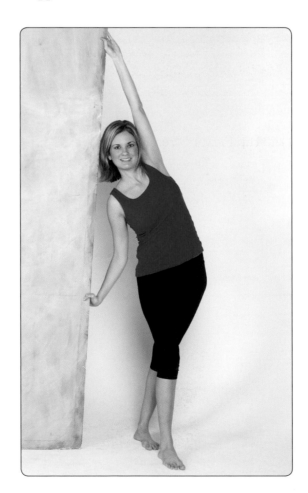

Duration and repetitions: Stretch each side for 10 to 15 seconds, and repeat the cycle 2 to 3 times at least once per day.

Tip: To maximize the effectiveness of this exercise, keep your pelvis tucked under and extend your torso upright from the thoracic spine and rib cage.

Precaution: If discomfort is felt in the lower back during this exercise, place the feet hip width apart rather than crossing them over each other.

Progress: Perform the Straight Arm Raise or the Lunge With Arm Raise.

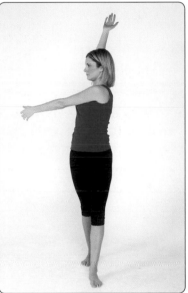

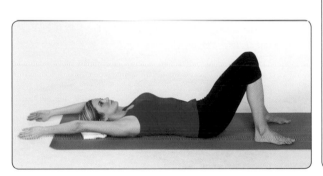

Regress: Perform the Hip Flexor Stretch (Frontal).

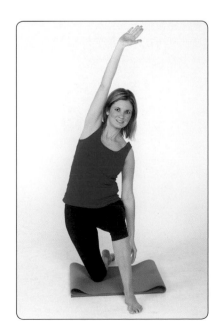

Chest Stretch

Area(s) of body: Thoracic spine and shoulder girdle

Imbalance(s): Excessive thoracic kyphosis, protracted shoulder girdle, elevated scapula, and internally rotated arms

Structures addressed: Stretches the pectorals; also activates and strengthens the rhomboids and lower fibers of the trapezius when contracted isometrically to assist with the exercise

Exercise benefits: Increasing the flexibility of the pectoral muscles and subsequently strengthening the shoulder retractors and depressors (e.g., rhomboids and lower trapezius) will help to retract and depress the shoulder blades, externally rotate the arms, and allow the thoracic spine to extend effectively.

How to perform

1. Stand about 2 feet away from a wall with the body turned 90 degrees away from the wall.
2. Reach your left hand behind your body, and place the palm flat on the wall.
3. Pull the left shoulder blade back and down to feel the stretch in the front of the left shoulder and chest.
4. Repeat on the opposite side.

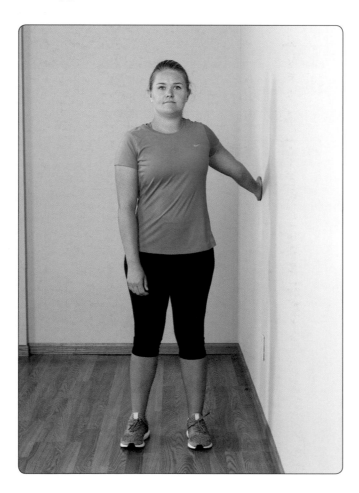

Duration and repetitions: Hold the stretch for 15 to 20 seconds, and repeat 2 to 3 cycles on each side at least once per day.

Tip: Massaging the pectoral muscles while performing this stretch will help increase the effectiveness of this exercise. This stretch can also be performed in a door frame.

Progress: Perform the Wave Goodbye or the Seated Row.

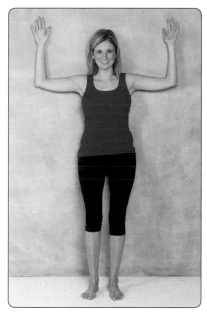 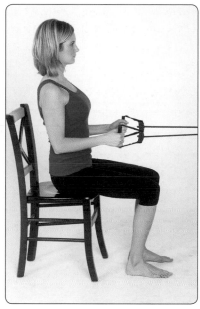

Regress: Perform Chest Massage.

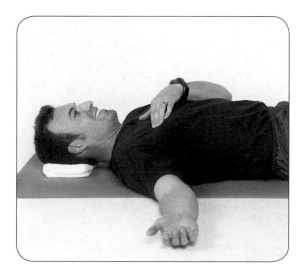

Biceps Stretch

Area(s) of body: Thoracic spine and shoulder girdle

Imbalance(s): Elevated scapula and protracted shoulder girdle

Structures addressed: Biceps muscles

Exercise benefits: Imbalances of the shoulder girdle can cause the biceps to become tight and restricted, thereby compounding movement issues in this area. Increasing the flexibility of these muscles (especially the biceps brachii, as it originates on the scapula) will enable the shoulder blades to retract and depress to achieve better alignment of the glenohumeral joint.

How to perform

1. Face away from a high countertop or a window sill; rotate one arm behind you and place your hand (thumb side down) on the surface, keeping the arm straight.
2. Pull your shoulder back and down and bend your knees until you feel a stretch in the biceps.
3. Repeat on the other side.

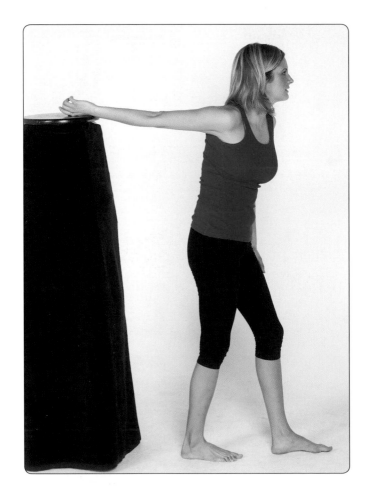

Duration and repetitions: Stretch each arm for 20 to 30 seconds at least once per day.

Tip: This exercise is great for people who have their elbows bent throughout the day, like those who type on a computer or drive for many hours.

Progress: Make a fist around the thumb and pronate the wrist (i.e., bend and turn it inward) to include the muscles and fascia of the forearm and wrist in this stretch.

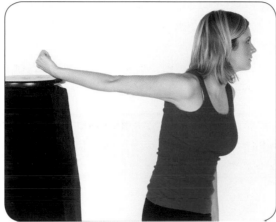

Regress: Perform the Tennis Ball on Biceps or the Lying Front of Shoulder Stretch.

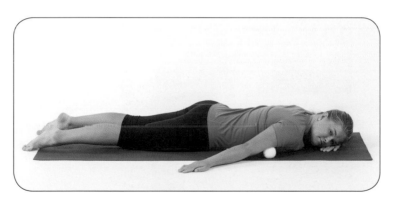

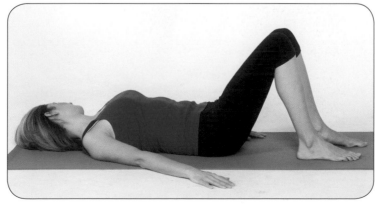

Why Stretch

Area(s) of body: Thoracic spine and shoulder girdle

Imbalance(s): Excessive thoracic kyphosis, elevated scapula, protracted shoulder girdle, and internally rotated arms

Structures addressed: Subscapularis and pectorals; also activates and strengthens the rhomboids, lower trapezius, infraspinatus, and teres minor

Exercise benefits: This exercise helps correct muscle imbalances in the thoracic spine, shoulder girdle, and arm (the glenohumeral joint) by stretching the chest and the front of the shoulder while strengthening the rhomboids, lower trapezius (traps), and external rotators of the shoulder and arm.

How to perform

1. Stand upright, with your pelvis tilted posteriorly and your arms externally rotated out to the sides.
2. Contract the rhomboids and external rotators of the arm to help pull the arms and shoulders back while activating the lower traps to help pull the shoulders down.

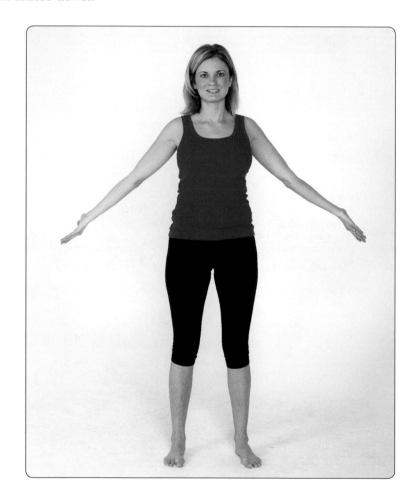

Duration and repetitions: Hold the stretch for 20 to 30 seconds, and repeat the cycle 2 to 3 times on each side at least once per day.

Tip: This stretch can also be done while seated at a desk chair by hanging the arms to the side.

Precaution: Keep your pelvis posteriorly tilted throughout this exercise to ensure that the movement is not initiated through the lower back.

Progress: Perform the Shoulder Retraction on Floor exercise.

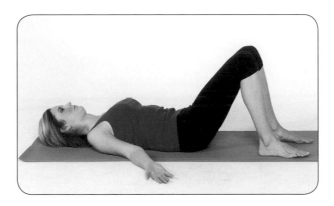

Regress: Perform the Front of Shoulder Massage or Chest Massage.

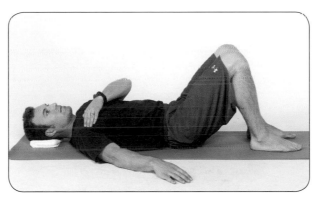

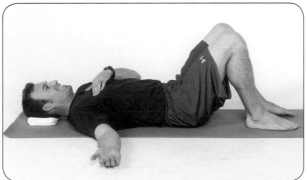

Lying Front of Shoulder Stretch

Imbalance(s): Protracted shoulder girdle, elevated scapula, and internally rotated arms

Structures addressed: Front of shoulder, pectorals, and biceps; also activates and strengthens rhomboids and lower trapezius

Exercise benefits: This exercise helps increase flexibility of the muscles in the front of the shoulder and arm. Increased flexibility in this area will enable the arm to rotate correctly in the shoulder joint while the scapula remains in the correct position on the rib cage.

How to perform

1. Lie on your back with knees bent; use a pillow to keep your head and neck neutral, if needed.

2. Place one arm slightly away from the body on the floor palm down; keep the arm straight.

3. Use the muscles that retract and depress the shoulder blades (the rhomboids and lower trapezius) to gently pull the shoulder back and down toward the floor until a stretch is felt in the front of the shoulder and the top of the arm.

4. A neck stretch can be incorporated into this exercise by turning your head away from the shoulder being stretched.

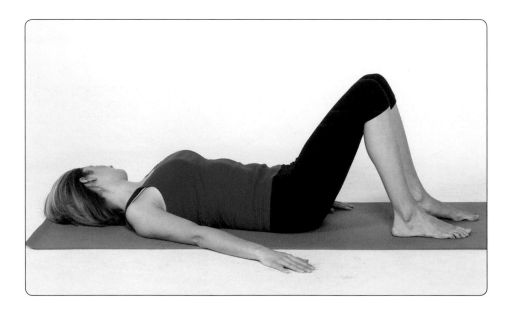

Duration and repetitions: Stretch each side for 15 to 20 seconds, and repeat the cycle 2 to 3 times at least once per day.

Tip: Massaging the front of the shoulder, chest, biceps, and forearm before performing this stretch is highly recommended to improve the effectiveness of this exercise.

Precaution: If pain is felt in the front of the shoulder, turn the palm slightly upward during this stretch.

Progress: Bend your elbow and place the hand of the side you are stretching under the lower back to increase the stretch.

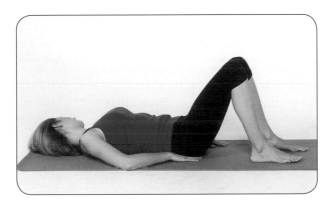

Regress: Perform the Front of Shoulder Massage or the Biceps Stretch.

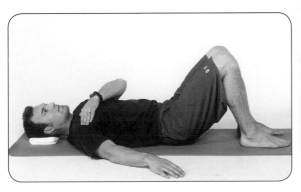

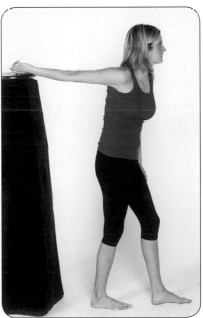

Neck Extensors Stretch

Area(s) of body: Head and neck

Imbalance(s): Excessive cervical lordosis

Structures addressed: Neck extensors; also strengthens the neck flexors

Exercise benefits: This exercise helps release tightness in the neck extensors caused by excessive cervical lordosis. This stretch can also be progressed to activate and strengthen the neck flexors.

How to perform

1. Place your hands on the crown of your head, keep your elbows together, and pull your shoulders down using the lower traps.

2. Pull your chin to your chest to feel the stretch in the back of the neck and shoulders.

3. This exercise can be performed either standing or while seated.

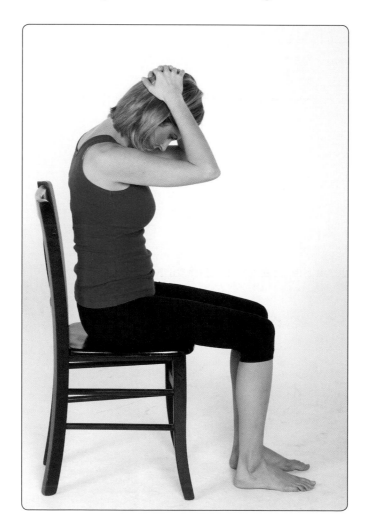

Duration and repetitions: Hold the stretch for 15 to 20 seconds, and repeat the cycle 2 to 3 times at least once per day.

Tip: The neck flexors can also be activated during this stretch (which will help relax the neck extensors) by dropping the arms and actively pulling your chin to your chest.

Precaution: Perform this exercise slowly. Discontinue immediately if any pain or discomfort is felt in the neck.

Progress: Perform Neck Flexion (Lying) or (Seated).

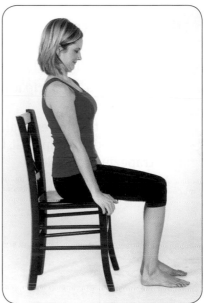

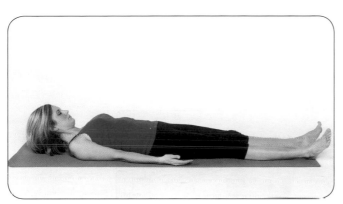

Regress: Perform the Theracane Back of Neck.

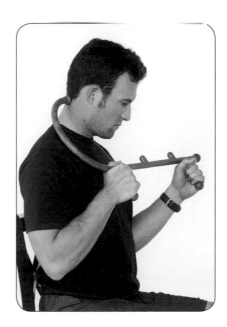

Palm on Wall Stretch

Area(s) of body: Thoracic spine and shoulder girdle, neck, and head

Imbalance(s): Internally rotated arms, protracted shoulder girdle, and elevated scapula

Structures addressed: Upper fibers of trapezius, biceps, and flexors of the hand and wrist; also activates and strengthens the rhomboids and the lower fibers of the trapezius

Exercise benefits: This exercise helps increase the flexibility of the muscles of the arm and shoulder while stabilizing the scapula to help improve the function of the glenohumeral joint and shoulder girdle.

How to perform

1. Stand beside a wall with your arm extended out to the side and your palm flat on the wall; spread your fingers slightly and hold the shoulder back and down.
2. Try to straighten your arm fully; do not let the shoulder come up and forward.

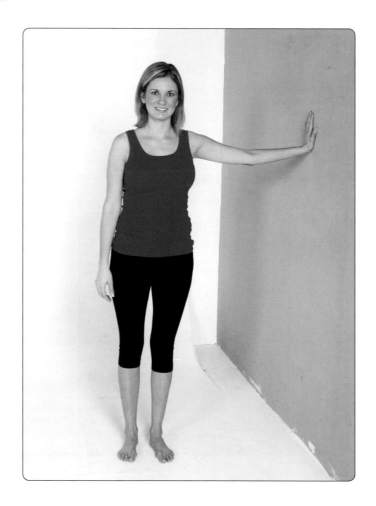

Duration and repetitions: Stretch each side for 15 to 20 seconds, and repeat the cycle 2 to 3 times on each side at least once per day.

Tip: This stretch may be felt in a number of places (i.e., hand, wrist, forearm, biceps, or the underside of the upper arm). Make a note of where the stretch is felt the most, and perform self-myofascial release techniques to help release those areas before repeating the stretch.

Progress: Rotate the arm forward (internally) while stabilizing the scapula.

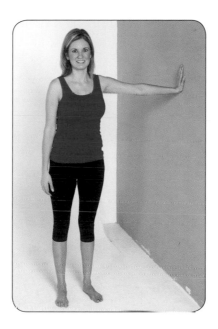

Regress: Turn your body toward the wall to decrease the stretch, or perform Forearm Massage.

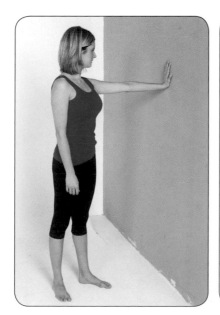
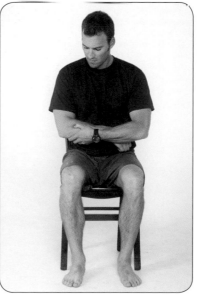

Forearm Stretch

Area(s) of body: Thoracic spine and shoulder girdle

Imbalance(s): Internally rotated arms, protracted shoulder girdle

Structures addressed: Forearm muscles

Exercise benefits: Increasing flexibility in the forearm and wrist will help the entire arm be able to function better without compensations occurring at the shoulder.

How to perform

1. Extend your arms out in front of your body; keep them straight, and cradle the back of one hand in the other.
2. Gently bend the wrist and fingers of the hand being held toward the torso until a stretch is felt in the outside of the forearm.

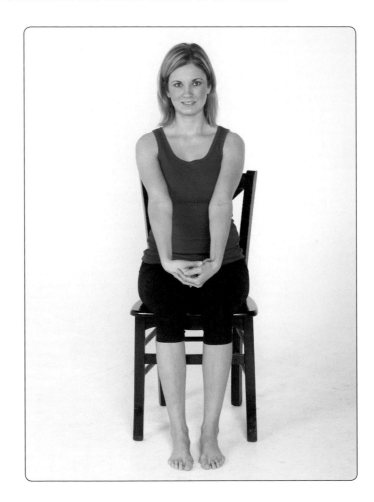

Duration and repetitions: Stretch each side for 20 to 30 seconds, and repeat the cycle 2 to 3 times at least once per day.

Tip: Keep your shoulders back and down to maximize the effectiveness of this exercise.

Progress: Rotate the forearm internally to increase the stretch.

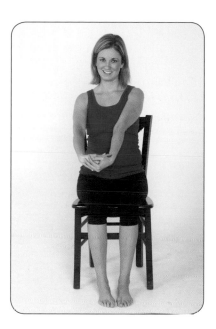

Regress: Perform Forearm Massage.

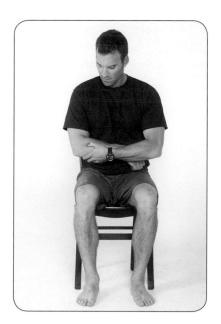

Wall Rotation Stretch

Area(s) of body: Entire kinetic chain

Imbalance(s): Lack of dorsiflexion, anterior pelvic tilt, excessive lumbar lordosis, excessive thoracic kyphosis, and protracted shoulder girdle

Structures addressed: Gastrocnemius, hip flexors, abdominals, pectorals, and latissimus dorsi; also activates and strengthens the gluteus maximus, spinal erectors, rhomboids, and lower fibers of the trapezius

Exercise benefits: This stretch mimics many body movements that are required for correct walking and running mechanics. It increases the flexibility of the ankle (to improve dorsiflexion), the flexibility of the hips (to improve pelvis and lumbar spine function), and the flexibility of the trunk and scapula (to improve spine and shoulder function). It is a great progression for combining and coordinating the entire kinetic chain.

How to perform

1. Stand sideways to a wall in a split stance with the foot that is closer to the wall forward.
2. Rotate the upper torso toward the wall, but keep the head, hips, legs, and feet facing straight forward.
3. Place both palms flat against the wall.
4. Hold the stretch without lifting the heels off the ground or shifting the spine or hips to the side.

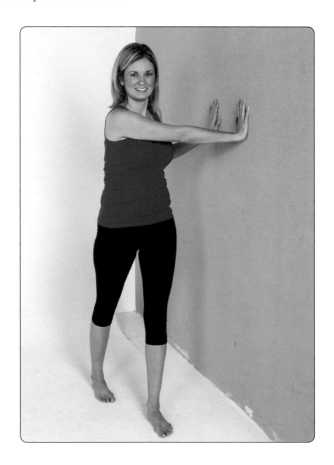

Duration and repetitions: Stretch each side for 15 to 20 seconds, and repeat the cycle 2 to 3 times at least once per day.

Tip: If there is difficulty remembering which foot to put forward when doing this stretch, simply mimic the movement of walking by rotating the torso and arms over the front leg.

Precaution: Holding your breath during this stretch may cause muscle cramping and tension around the torso. It is important to relax and breathe continuously when performing this exercise.

Progress: Perform the Lunge To Step Up (with Rotation).

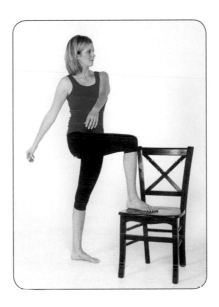

Regress: Perform the Hip Flexor Stretch (Transverse) or Two Tennis Balls on Upper Back.

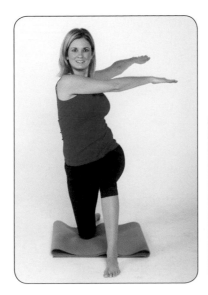

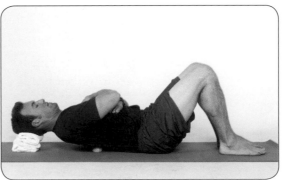

Review of Key Points

Stretching exercises are introduced into a corrective exercise program once the client has performed the self-myofascial release techniques required to rejuvenate and regenerate unhealthy muscles and fascia.

- Stretches introduce range of motion to joints, muscles, and other soft tissues in preparation for the strengthening phase of a corrective exercise program.

- Introduce stretching exercises gradually into a client's program. Previous experiences of pain, muscle tension, joint inflammation, guarding, and movement restrictions can all influence the types and intensity of stretches needed.

- There are many ways to regress and progress a client's stretching program, such as adding or removing balance aids and incorporating or excluding other body parts.

- Use your knowledge of functional anatomy to select appropriate stretches, and teach clients where they should feel each stretch.

- Use stretching cautiously with clients who have chronic musculoskeletal imbalances, arthritis, osteoporosis, or a history of steroid use, or who have recently had surgery or an injury.

- Do not try to stretch tissues surrounding a broken bone, areas that have sustained trauma, or joints or soft tissues that are acutely inflamed.

Self-Check

It is crucial to know how and when to progress a client's corrective exercise program from self-myofascial release techniques to stretching exercises. Following are examples of musculoskeletal problems and appropriate self-myofascial release techniques. In the second column, identify a suitable stretching exercise for each client to progress to, and briefly explain why you selected that stretch. The first situation has been completed as an example.

Client situation/imbalance with appropriate self-myofascial release technique identified	Recommended stretch
A client has pain at the front of her ankle when she walks long distances. Your assessment reveals that she has limited dorsiflexion. She has been performing a Calf Massage.	Calf Stretch (standing). Increasing flexibility of the calf muscles in a weight-bearing situation will enable the lower leg to come forward over the foot and improve the client's ability to dorsiflex, thereby eliminating pain in the front of her ankle when she walks.
A client experiences neck pain at the end of a long day sitting at his computer. Your assessment reveals that he has excessive cervical lordosis. He has been performing Theracane on Back of Neck.	
A client gets pain on the inside of her right knee after she plays tennis. Your assessment reveals that she has overpronated feet. She has been performing the Golf Ball Roll.	
A client complains of lower back pain after playing golf. Your assessment reveals that he has an anterior pelvic tilt. He has been performing the Foam Roller on Gluteal Complex.	

CHAPTER 21

Strengthening Exercises

Strengthening exercises are the ultimate progression of a client's corrective exercise program. They are only introduced after the regular application of stretching and self myofascial release techniques to soft tissue structures (Clark and Lucett 2011; Price 2013; Price and Bratcher 2010). Strengthening exercises help recondition, retrain, and build up soft tissue structures that have been hampered by imbalances. The goal is to retrain the neuromuscular, myofascial, and musculoskeletal systems to correct problems and safeguard the body from future harm (Hoffman 2014; Houglum 2016).

Selecting, designing, progressing, and regressing a corrective strengthening program appropriately will help improve stability, increase mobility, and restore coordination to previously painful and injured parts (McGill 2016; Price and Bratcher 2010). Musculoskeletal imbalances can lead to compensations and dysfunctional movement patterns that will affect how people perform their strengthening exercises (Clark and Lucett 2011). So you must choose exercises that are within your clients' abilities and make sure that they do them correctly. Otherwise, existing musculoskeletal imbalances could be exacerbated, or the wrong soft tissue structures could be stimulated (Price and Bratcher 2010).

STRENGTHENING EXERCISE QUICK TIPS

Following is a recap of strategies that you can use to introduce your clients to strengthening exercises.

- While it is extremely important to make sure clients perform their exercises correctly and safely, give them the latitude to make small mistakes when they first try a new exercise. This will enable you to offer feedback and help them to learn how to correct their technique and make future improvements (Coyle 2009).

- Use visual, verbal, and kinesthetic teaching cues to adapt your instruction style to your clients' learning styles (Wrisberg 2007).

- Always explain why you are recommending a particular strengthening exercise. Emphasize how each strengthening exercise builds on the self-myofascial release techniques and stretching exercises a client has already performed.

- Regress a strengthening exercise if a client experiences discomfort performing the movement, has difficulty performing the exercise correctly, or experiences excessive soreness after a session (Bryant and Green 2010).

- Regress a strengthening exercise by introducing a less challenging movement, incorporating props such as balance aids, or revisiting a self-myofascial release or stretching exercise.

- Progress a strengthening program if a client has reached a certain level of proficiency, needs to combine exercises to save time, or has made more ambitious goals.

- Progress a strengthening exercise by introducing a more dynamic movement, using fewer props, adding external loads to the movement, or incorporating multiple planes of movement (Magee, Zachazewski, and Quillen 2007; Price and Bratcher 2010).

Reminder

Review the comprehensive information on teaching tips, progressions and regressions, and when *not* to use strengthening exercises provided in chapter 17 before introducing any of the exercises in this chapter into a client's corrective exercise program.

STRENGTHENING EXERCISE LIBRARY

The strengthening exercises highlighted in this chapter are designed to be progressive (i.e., from isolated to integrated, concentric to eccentric, single joint to multijoint, one plane to multiple planes, and open chain to closed chain) and easy to perform in a gym setting, at home, at the office, or when traveling, with little or no equipment required.

Big Toe Pushdowns

Area(s) of body: Feet and ankles, knees

Imbalance(s): Overpronation, valgus knee position, and lack of dorsiflexion

Structures addressed: Structures that make up the medial longitudinal arch of the foot, specifically flexor hallucis longus

Exercise benefits: Habitual overpronation can put excessive stress on the structures of the medial side of the foot and ankle, particularly the medial longitudinal arch. This exercise strengthens the structures that help support this arch to help the foot resist overpronation, promote dorsiflexion, and slow down the knee as it moves toward the midline of the body.

How to perform

1. Stand with your feet facing forward, and raise the medial longitudinal arch to create a neutral position of the feet and ankles (i.e., the weight will shift slightly toward the outside of the foot).

2. Align the toes so they are straight, and push the big toe down toward the floor without "scrunching" the other toes.

3. Perform this exercise isometrically at first, then add movement by gently rocking forward and backward, using the big toe as a braking mechanism to control the body weight as it moves over the foot.

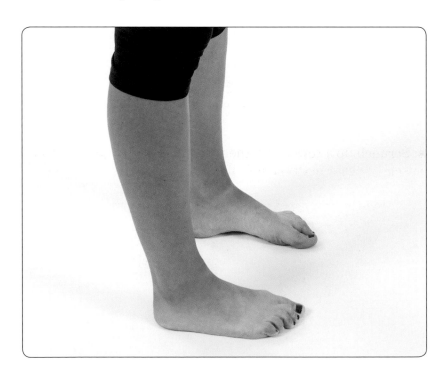

Duration and repetitions: Perform an isometric contraction for 20 to 30 seconds, and repeat 2 to 3 times at least once per day, progressing to dynamic movements of 10 to 15 repetitions.

Tip: When you perform this exercise correctly, you should feel the muscles under the arch working as the big toe is pushed down.

Precaution: Progress this exercise gradually to avoid overtaxing the muscles because this could lead to cramping.

Progress: Rock the body back and forward over the feet.

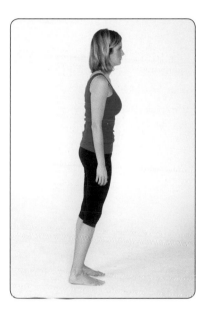

Regress: Scrunch up a towel with the toes to help activate the flexor hallucis longus muscle or perform the Golf Ball Roll.

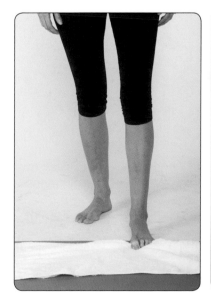 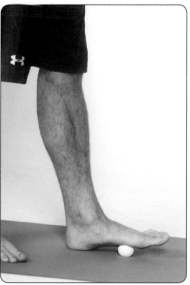

Lying Pelvic Tilt

Area(s) of body: Lumbo-pelvic hip girdle

Imbalance(s): Anterior pelvic tilt, excessive lumbar lordosis

Structures addressed: Rectus abdominis, gluteus maximus, and hamstrings

Exercise benefits: This exercise helps to strengthen muscles that flex the lumbar spine and posteriorly rotate the pelvis, for the purpose of helping to mobilize this area and promote better movement.

How to perform

1. Lie on the floor with your knees bent.
2. Flatten your lower back by tilting the pelvis under, and contract the abdominals to pull the pubic bone up toward the bottom of the rib cage.
3. Do not let the shoulders and upper back round off the floor as the pelvis is tilted.

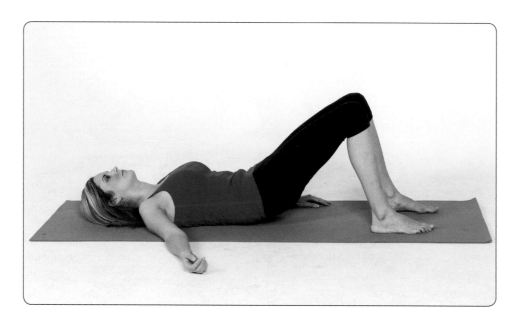

Duration and repetitions: Perform 10 to 15 repetitions at least once per day.

Tip: Do not let the pelvis anteriorly rotate as the tailbone comes off the ground.

Precaution: Perform this exercise gently and slowly at first to help the structures of the lower back to adapt.

Progress: Perform the Gluteal Activation Over Ball or the Butt Lift.

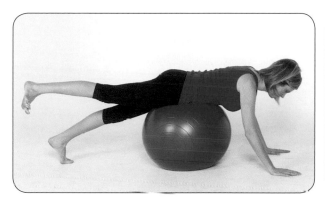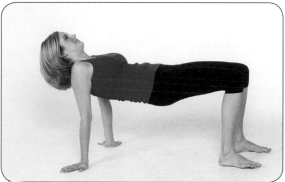

Regress: Massage the glutes with a tennis ball or foam roller, or perform the One Tennis Ball on Lower Back.

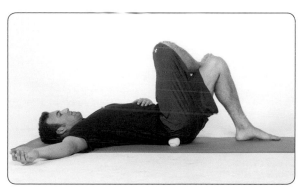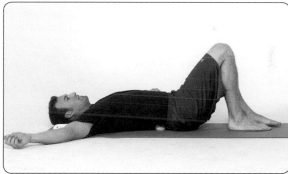

Duck Stand

Area(s) of body: Feet and ankles, knees, lumbo-pelvic hip girdle

Imbalance(s): Overpronation, valgus knee position, anterior pelvic tilt, and excessive lumbar lordosis

Structures addressed: Gluteus maximus, iliotibial band, rectus abdominis, and posterior fibers of gluteus medius

Exercise benefits: This exercise helps strengthen the muscles that assist with rotating the legs outward (thus raising the arches of the feet and aligning the knee with the feet and ankles) and tilting the pelvis posteriorly. It also helps flex the lumbar spine to decrease lumbar lordosis.

How to perform

1. Begin by standing on both feet with your heels together and your feet and legs rotated out like a duck.
2. Tilt the pelvis posteriorly (i.e., tuck it under), and contract the gluteus maximus muscle to further rotate the legs outward.
3. As the legs rotate outward, feel the arches of the feet rise up and the weight shift to the outsides of the feet and toward the heels.

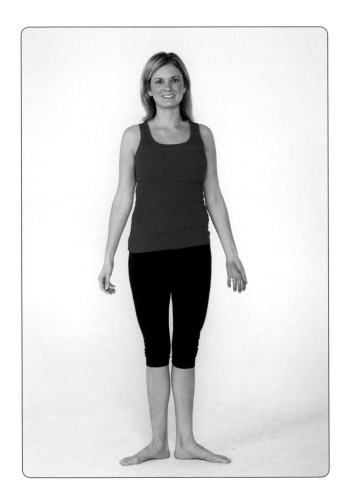

Duration and repetitions: Hold the contraction isometrically for 15 to 20 seconds, and repeat the cycle at least 3 times once per day.

Tip: Drive your heels into the ground, and keep your torso erect.

Precaution: If you have discomfort in your knees, straighten your feet so that they are not turned out so much. If pain persists, stop performing the exercise.

Progress: Perform Big Toe Pushdowns dynamically or the Gluteal Activation Over Ball.

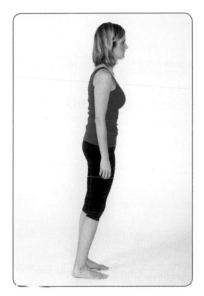
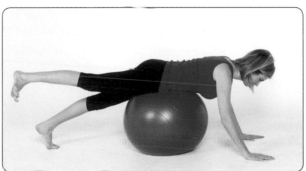

Regress: Perform the Lying Pelvic Tilt or the Foam Roller Gluteal Complex.

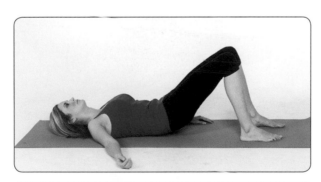

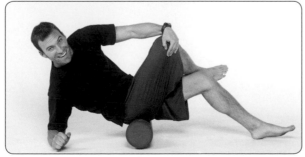

Gluteal Activation Over Ball

Area(s) of body: Lumbo-pelvic hip girdle

Imbalance(s): Overpronation, valgus knee position, anterior pelvic tilt, and excessive lumbar lordosis

Structures addressed: Gluteus maximus, gluteus medius, and gluteus minimus

Exercise benefits: This exercise helps strengthen the glutes and retrain the lumbo-pelvic hip girdle so that the hip and leg complex can go into extension (i.e., take the leg behind the body) without "cheating" by anteriorly tilting the pelvis or overarching the lower back.

How to perform

1. Lie on top of a stability ball with the pelvis in the center of the ball, hands resting on the floor and eyes looking down to avoid excessive arching of the neck.
2. Rest one foot on the ground to stabilize the body as the pelvis is tilted posteriorly to flex the lumbar spine.
3. Dorsiflex the other foot and rotate the leg outward, keeping that leg straight.
4. Slowly lift the straight leg up and tilt the pelvis to activate the glutes and keep the lower back from arching.
5. Lower the leg back down a few inches, and then raise it again.
6. Repeat on the opposite side.

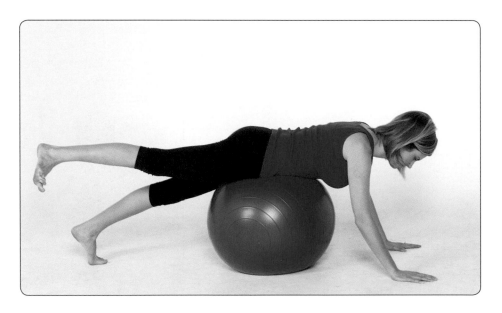

Duration and repetitions: Perform 10 to 15 repetitions on each side at least once per day.

Tip: Most people with lumbar lordosis will try to lift the leg by arching the lower back, so watch for this compensation. Also, rotating the lifting leg inward and outward will strengthen different fibers of the gluteal muscles.

Precaution: Do not try to move the leg by rotating or tipping the pelvis to one side.

Progress: Perform the Butt Lift.

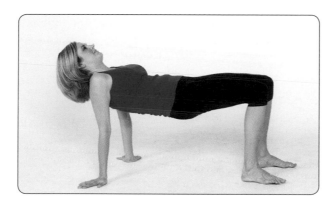

Regress: Perform Lying Pelvic Tilt or Duck Stand.

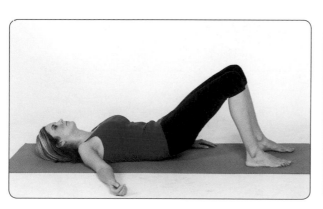

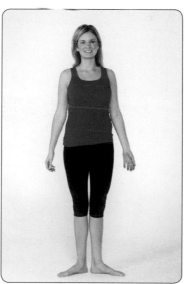

Butt Lift

Area(s) of body: Feet and ankles, knees, lumbo-pelvic hip girdle

Imbalance(s): Overpronation, valgus knee position, anterior pelvic tilt, and excessive lumbar lordosis

Structures addressed: Gluteus maximus, rectus abdominis, and erector spinae

Exercise benefits: Strengthening the glutes and spinal erectors and teaching the hip and leg complex to extend correctly will train the entire lumbo-pelvic hip girdle to move more effectively without compensating.

How to perform

1. Sit on the floor with knees bent and hands placed behind your body.
2. Align your feet forward with the arches lifted.
3. Posteriorly tilt the pelvis to move it into a neutral position as the hips are lifted off the floor.
4. Lift through the shoulders to keep your chest up, and keep your chin tucked as the hips are raised.
5. Slowly lower the hips without touching your butt to the floor while maintaining a neutral pelvic position throughout.

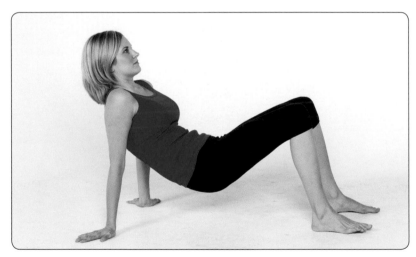

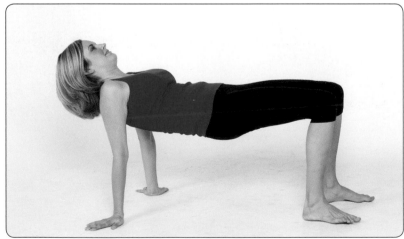

Duration and repetitions: Perform the exercise isometrically at first, holding the up position for 15 to 20 seconds. Progress to 10 to 12 repetitions once per day.

Tip: If a client has shoulder or wrist problems, use a stability ball to support the head and shoulders during this exercise.

Precaution: Most people with an anterior pelvic tilt and excessive lumbar lordosis will overarch their backs as they lift the hips during this exercise. Coach these clients to maintain a neutral pelvic position throughout the exercise by posteriorly tilting the pelvis.

Progress: Perform the Lunge With Knee Pull.

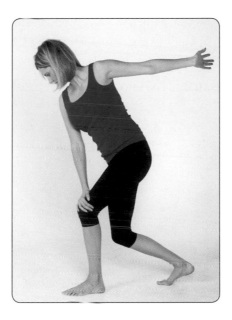

Regress: Perform the Lying Pelvic Tilt or the Gluteal Activation Over Ball.

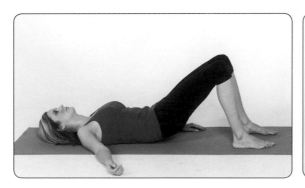 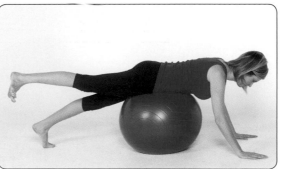

Side Lying Leg Lift

Area(s) of body: Feet and ankles, knees, lumbo-pelvic hip girdle

Imbalance(s): Overpronation, valgus knee position, and anterior pelvic tilt

Structures addressed: Abductor muscles and deep hip rotators

Exercise benefits: This exercise helps to stabilize the pelvis and promote a more neutral position for the hip, thereby creating better alignment and movement of the lumbo-pelvic hip girdle, legs, knees, and feet.

How to perform

1. Lie on your side with a half foam roller or pillow under your neck to keep the head in line with the spine.
2. Straighten the bottom leg, rest the instep of the top foot on the calf of the bottom leg, and lower the knee toward the ground.
3. Posteriorly rotate the pelvis, keeping the hips stacked vertically on top of each other.
4. Slowly lift the top knee up and down without arching the lower back, hiking the hip, or anteriorly rotating the pelvis.

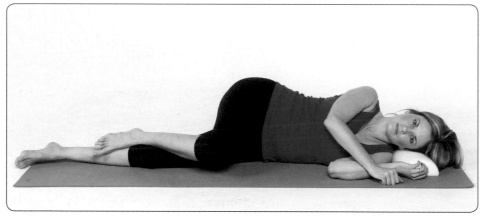

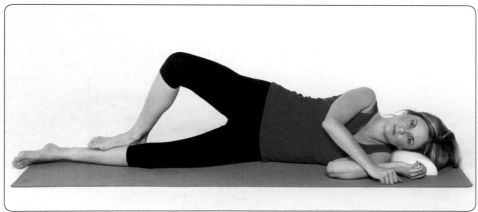

Duration and repetitions: Perform the exercise isometrically at first by lifting and holding the leg in the top position for 20 to 30 seconds and repeating 2 to 3 times. Progress to 10 to 12 repetitions once per day.

Tip: If clients do not feel the contraction in the sides of their glutes, gently add resistance to the lowering (eccentric) phase of the movement to help activate those muscles.

Precaution: Watch for the following three compensations during the leg lifting phase of this exercise: hiking of the hip, anteriorly rotating the pelvis, and rotating the torso.

Progress: Perform the Lunge With Side Reach.

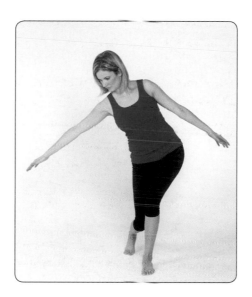

Regress: Perform the Abductor Stretch or Duck Stand.

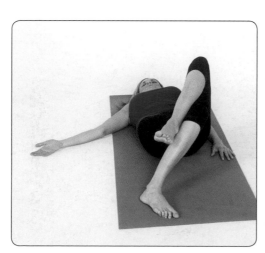 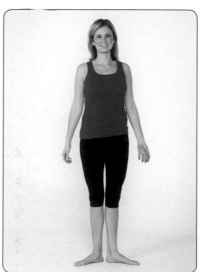

Shoulder Retraction on Floor

Area(s) of body: Thoracic spine and shoulder girdle

Imbalance(s): Excessive thoracic kyphosis, protracted shoulder girdle, elevated scapula, and internally rotated arms

Structures addressed: Rhomboids, trapezius (middle and lower fibers), thoracic extensors, infraspinatus, and teres minor

Exercise benefits: This exercise helps to strengthen the muscles that extend the thoracic spine and retract and depress the scapula. It also strengthens the rotator cuff muscles that help to externally rotate the arm and position the humerus correctly in the glenohumeral joint.

How to perform

1. Lie on your back with knees bent and your head on a pillow or folded towel (if needed) to make sure the neck is in a neutral position.

2. Place your arms out to the sides abducted approximately 45 degrees away from the body, with palms facing up.

3. Pull your shoulders back and down to the floor, keeping the pelvis posteriorly rotated to ensure that your lower back stays in contact with the floor and does not arch during the movement.

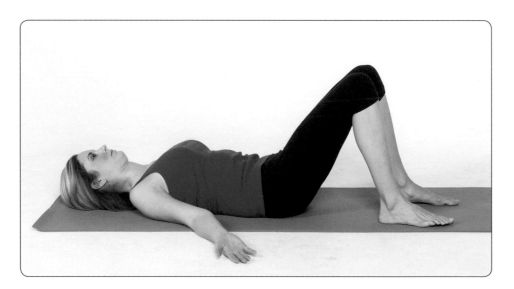

Duration and repetitions: Perform an isometric contraction for 20 to 30 seconds 2 to 3 times per day.

Tip: If a client cannot feel the muscles that retract and depress the shoulder blades activate, use another strengthening exercise like the Seated Row or the Straight Arm Pulldown (detailed later in this chapter) to help activate them, and then return to this exercise.

Progress: Perform The Flasher or The Wave Goodbye.

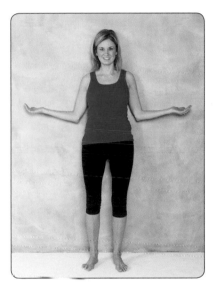 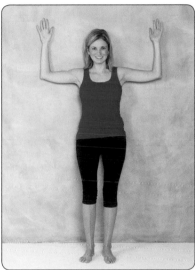

Regress: Perform the Why Stretch or the Front of Shoulder Massage.

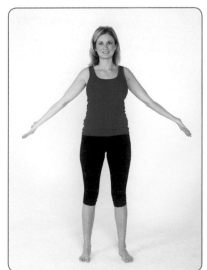 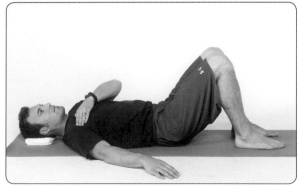

Straight Arm Pulldown

Area(s) of body: Thoracic spine and shoulder girdle, head and neck

Imbalance(s): Elevated scapula and protracted shoulder girdle

Structures addressed: Trapezius muscle (lower fibers) and rhomboids

Exercise benefits: This exercise helps strengthen the lower fibers of the trapezius to help depress the scapula and pull it closer to the spine. Also, if the lower fibers of the trapezius are strong and active, it can take stress off the upper fibers, where many people hold excessive tension.

How to perform

1. Sit on a gym ball or on the seat of a lat pulldown machine, and reach up to grasp the bar or handles of suspended tubing.
2. Pull the shoulder blades back and down without bending the arms (this uses the lower traps and rhomboids).
3. Do not engage the lats by bending the arms.

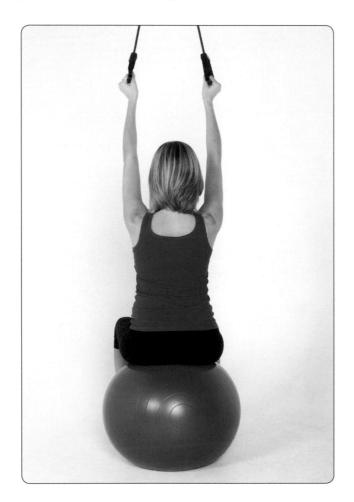

Duration and repetitions: Perform an isometric contraction for 20 to 30 seconds, and repeat 2 to 3 times before progressing to dynamic movements of 10 to 15 repetitions.

Tip: If there is difficulty in performing this movement or in being aware of the lower fibers of the trapezius contracting, do one arm at a time first to help you to feel the muscles that should be working.

Progress: Perform the Straight Arm Raise

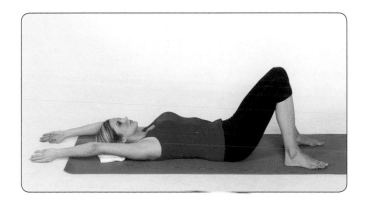

Regress: Perform the Tennis Ball Around Shoulder Blade.

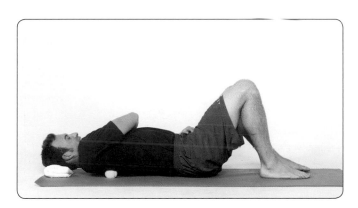

Seated Row

Area(s) of body: Thoracic spine and shoulder girdle, neck and head

Imbalance(s): Excessive thoracic kyphosis, protracted shoulder girdle, elevated scapula, internally rotated arms, and forward head

Structures addressed: Erector spinae group, rhomboids, trapezius, latissimus dorsi

Exercise benefits: This exercise helps strengthen the muscles that keep the thoracic spine erect and pull the head back as well as those muscles that retract, depress, and stabilize the shoulder blades. Strengthening these muscles can have a positive impact on the head and neck, thoracic spine, shoulder girdle, and arms.

How to perform

1. Sit up straight on a chair or rowing machine.
2. Grasp the handles of an elastic tube or the rowing machine and pull them toward your torso in a rowing motion.
3. Keep your shoulders back and down, and do not arch your lower back excessively during the movement.
4. Keep your head in line with the spine, and keep your chin tucked in.
5. Return the handles to the starting position and repeat without leaning forward.

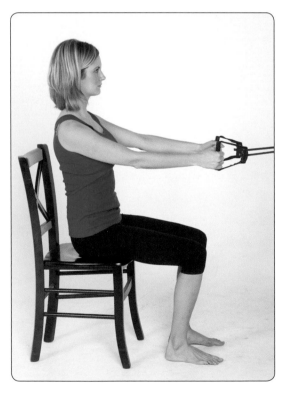 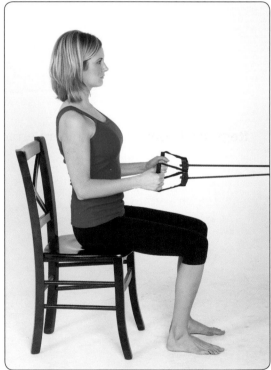

Duration and repetitions: Perform an isometric contraction for 10 to 15 seconds, and repeat 2 to 3 times before progressing to dynamic movements of 10 to 15 repetitions.

Tip: When the elbows come in line with the sides of the ribcage, stop pulling. Going farther back may cause the shoulder blades to elevate, and this will defeat the purpose of the exercise.

Precaution: Coach clients to bend at the hips as they reach forward to avoid excessive rounding of the spine.

Progress: Perform this exercise standing.

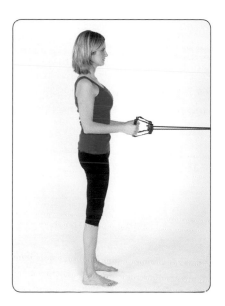

Regress: Perform the Shoulder Retraction on Floor.

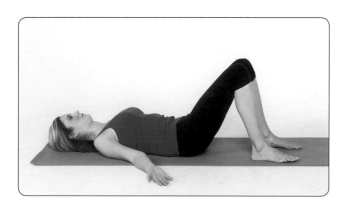

The Flasher (Lying)

Area(s) of body: Thoracic spine, shoulder girdle

Imbalance(s): Excessive cervical lordosis, forward head, excessive thoracic kyphosis, protracted shoulder girdle, elevated scapula, and internally rotated arms

Structures addressed: Erector spinae group, muscles that flex the neck, muscles that retract the head (when performed standing), infraspinatus, teres minor, rhomboids, and trapezius

Exercise benefits: This exercise strengthens the muscles that keep the torso and head erect, retract and depress the shoulder blades, and externally rotate the arm. It also stretches the muscles in the front of the chest and shoulder.

How to perform

1. Lie on your back with your arms bent, elbows close to the sides, and fingers pointing toward the ceiling, using a pillow to support your head if needed.
2. Pull the shoulder blades back and down.
3. Externally rotate the arms by bringing the backs of the hands toward the floor.
4. The movement should be felt between the shoulder blades and in the backs of the arms near the top of each arm.

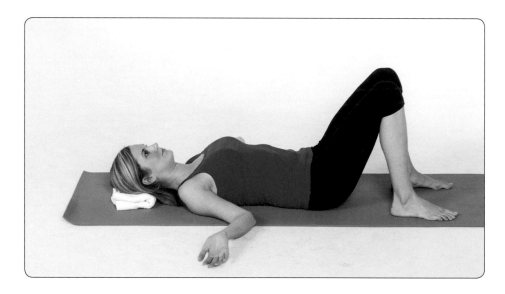

Duration and repetitions: Perform the exercise isometrically at first, holding the contracted position for 15 to 20 seconds and repeating 2 to 3 times. Progress to 10 to 15 repetitions for 2 to 3 sets, 3 to 4 times per week.

Tip: To achieve better full-body posture during this exercise, teach clients to do it while standing against a wall. Coach them to obtain a neutral foot position, posteriorly rotate the pelvis, stand erect, and tuck their chins in before and throughout the movement.

Precaution: If discomfort is felt at the front of the shoulder, raise the elbows off the floor with a rolled-up towel; check for proper technique, and regress the exercise if necessary.

Progress: Perform this exercise standing, or add resistance with an exercise band.

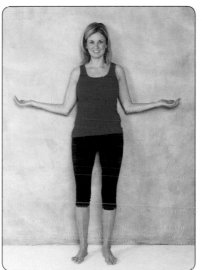 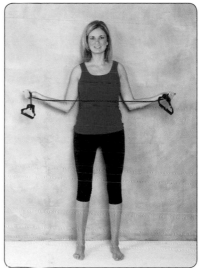

Regress: Perform this exercise one side at a time while lying on the ground, placing a pillow under the elbows and a foam roller to the side of the shoulder to decrease the range of motion required before the back of the hand makes contact with the roller.

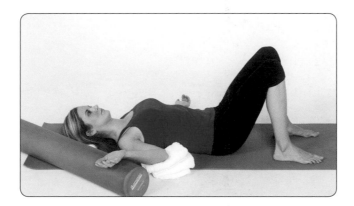

The Wave Goodbye (Lying)

Area(s) of body: Thoracic spine, shoulder girdle

Imbalance(s): Excessive cervical lordosis, excessive thoracic kyphosis, internally rotated arms, protracted shoulder girdle, and elevated scapula

Structures addressed: Erector spinae group, muscles that flex the neck, muscles that retract the head (when performed standing), infraspinatus, teres minor, rhomboids, and trapezius

Exercise benefits: This exercise helps strengthen the muscles that externally rotate the arm and stabilize the scapula while the spine and head are in proper alignment.

How to perform

1. Lie on the floor with the lower back flat to the floor with elbows raised to shoulder height and bent, palms facing the feet, and fingers pointing toward the ceiling, using a pillow to support the head and neck if needed.

2. Pull your shoulder blades back and down to the floor, tucking your chin in so that the neck does not arch backward to the floor.

3. Slowly press the backs of your hands against the floor, keeping your shoulders back and down.

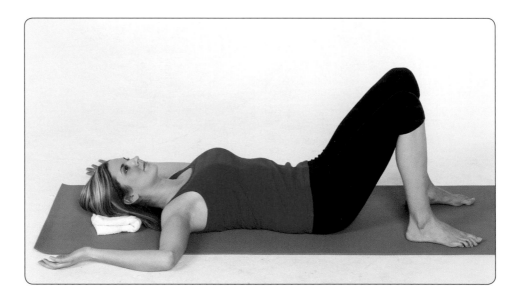

Duration and repetitions: Perform the exercise isometrically, holding the contracted position for 15 to 20 seconds and repeating 2 to 3 times. Progress to 10 to 15 repetitions for 2 to 3 sets, 3 to 4 times per week.

Tip: Keep the pelvis posteriorly rotated throughout to stop the lower back from overarching and to engage the thoracic extensors.

Precaution: Clients who have excessive thoracic kyphosis may shrug their shoulders as they rotate their arms. Coach them to engage their lower traps to help depress their shoulder blades.

Progress: Perform this exercise standing, or add resistance with tubing. Clients should be able to complete 10 to 15 repetitions with good form before adding resistance.

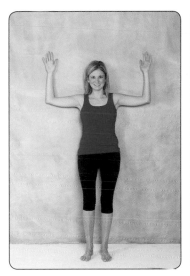 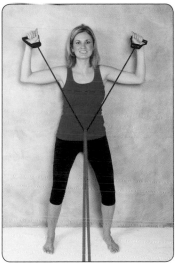

Regress: Use a pillow to support the elbows and a foam roller above the head to decrease the range of movement needed, or perform the Theracane on Trapezius.

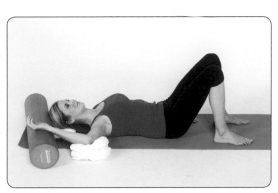 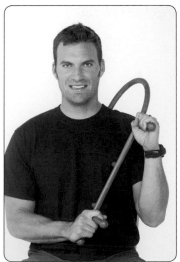

Straight Arm Raise (Lying)

Area(s) of body: Thoracic spine, shoulder girdle

Imbalance(s): Excessive thoracic kyphosis, elevated scapula

Structures addressed: Erector spinae group, muscles that flex the neck, muscles that retract the head (when performed standing), rhomboids, and trapezius

Exercise benefits: This exercise teaches clients to engage their thoracic extensors and disengage their lumbar extensors to encourage better thoracic extension and discourage excessive lumbar lordosis. It also strengthens the muscles that stabilize the scapula to prevent excessive "shrugging" when using the arms.

How to perform

1. Lie on the floor with your knees bent, your arms by your sides, and your pelvis posteriorly rotated.
2. Slowly raise your arms up over your head, keeping the arms straight and keeping the muscles that stabilize the shoulder blade engaged.
3. Make sure the lower back does not arch excessively during the movement.

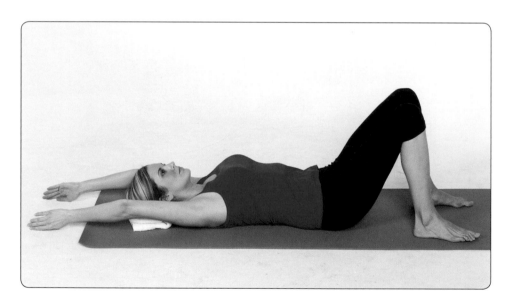

Duration and repetitions: Perform this exercise isometrically at first, holding the raised arm position for 10 to 15 seconds, and repeat 2 to 3 times. Progress to 10 to 15 repetitions raising and lowering the arms for 2 to 3 sets, 2 to 3 times per week.

Tip: Many people may arch their backs excessively when lifting their arms over their heads. Coach them to keep the pelvis posteriorly tilted and to extend the spine using their upper back muscles (thoracic extensors).

Precaution: Two compensations to watch for when clients perform this exercise are shrugging the shoulders and bending the arms. Regress this exercise when needed to ensure correct technique.

Progress: Perform this exercise standing, or perform the Back Step With Arm Raise.

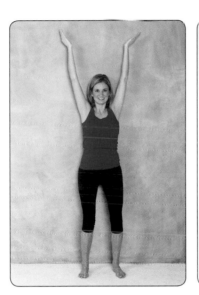
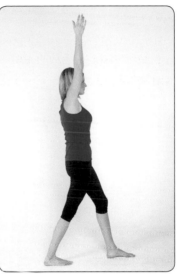

Regress: Use a foam roller above your head to decrease the amount of movement needed, or perform the Front of Shoulder Massage.

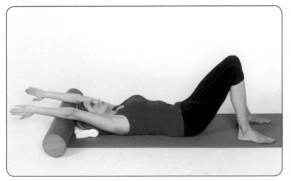
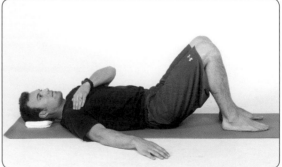

Neck Flexion

Area(s) of body: Neck and head

Imbalance(s): Excessive cervical lordosis, forward head

Structures addressed: Muscles that flex the neck and retract the head

Exercise benefits: This exercise helps strengthen the muscles that help pull the head back while keeping the eyes parallel to the horizon to reduce unnecessary stress caused by excessive cervical lordosis and a forward head.

How to perform

1. Stand against a wall, or sit in a chair with torso erect (do not overarch lower back).
2. Pull your chin in and your head back to lengthen the back of the neck.
3. Keep your shoulders back and down and your pelvis tucked throughout the exercise.

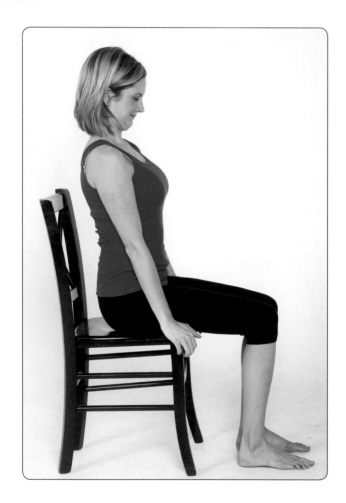

Duration and repetitions: Perform this exercise isometrically at first, and hold the position 10 to 15 seconds and repeat 2 to 3 times. Progress to 6 to 10 repetitions at least once per day.

Tip: This exercise can be performed at the office, while driving, or at any time to help keep the muscles of your neck strong, flexible, and mobile.

Progress: Perform this exercise while lying down.

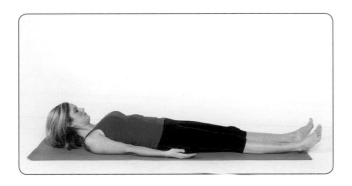

Regress: Use heat, or perform the Theracane on Back of Neck.

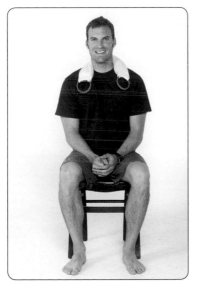
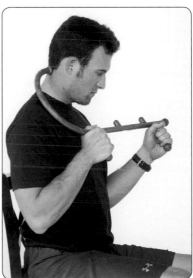

Extension Crunch

Area(s) of body: Thoracic spine, shoulder girdle

Imbalance(s): Excessive lumbar lordosis, excessive thoracic kyphosis, and excessive cervical lordosis

Structures addressed: Rectus abdominis, muscles that flex the neck, muscles that retract the head, and the extensor muscles of the thoracic spine

Exercise benefits: This exercise strengthens the rectus abdominis to rotate the pelvis posteriorly and to help flex the lumbar spine. It also strengthens the muscles that flex the neck (while keeping the head back), and it trains the rectus abdominis to work eccentrically to train the thoracic spine to extend correctly.

How to perform

1. Lie back over a stability ball with your feet up against a wall or your heels on a table.
2. Place your hands behind your head to support your neck.
3. Posteriorly tilt the pelvis while keeping your shoulders down, your head back, and your chin tucked in.
4. Gently lie back over the ball, pulling the thoracic spine into extension while keeping the pelvis posteriorly tilted.
5. Once you are comfortable with this position, lift your torso slightly and then lower your upper back and head as far back as possible (without arching the lower back or neck).

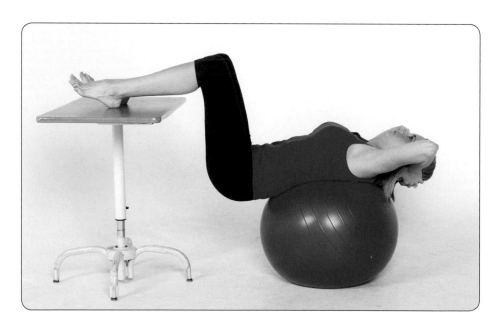

Duration and repetitions: Perform this exercise isometrically at first, holding the pelvis up while extending the thoracic spine over the ball for 15 to 20 seconds. Progress to 8 to 10 repetitions of slightly lifting and lowering the torso for 2 to 3 sets, 3 to 4 times per week.

Tip: Hold the ball for clients so they do not feel too unstable.

Precaution: If the lower back gets tight or painful during the exercise, it means that the client is trying to extend over the ball using the lumbar spine and not extending the thoracic spine correctly. If this occurs, coach the client in the correct technique. If pain persists, discontinue this exercise.

Progress: Increase the distance between the ball and the wall to increase difficulty or perform repetitions.

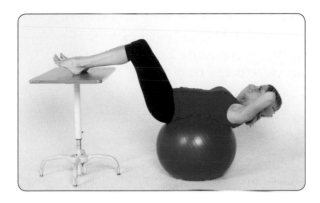

Regress: Perform the Abdominal Massage.

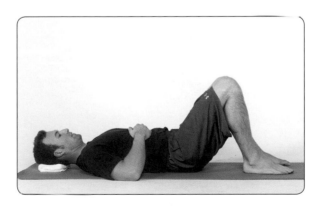

Back Step With Arm Raise

Area(s) of body: Entire kinetic chain

Imbalance(s): Lack of dorsiflexion, anterior pelvic tilt, excessive lumbar lordosis, and excessive thoracic kyphosis

Structures addressed: Hip flexors, gastrocnemius, rectus femoris, rectus abdominis, erector spinae group, and muscles of the shoulder complex

Exercise benefits: This exercise strengthens the muscles that help extend the thoracic spine and stabilize the scapula while simultaneously stretching the abdominal, hip flexor, and calf muscles so that the legs, hips, and spine can move together into extension without overarching the lower back.

How to perform

1. Stand with both feet facing forward and your pelvis tucked under.
2. Step back with your right leg while raising your right arm over your head.
3. Do not excessively shrug the shoulder of the arm being raised.
4. Complete the movement on the right side by stepping forward with the right leg while bringing the arm down; then step backward with the left leg and raise the left arm to perform the movement on the left side.
5. Repeat on both sides.

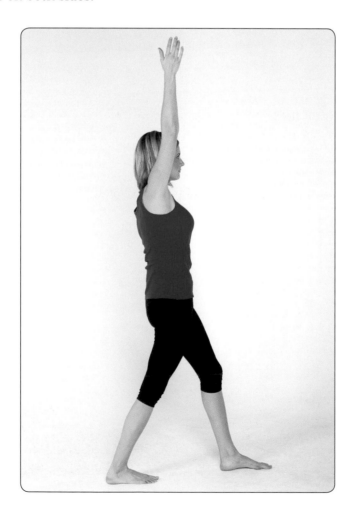

Duration and repetitions: Perform the exercise isometrically at first, holding the arm up and leg back position for 10 to 15 seconds. Progress to dynamic movements of 10 to 12 repetitions on both sides 2 to 3 times per week.

Tip: If a client has difficulty performing this movement correctly, check the flexibility of the gastrocnemius, abdominals, and hip flexor muscles, and address any issues you find with myofascial release or isolated stretching exercises.

Precaution: If clients experience lower back pain when performing the exercise, simply instruct them to take a smaller step backward, and ensure that they tilt the pelvis correctly during the movement.

Progress: Perform the Lunge With Arm Raise.

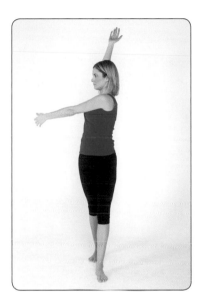

Regress: Perform the Standing Straight Arm Raise or Abdominal Massage.

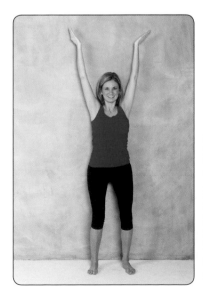

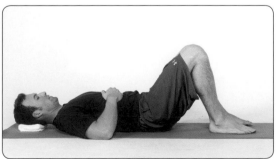

Lunge With Knee Pull

Area(s) of body: Entire kinetic chain

Imbalance(s): Overpronation, lack of dorsiflexion, valgus knee position, tracking problems of the knee, excessive thoracic kyphosis, and anterior pelvic tilt

Structures addressed: Works the entire kinetic chain, but focuses on the gluteal muscles, quadriceps group, adductors, erector spinae group, and the muscles of the lower leg and foot

Exercise benefits: This exercise focuses on eccentrically strengthening the gluteal muscles, quadriceps, and muscles of the calf and foot. Strengthening these muscles in this manner enables them to help slow down the knee as it moves forward and toward the midline. Strengthening the gluteal muscles also helps to stabilize the pelvis and lower back. When performed with rotation, this exercise also helps to mobilize the thoracic spine and to strengthen the muscles of the back.

How to perform

1. Step forward into a gentle lunge, making sure both feet are facing forward.
2. Bend at the hips, and grab the front knee with the opposite hand.
3. Pull the pelvis of the front leg back toward the back foot while pulling the front knee toward the midline of the body.
4. Allow the foot to pronate, but use the flexor hallucis longus (i.e., push the big toe down) to help stabilize the front foot and prevent overpronation.
5. Keep the spine straight—lean forward at the hips and do not round the spine—until you feel the glute on the leg that is forward activate.

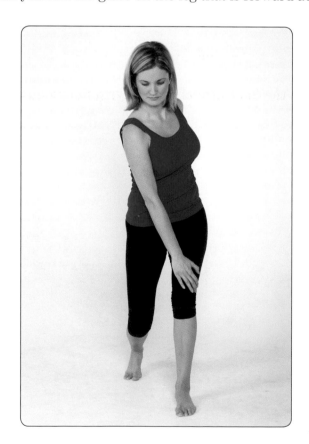

Duration and repetitions: Perform this exercise isometrically at first, holding the lunge position for 5 to 10 seconds, and repeat 2 to 3 times. Progress to dynamic movements of 8 to 12 repetitions on both sides 2 to 3 times per week.

Tip: Rotating the torso back and away from the front leg will also help activate the glute.

Precaution: If clients experience pain in their lower back or knees, regress to a suitable self-myofascial release or stretching exercise.

Progress: Rotate the torso farther away from the front leg, and extend the arm on the same side as the front leg behind you.

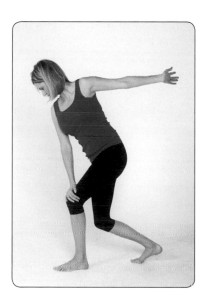

Regress: Perform the Glute Stretch or the Lying Rotation Stretch.

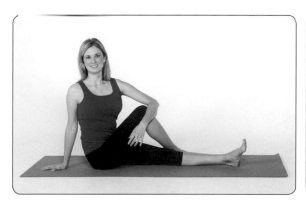

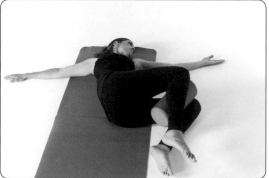

Lunge With Arm Raise

Area(s) of body: Entire kinetic chain

Imbalance(s): Overpronation, lack of dorsiflexion, valgus knee position, tracking problems of the knee, anterior pelvic tilt, excessive lumbar lordosis, and excessive thoracic kyphosis

Structures addressed: Works entire kinetic chain but focuses on gluteal muscles, hip flexor group, quadriceps group, adductors, abdominals, erector spinae group, obliques, and muscles of the lower leg and foot

Exercise benefits: This exercise helps retrain the major muscles and structures of the body to transition correctly from flexion to extension as the hips, spine, and torso rotate. Learning to coordinate these movements correctly will address nearly all of the most common musculoskeletal imbalances.

How to perform

1. Step forward into a gentle lunge, leaning forward and rotating slightly to reach the arm opposite the leg that is forward, across toward the front knee, while reaching the other arm backward.

2. Return from the lunge, rotating the torso upright and back.

3. Raise the same arm that was previously reaching forward above the head and behind the body without shrugging the shoulder, while rotating the opposite arm across the torso.

4. Try to keep the feet facing forward throughout this exercise; reposition them to face forward as needed.

5. Repeat the movement, rotating down and forward to up and back.

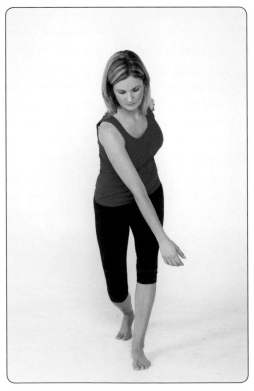 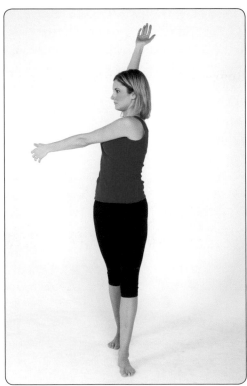

Duration and repetitions: Perform 10 to 15 repetitions on both sides once per day. (Increase to 2 to 3 sets of 8 to 12 repetitions as a client's ability improves, but decrease the frequency that this exercise is performed to allow adequate rest and recovery between sessions.)

Tip: This exercise is an integration of many exercises previously learned. If a client has difficulty with any part, simply break this exercise down into its parts and perform them separately. For example, performing the Lunge With Knee Pull will help with the forward lunge part of the exercise, and performing the Step Back With Arm Raise will help with the second part.

Progress: Perform the exercise holding light dumbbells.

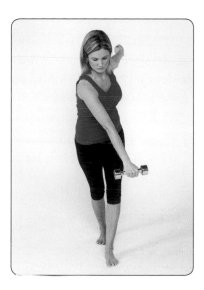

Regress: Perform the Straight Arm Raise or the Foam Roller Hip Flexors.

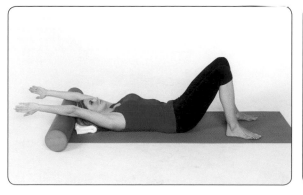 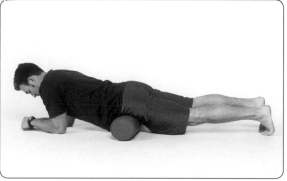

Lunge With Side Reach

Area(s) of body: Entire kinetic chain

Imbalance(s): Overpronation, valgus knee position, tracking problems of the knee, anterior pelvic tilt, and excessive lumbar lordosis

Structures addressed: Works the entire kinetic chain, but focuses on the muscles that slow down the legs, pelvis, and spine as they move laterally

Exercise benefits: This exercise eccentrically strengthens the muscles that help slow down the pelvis, leg, and spine as they move from side to side. It also helps mobilize and strengthen the muscles that control the movement of the pelvis and spine to mitigate compensation patterns, such as an anterior pelvic tilt and excessive lumbar lordosis.

How to perform

1. With both feet facing forward, lunge forward gently with the left foot while reaching the right arm out toward the right side.
2. During the lunging movement, push the left hip to the left (i.e., away from the right hand) to help keep the body balanced over its center.
3. During this movement, let the left leg move in toward the midline of the body.
4. Stand up to return to the starting position, and reach with the right arm over the head toward the left, pushing the hips toward the right side of your body.
5. Repeat the movement, transitioning from side lunge to overhead reach.

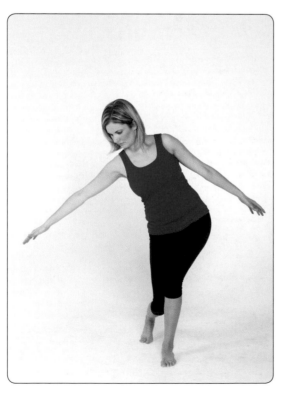
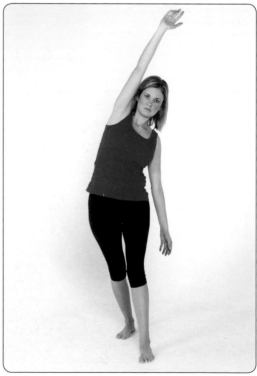

Duration and repetitions: Perform 10 to 15 repetitions on both sides once per day. (Increase to 2 to 3 sets of 8 to 12 repetitions as a client's ability improves, but decrease the frequency that this exercise is performed to allow adequate rest and recovery between sessions.)

Tip: Placing the left hand on the left-side gluteal complex (if the right hand is reaching out to the right side) at the beginning of this exercise will enable clients to feel if the abductor muscles are activating correctly. If they are deficient in any way you will need to regress this exercise to activate these muscles (e.g., perform the Side Lying Leg Lift).

Progress: Perform the exercise holding light dumbbells.

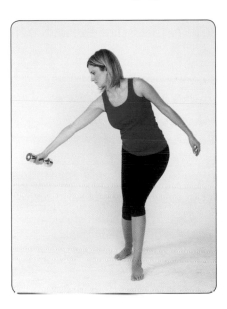

Regress: Use a balance aid or perform the Side Lying Leg Lift.

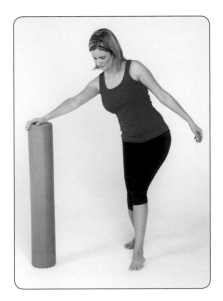

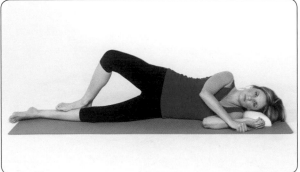

Side Lunge With Rotation

Area(s) of body: Entire kinetic chain

Imbalance(s): Overpronation, valgus knee position, tracking problems of the knee, anterior pelvic tilt, excessive lumbar lordosis, and excessive thoracic kyphosis

Structures addressed: Works the entire kinetic chain, but focuses on gluteal muscles, quadriceps group, adductors, erector spinae group, obliques, and muscles of the lower leg and foot

Exercise benefits: This exercise focuses on retraining and strengthening the muscles that help stabilize the leg and pelvis as weight is transferred from one side of the body to the other. It also helps mobilize and strengthen the structures of the spine so it can rotate correctly.

How to perform

1. Stand with your feet facing forward and about 24 to 36 inches (60 to 90 cm) apart.
2. Transfer your weight onto one leg, bending the ankle, knee, and hip on that side to perform a squat.
3. Rotate the arms and torso over the weight-bearing leg during the squat.
4. Return to the standing position and repeat on the other side, learning to transfer weight from side to side as the trunk rotates.

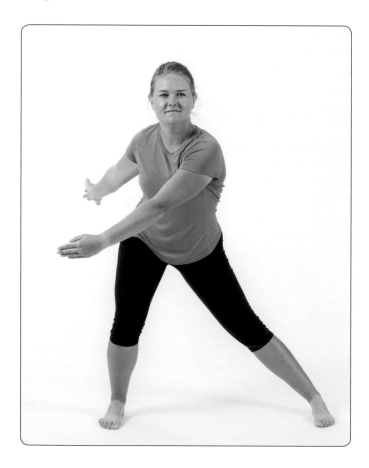

Duration and repetitions: Perform 10 to 15 repetitions at least once per day. (Increase to 2 to 3 sets of 8 to 12 repetitions as a client's ability improves, but decrease the frequency that this exercise is performed to allow adequate rest and recovery between sessions.)

Tip: Coach clients to imagine that they are ice skating as they transfer weight from side to side to help them visualize or feel the desired movement.

Precaution: If clients complain of back or knee pain when performing this exercise, coach them to place their hands on a balance aid in front of them and only to incorporate the torso rotation when they are ready to progress.

Progress: Perform with one leg at a time, with the opposite leg on a gym ball.

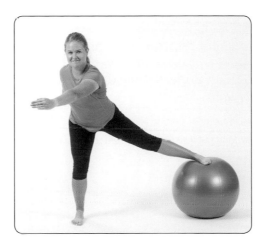

Regress: Perform the Lying Rotation Stretch or the Side Lying Leg Lift

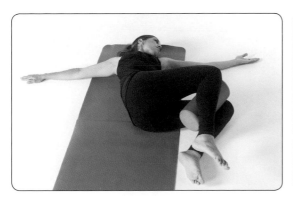
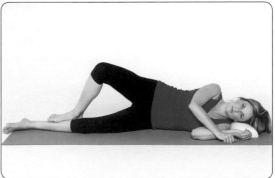

The Pivot

Area(s) of body: Feet and ankles, knees, and lumbo-pelvic hip girdle

Imbalance(s): Overpronation, valgus knee position, anterior pelvic tilt, and excessive lumbar lordosis

Structures addressed: Works the entire lower kinetic chain but focuses primarily on the gluteal muscles, the hip flexor group, the quadriceps group, the adductors, and the muscles of the lower leg and foot

Exercise benefits: This exercise helps strengthen all the muscles of the lower body that slow down pronation of the foot, internal rotation of the leg, and flexion of the hips.

How to perform

1. Stand on the left foot, making sure that it is aligned forward.
2. Keep the torso straight, and do not lean to the side.
3. Lift the right knee and hike the right side of the pelvis to help activate the left glute (which will help bring the left foot, leg, and hip into better alignment).
4. Gently bend the left hip, knee, and ankle, and pivot your raised leg down and backward, letting the left knee shift in toward the midline of the body and the right leg drop and rotate behind the body.
5. Use the glutes, quadriceps, and muscles of the feet to slow down the left knee as it bends and the leg and ankle as they rotate inward.
6. Return to the standing position balanced on the left leg with the right knee raised up and forward.

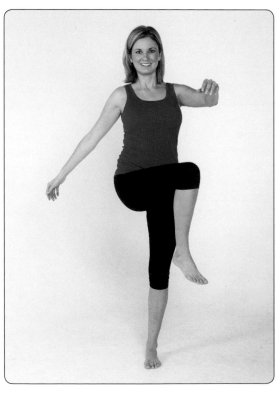
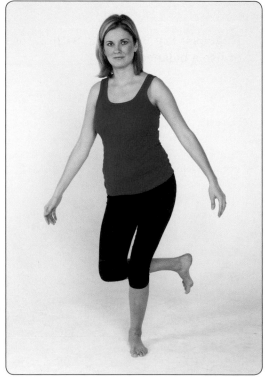

Duration and repetitions: Perform the exercise isometrically at first holding the starting position balanced over the left leg with the right knee up and forward to activate the gluteal muscles. Progress to completing the entire movement for 8 to 12 repetitions on both sides for 2 to 3 sets, 2 to 3 times a week.

Tip: The pivoting movement should be controlled by the muscles of the hips, legs, and feet so that the ankle and knee do not get overly stressed.

Precaution: If pain or discomfort is felt in the knee, stop immediately and regress to an easier exercise.

Progress: Perform the Lunge To Step Up.

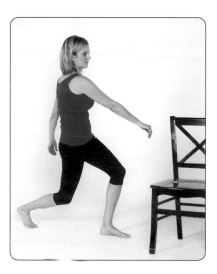

Regress: Tap the ground with the other foot as it goes back to maintain balance, or use a balance aid.

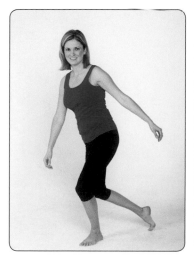 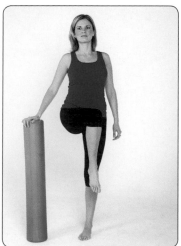

Lunge to Step Up

Area(s) of body: Entire kinetic chain

Imbalance(s): Overpronation, lack of dorsiflexion, valgus knee position, tracking problems of the knee, anterior pelvic tilt, excessive lumbar lordosis, and excessive thoracic kyphosis

Structures addressed: Works the entire kinetic chain, including the gluteal muscles, the hip flexors, the quadriceps group, the adductors, the erector spinae group, the obliques, and muscles of the lower leg and foot

Exercise benefits: This exercise mimics gait to help strengthen all the muscles that both create and slow down hip flexion and hip extension while keeping the feet, legs, pelvis, and spine stable and functioning correctly.

How to perform

1. With both feet facing forward, step backward into a lunge, tilting the pelvis under on the back leg and keeping the spine upright to prevent the lower back from arching too much.

2. Stand up out of the lunge, lifting the back leg off the ground, and placing the foot of the back leg on a step or a stool placed in front at about knee height.

3. Take the foot off the stool and step back into the lunge to repeat.

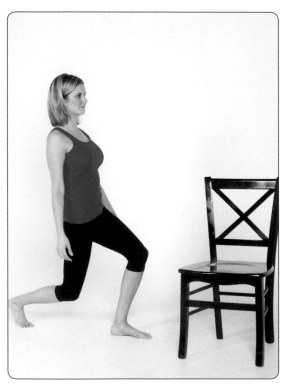
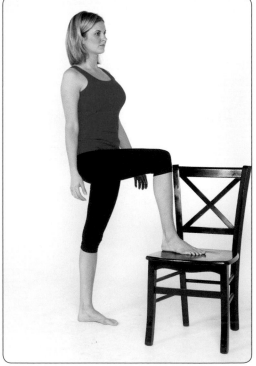

Duration and repetitions: Perform 10 to 15 repetitions on both sides once per day. (Increase to 2 to 3 sets of 8 to 12 repetitions as a client's ability improves, but decrease the frequency that this exercise is performed to allow adequate rest and recovery between sessions.)

Tip: Clients should feel the glutes and muscles of the front leg and the hip flexors of the back leg load eccentrically as they lunge down. Coach them to keep their feet facing forward to ensure that their legs, hips, and pelvis are aligned correctly.

Progress: Rotate the torso over the front leg as the hip flexes and extends (i.e., swing the arms from side to side).

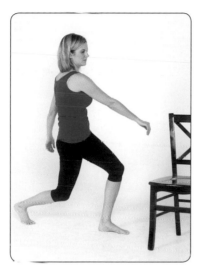 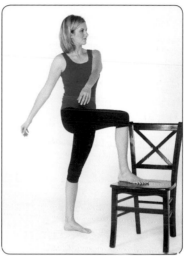

Regress: Perform the Lunge With Knee Pull or the Wall Rotation Stretch.

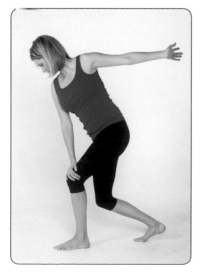 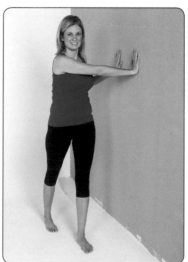

Sumo Squat With Rotation

Area(s) of body: Entire kinetic chain

Imbalance(s): Overpronation, valgus knee position, tracking problems of the knee, anterior pelvic tilt, excessive lumbar lordosis, and excessive thoracic kyphosis

Structures addressed: Works the entire kinetic chain, but focuses on the gluteal muscles, the hip flexor group, the quadriceps group, the adductors, the erector spinae group, the obliques, the rhomboids, the trapezius, the rotator cuff group, and muscles of the lower leg and foot

Exercise benefits: This exercise is designed to help strengthen the muscles around the lumbo-pelvic hip girdle to enable the body to transfer weight from side to side as the hip rotates internally and externally and as the spine flexes and extends. Retraining the body to coordinate these movements correctly will help address many of the common musculoskeletal imbalances of the feet, legs, hips, pelvis, and spine.

How to perform

1. Stand on the left leg with the right knee raised and the left arm up.
2. Hike the right side of the pelvis slightly to ensure that the left side of the pelvis is stacked correctly over the left leg and that the left glutes are activated.
3. Rotate the pelvis and torso to the right, using the muscles in the left foot, leg, and glutes to slow down the left leg and the body as they rotate.
4. Place the right foot on the ground behind the body and squat, allowing the spine to round as the left arm reaches between the legs toward the right heel.
5. Return to the standing position balanced on the left leg and repeat the movement, performing a rotating squat with a reach between the legs.
6. Repeat on the opposite side.

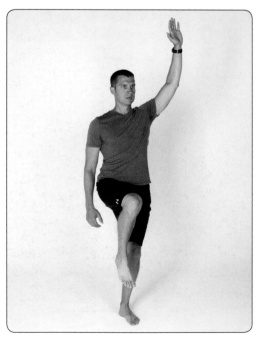 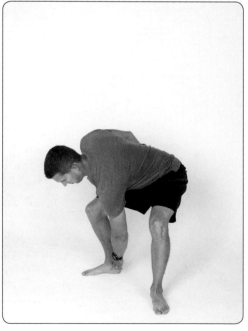

Duration and repetitions: Perform 10 to 12 repetitions on both sides once per day. (Increase to 2 to 3 sets of 6 to 10 repetitions as a client's ability improves, but decrease the frequency that this exercise is performed to allow adequate rest and recovery between sessions.)

Tip: This exercise is an integration of many exercises previously learned. If a client has difficulty with any part, simply break this exercise down into its parts and perform them separately. For example, The Pivot will help with the single-leg stand position, and the Side Lunge With Rotation will help strengthen the muscles that enable the body to transfer weight from side to side.

Progress: Perform the exercise holding a medicine ball.

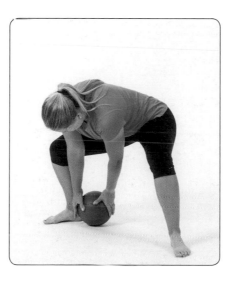

Regress: Perform the Lower Back Stretch or The Pivot

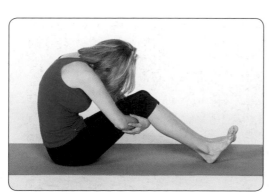

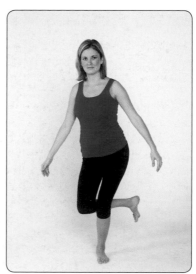

Now that we have concluded this final chapter in the corrective exercise library, you can appreciate the importance of knowing how and when to progress a client's program to meet her needs and abilities. The series of videos that follow is designed to help you better understand this concept, and observe this process with a client. The gluteal complex has been selected as an example of how to progress a series of corrective exercises designed to target a specific muscle group.

 Go to the online video and watch video 21.1, where Justin talks about the exercise rationale for targeting the glutes.

 Go to the online video and watch video 21.2, where Justin gives coaching and cueing tips for the Foam Roller Gluteal Complex.

Go to the online video and watch video 21.3, where Justin gives coaching and cueing tips for the Glute Stretch.

Go to the online video and watch video 21.4, where Justin gives coaching and cueing tips for the Gluteal Activation Over Ball.

Go to the online video and watch video 21.5, where Justin gives coaching and cueing tips for the Lunge With Knee Pull.

Review of Key Points

Strengthening exercises are the ultimate goal of a corrective exercise program, and they are crucial to ensuring that the underlying causes of your client's musculoskeletal imbalances are addressed effectively. Strengthening exercises are introduced after the regular application of self-myofascial release techniques and stretching exercises, and they should be gradually progressed based on a client's needs, abilities, and goals.

- Adding appropriate strengthening exercises to a client's program will help improve stability, increase mobility, and restore coordination.
- Clients with existing musculoskeletal imbalances may perform complex strengthening movements incorrectly and make their condition worse. Watch them closely as they perform these exercises, and regress the exercises when appropriate.
- Always regress a strengthening exercise if a client complains of pain or discomfort.
- Removing or adding balance aids and incorporating or excluding other body parts are effective ways to progress or regress strengthening exercises.
- Using visual, verbal, and kinesthetic teaching cues will help you accommodate the learning styles of different clients.
- Do not use strengthening exercises on tissues that surround or cross a fracture site, tissues that have recently had an acute injury or surgery, or an area that has sustained trauma.
- Obtain clearance from a licensed medical professional before adding strengthening exercises for clients who have a history of chronic illness or musculoskeletal imbalances, neuromuscular disease, rheumatoid arthritis, or severe osteoarthritis.

Self-Check

The appropriate progression and regression of strengthening exercises is important to ensuring that they are safe, do not exacerbate imbalances, and advance your clients toward their goals. The first column in the following chart contains a list of strengthening exercises. In the second and third columns, identify an appropriate progression and regression for each exercise in the first column. An example has been provided for you.

Strengthening exercise	Progression	Regression
Sumo Squat With Rotation	Perform exercise holding a weight like a medicine ball	Lower Back Stretch
Lunge With Knee Pull		
Butt Lift		
Gluteal Activation Over Ball		
Side Lunge With Rotation		
Wave Goodbye (performed lying down)		
Straight Arm Raise (performed standing)		
Side Lunge With Reach		

Part V

Corrective Exercise Program Design

In part V, you will learn about corrective exercise program design and how to develop fruitful client relationships. The detailed knowledge you gained from parts III and IV about the specific corrective exercises will prove invaluable as you now cultivate real client relationships and corrective exercise programs.

Part V will teach you to understand how prospective clients behave and what motivates them to consider your services. You will learn how to handle initial contacts, and you will learn techniques for structuring consultations that encourage them to sign up for your services. You will also discover how to tailor your teaching style during corrective exercise sessions to meet the needs of individual clients.

In addition to teaching you how to conduct effective consultations and exercise sessions, part V will teach you ways to use both your technical talents and your communication skills to conduct successful programs. A comprehensive case study is also included to help you understand how the assessment and program design process can be implemented seamlessly when working with a real client.

CHAPTER 22

Building Successful Client Relationships

Designing effective corrective exercise programs requires you to apply your technical skills. However, an equally important aspect of program design involves forming productive working relationships with clients. This requires you to evaluate a client's motivations for seeking out your help and to adapt your communication, teaching, and coaching strategies for each person. Understanding the needs of clients is important to ensuring the success of your corrective exercise programs (Price and Bratcher 2010).

UNDERSTANDING BASIC MOTIVATIONS AND BEHAVIOR

There are two main reasons why clients who suffer from the effects of musculoskeletal imbalances seek help from allied health and fitness professionals.

1. They lack the knowledge (or the time required to gain the knowledge) they need to resolve the problem on their own. Clients may not be aware of what is causing their problems or what techniques can help solve them.

2. They lack confidence in their own abilities. This lack of confidence, which is usually linked to their lack of knowledge, often results from a

bad experience with exercise or with another fitness professional in the past. This fuels their anxiety and their fear of failure about engaging in a program of regular exercise (Caissy 1998).

These psychological factors can present a challenge for you if you do not address them properly when building client relationships.

To develop an effective working relationship with a client who lacks knowledge or confidence, you must understand some basic principles about human interaction and behavior. There are some fundamental dynamics that exist whenever a relationship is created between two parties, particularly in those relationships where one party is seeking help or advice from the other. In this type of relationship, each person assumes a role, either as the expert or as the subordinate, based on whether one is the person providing assistance or the person being assisted (Bandura 1986).

This chapter will briefly address the major components of an expert–subordinate relationship so that you can learn to manage them to create productive client relationships. They will also be highlighted in later chapters to help you understand the intricacies of such relationships and how you can use appropriate coaching, communication, and teaching skills to achieve positive outcomes for your programs.

HOW ROLES AFFECT BEHAVIOR

When clients seek your help to address their musculoskeletal imbalances, they will naturally view you as the expert in this field. They will assume the role of subordinates who will rely on you to provide the guidance and direction they need to resolve their issues (Altman, Valenzi, and Hodgetts 1985). This assumption of roles (and of the behavior that is expected from each party) is fraught with potential problems. While you are a specialist in the area of musculoskeletal assessment and corrective exercise, immediately assuming the role of expert will reinforce clients' perception that you (and you alone) are responsible for fixing their problems. This will hamper your ability to help your clients to learn and to gain self-confidence, because they are now relying on you to take control of every aspect of their program. They may act in very distinctive ways by not speaking up, becoming disinterested, blaming you when things are not working out as expected, and ultimately dropping out of the program. In short, if clients view you as the expert with all the answers, your ability to encourage them to participate, learn, build confidence in themselves, and adhere to their programs will be greatly diminished (Tyler, Kramer, and Oliver 1999; Williams 1993).

By the same token, clients who assume the role of subordinates will usually do whatever the expert tells them to do, often without question. You may have seen this yourself when observing another personal trainer or fitness professional working with a client. You may have seen a trainer's clients lift weights that are too heavy for them or perform exercises that are unsafe or beyond their abilities because the trainer instructed them to do so. This happens because the clients believe it is not their place to question the expert. While you may wish to have clients follow your instructions without question, this kind of relationship means that if anything goes wrong, the clients will blame you. They will think you should have known better (Tyler, Kramer, and Oliver 1999).

In addition to being aware of how clients view each of your roles, there are several other elements that factor into accurately shaping their expectations. The activities they engage in, any past injuries, surgeries, or diseases they may have had, their adherence to performing their homework, and their mindset about their musculoskeletal health and your ability to help them can all limit progress or hinder goal attainment. Therefore, to achieve their goals of becoming pain-free and functional again, clients' relationships with you must be developed to make them responsible for program outcomes, accountable for their own actions, and full participants in everything that contributes to program success.

ENCOURAGING CLIENT PARTICIPATION

You can help clients assume a sense of empowerment for the outcomes of their programs in two distinct ways:

1. Educate them.
2. Get them to take personal responsibility.

EDUCATION

Since most clients don't know how to help themselves overcome their musculoskeletal imbalances, teaching them about their bodies is an effective way to encourage their participation. Specifically, you can

- explain how each part of the body works individually and with other parts,
- show them what musculoskeletal imbalances they are experiencing,
- discuss how these imbalances affect their muscles and other soft tissues,
- talk about what they can do to overcome these limitations, and
- examine what they might be doing that could affect the progress of their program.

Once clients begin to understand why they experience pain or movement restrictions, and what may be contributing to their problems (e.g., sitting at a desk for eight hours or wearing high-heeled shoes), they become more aware of the things they are doing (or not doing, as the case may be) that might be problematic. This will strengthen their desire to do things differently (Reeve 2015).

RESPONSIBILITY

You can encourage clients to take responsibility for the success of their programs by encouraging them to ask questions, contribute ideas, and offer information when you discuss their programs. This will help them feel that they are important to the process, and it will bolster their confidence and self-esteem. The more a client's self-reliance grows, the more he will contribute to planning the exercise program and the better his adherence will be (American College of Sports Medicine 2014). When used consistently, these communication and program design techniques will have a cascading effect on a client's behavior; ultimately, he will feel personally responsible for achieving his goals. Encouraging his participation in program design will also have a direct impact on his mindset, his physical and mental efforts, and his level of attainment.

FUNCTIONING AS A FACILITATOR

Shaping client expectations and encouraging client participation also require you to redefine the part you play in program design. You may initially assume an authoritative role in client relationships. However, you too must adjust your approach. The simplest and most effective way to do this is to view your role as that of a facilitator rather than an expert. This subtle but important shift helps promote teamwork from the outset.

You can strengthen your role as a facilitator during consultations and assessments by asking open-ended questions and paying attention to clients' verbal and nonverbal responses. Active listening (i.e., paying attention to clients' body language, having empathy for their situations, and not just waiting for them to finish talking so you can say what you want to say) will also enable you to help clients to identify strategies or changes they need to make on their own to improve their condition (Brockbank and McGill 2006; Bryant, Green, and Newton-Merrill 2013; Price 2012). Specific communication strategies for initial consultations and exercise sessions will be discussed in detail in chapters 23 and 24.

While it may be easier and less time consuming to direct clients to a specific course of action because you as a professional know what will help them, their motivation and ultimate success depend on their making their own decisions. Involving them in designing their own programs is important to shaping their expectations and behavior, and it will help them to understand what you can both achieve by working together. While you *are* a source of professional knowledge and guidance, it is not your job to solve all of a client's problems. Be aware of any tendency you may have to try to step in and fix things when clients share their stories and complaints. This type of response only positions you as an expert, not a facilitator. As you listen to clients share their concerns, and as you ask follow-up questions, you can reduce their anxiety and encourage them to take responsibility for the things they have identified that are influencing their musculoskeletal health (Schwarz 2017).

As you talk or work with clients, issues that may affect their progress, such as depression, anxiety disorders, or other psychological conditions, may come to light. It is not within your scope of practice to diagnose or treat any psychological or medical condition, but you should have a referral system in place to qualified doctors and mental health practitioners who can assist clients when appropriate. (More information in this topic appears in chapter 28, Scope of Practice, Networks, and Referrals.)

Go to the online video and watch video 22.1, where Justin talks about empowering clients for program success.

Review of Key Points

In order to design successful corrective exercise programs, you must understand basic human behavior and motivations in addition to having skills in assessment, anatomy, and exercise.

- There are two main reasons why people with musculoskeletal imbalances seek assistance from fitness professionals:
  1. They lack the knowledge needed to resolve problems on their own.
  2. They lack confidence in their own ability to alleviate their condition.

- Understanding basic human dynamics and behavior can help you to educate clients and build their confidence, thereby validating their decision to seek your help.

- When clients approach fitness professionals for help, they typically assume the role of someone subordinate to the fitness professional's expertise. The assumption of subordinate and expert roles affects the way each party views the actions and responsibilities of the other.

- To avoid the potential pitfalls of a subordinate-and-expert relationship, view your role as that of a facilitator instead of an authority figure. Help your clients to understand the basic principles of designing a corrective exercise program.

- By adopting a facilitator approach, you can develop a teamwork approach to working with clients on their programs.

- Requiring or encouraging clients to contribute ideas and suggestions from the outset will help build their confidence. As their confidence grows, clients will get more involved in the process, and they will feel a sense of responsibility for program outcomes.

Self-Check

There are many ways you can improve your abilities as a facilitator in your client relationships. Consider the attributes and skills that follow, and put a check mark next to those items you think are important to develop or possess in your efforts to build better client relationships.

Skills and knowledge	Important	Not important
The ability to remain focused on a client's long-term objectives and outcomes		
Skill at creating prepackaged corrective exercise programs and solutions		
The ability to defend your recommendations if a client becomes upset during a consultation or session		
Above-average listening skills		
Open and direct verbal communication skills		
A willingness to concede to anything and everything a client wants		

Skills and knowledge	Important	Not important
Being accessible to clients (within reason) as it pertains to their exercise programs		
Being able to provide consistent information, service, and feedback to clients		
A steadfast devotion to your own ideas and views of corrective exercise		
The ability to plan ahead and foresee obstacles		
The ability to understand that client anxiety may sometimes be expressed as anger, defiance, or tearfulness		
The ability to understand how the assumption of typical roles in a trainer-and-client relationship can affect program outcomes		

CHAPTER 23

Conducting Consultations

In chapter 22, you learned about the motivations and psychological traits that can affect behavior as you and your clients meet to address their musculoskeletal concerns. Understanding that your client might view this experience very differently than you do will encourage you to communicate as clearly as possible at every stage of the consultation process. Trying to understand your client's perspective will also help you to build trust, avoid mistakes, and increase the likelihood that a prospect will sign up to use your services.

FIRST CONTACT

As with any situation where two parties are involved, there are always different ways of seeing, feeling, communicating, and interpreting the first contact with each other. The following section will explore the elements of this interaction from a typical client's perspective and then from yours. It will also cover practical considerations and tips for success during this initial contact so that the client will set up an appointment and give you the opportunity to perform a complete in-person assessment.

CLIENT'S PERSPECTIVE

When prospective clients first inquire into your services, it is likely they have tried and failed to improve their conditions with the help of other health and fitness professionals, especially if they have had the problems for some time (Boyes 2015). Therefore, while they may be hopeful, they may doubt that you can help them. If they cannot participate in activities they enjoy because of pain or dysfunction, they might fear that they will never be able to do them again. Their anxiety may have been compounded by misinformation they gathered online (Simpson, Neria, Lewis-Fernández, and Schneier 2010).

Most potential clients will also be apprehensive about meeting with you to discuss their situation. You can begin to allay their fears by responding to their initial inquiries by telephone rather than by email or texting. Talking with a person, rather than communicating electronically, helps a potential client feel more comfortable about meeting you.

YOUR PERSPECTIVE

While a potential client will probably be anxious about contacting you for assistance, your reaction will probably be excitement that you may be getting another customer. You may also feel nervous about meeting a new person and persuading her to sign up for your services. This combination of excitement and nervousness can sometimes make you do things you would not normally do when speaking with clients, like talking too much in an effort to establish your worth, using technical jargon, or making assumptions about her condition before you have even met her (Donaldson 2007).

In order to quell your own anxieties when first contacting a prospective client, keep the initial conversation simple, and refrain from talking about yourself too much. Once the person has summarized her problem, suggest that she make an appointment for a consultation so you can assess her and make an informed decision about whether you can help her.

PRACTICAL CONSIDERATIONS FOR INITIAL CONTACT

There are many things to keep in mind so that your initial contact with a client can be a positive experience.

GATHERING ESSENTIAL INFORMATION

During your initial conversation about an in-person consultation, you must exchange certain basic information:

- Ask for (and record) the prospective client's full name, contact details, and general reason for wanting to meet with you.
- Discuss what the client can expect during the consultation and assessment process and what he should wear.
- Provide your telephone number and clear directions on how to get your facility.
- Confirm the time and date of the appointment before ending the conversation.
- Send a follow-up email containing the details of the appointment and directions to the meeting (Price and Bratcher 2010).

CHARGING FOR CONSULTATIONS

During your initial conversation, you should tell the prospective client whether the consultation and assessment session is complimentary or a paid service. If a person is coming to see you specifically for help with a musculoskeletal issue, it may be best to provide the initial consultation and assessment free of charge. Otherwise, a prospective client who has had unsuccessful experiences with other health and fitness professionals may think that you, too, are just out to take his money. However, if you are willing to take the time to speak to him on the telephone and then conduct a full, complimentary verbal, visual, and hands-on assessment, he will be more likely to trust you and your skills. As your reputation in the field of corrective exercise grows, you will receive more referrals. At that point, you may decide to start charging for consultations since most of your referrals will come from sources the potential client trusts, such as friends, family members, a peer, or a work colleague, and there will be less need for persuasion (Bly 1991).

VERBAL ASSESSMENT PROCESS

The following section will explore the elements of the verbal portion of the in-person consultation and assessment process from a typical client's perspective and then from your perspective. It will also cover practical considerations and tips for success during the verbal assessment.

CLIENT'S PERSPECTIVE

When a prospective client arrives for her appointment with you, she might expect to be greeted by a receptionist. While this type of setup may provide a professional air (and be more convenient for you), having to interact with another stranger upon arrival often adds to the client's nervousness. Therefore, whenever possible, greet the prospective client yourself when she arrives. This allows you to introduce yourself, and it makes her feel more relaxed (since she will recognize you from having spoken on the phone). If you are busy working with another

---

First Contact: Keys to Success

- It is not uncommon for potential clients to ask you to venture a guess about their particular musculoskeletal issue over the telephone or before you have performed a complete in-person structural assessment. Never do this—it is unwise, unprofessional, and potentially sets you up for failure if your assumptions are incorrect.
- If possible, avoid discussing fees until after the initial consultation so you can demonstrate your skills and establish the value of your program first.

Obviously, if you are asked directly for a schedule of fees, it is appropriate to state your rates.

- Keep the first contact on the telephone brief and professional because it will convey that you are a valued expert whose time is respected.
- If a prospective customer was referred to you by a current client, you may acknowledge that you know that client. However, never discuss the details of the referring party's problems or program.

client when the new person arrives, you should still acknowledge her presence and let her know that you will be with her shortly (Price and Bratcher 2010). Personally acknowledging prospective clients on arrival also helps to cultivate a more positive attitude about the consultation.

Prospective clients may assume that they will be asked to complete some lengthy paperwork and then told to sit and wait. This can be frustrating, especially for someone whose musculoskeletal pain makes it uncomfortable to sit for prolonged periods. While some paperwork may be needed before the consultation begins, limit this to a short intake form that asks for the client's basic information. You can gather more detailed information about their condition and their history during the verbal consultation, and again when they agree to sign up for your services. Showing consideration by limiting the initial paperwork conveys empathy, and this positive feeling will carry over into the assessment process (Price 2012).

Once the verbal consultation begins, the potential client will experience many emotions, and these may be expressed in various ways. Typically, an anxious client will

- feel nervous or self-conscious that his body and lifestyle are being scrutinized,
- be reluctant to speak and to share pertinent information,
- talk nonstop or speak very quickly, making it difficult for you to glean important data, and
- give nonverbal indications of nervousness such as crossing his arms or legs, fidgeting, looking away, or turning his body away (Griffin 2006).

Being aware of these clues can help you to detect when a person is feeling uneasy and should prompt you to change your own behavior to make the experience more positive and less stressful for the prospective client.

YOUR PERSPECTIVE

While a prospective client may be expected to feel nervous during the in-person consultation, you may also feel apprehensive about the meeting. If a prospective client arrives very early for the consultation and you are with another client, for example, you may get anxious about the new person watching you work. As a result, you may interact differently with the client you are currently helping. Be aware of your own tendencies when you are nervous, and refocus on the task at hand. This will result in a better experience for everyone.

On the other hand, if a prospective client is late for an appointment, you may worry that you will not be able to finish the assessment and consultation before your next scheduled client arrives. In that case you can tell the prospective client when she arrives that you have another appointment directly after hers. This will enable you to adjust your meeting strategy and let the client know when to expect the consultation to end (Price and Bratcher 2010).

Occasionally, your own experiences and biases may surface upon meeting a new client face-to-face. This can affect the way you interact with that person (Sternberg, Roediger, and Halpern 2007). For example, if you have little empathy for extremely overweight people, you may not be sympathetic when an obese person tells you about his musculoskeletal discomfort. Alternatively, you might make assumptions based on clothing or appearances about whether a person can afford your rates. Every potential client deserves your full respect and attention. It is your responsibility to be aware of your own preconceptions so they do not affect the way you communicate with prospective clients.

PRACTICAL CONSIDERATIONS FOR THE VERBAL ASSESSMENT

There are many aspects of the verbal assessment that must be taken into account to ensure a smooth and productive experience.

CONSULTATION AREAS

During the verbal assessment you will discuss a variety of topics, some of which may be personal. It is essential to use a quiet place to conduct this part of the consultation so the client can feel comfortable answering your questions. If possible, arrange the consultation space in a way that signifies that you and the client are equals; move your chair around from behind your desk, or choose a couch or bench where you both can sit together (Griffin 2006).

RAPPORT BUILDING

Establishing rapport quickly with a prospect will increase the likelihood that the verbal assessment will go well.

- Make direct eye contact, and make sure that your body language, tone of voice, and spoken words are in harmony. If your words are positive, but your body language is closed off or you avoid eye contact when speaking, potential clients will get mixed messages that may erode your credibility (Griffin 2006).

- Begin the consultation with an open-ended question, such as, "How can I help you?" Open-ended questions let clients answer in a way that is comfortable for them, enabling them to control the opening subject matter.

- As the person gains confidence during the discussion, begin to ask closed-ended questions, such as, "Do you have pain in your feet?" in order to get more specific information (Friesen 2010).

GUIDING THE CONVERSATION

When you ask an open-ended question at the beginning of the assessment, the client may tell you about discomfort she has in a certain part of her body, such as her lower back. Once you have talked about this issue, use the Client Assessment Diagram (CAD) to steer the conversation toward the topics you need to complete the evaluation (Price and Bratcher 2010). For example, you can guide the conversation by asking, "Have you ever experienced other pains in your body such as your knees?" Even if the prospective client does not mention previous or current pains, it is necessary to ask about pain and function for every part of the body. Doing so may remind her of past incidents, such as broken bones, surgeries, or accidents, that can affect the success of her program (Petty and Moore 2002).

As the assessment continues, the prospective client may reveal that someone she knows had similar issues that required drastic measures to resolve, such as a friend who had a hip replacement. Address these anxieties head-on by reminding her that you will be performing a thorough physical evaluation of her entire body following the verbal assessment, and you will be offering corrective exercise solutions. Acknowledging clients' concerns in this manner keeps the verbal assessment going while also helping turn their fears into hope for the future (Price and Bratcher 2010).

CONTEMPLATING SOLUTIONS AND GAUGING COMMITMENT

During the verbal assessment, you will ask about any activities or exercises the person is currently using to try to deal with their limitations or their pain. This type of information will help you gauge whether the client has already created some form of disciplined approach and time commitment to resolving the problem. It will also provide you with an opportunity to evaluate the client's prior experience(s) with other health and fitness professionals and whether she is genuinely ready to participate in a corrective exercise program (Price and Bratcher 2010).

Verbal Assessment: Keys to Success

- If clients must wait before the assessment begins, make sure they feel comfortable in the interim by offering them water and directions to the rest rooms or changing facilities.

- Using technical jargon or talking too much can make a client feel overwhelmed. Be conscious of this as you conduct the assessment (Donaldson 2007).

- Refrain from getting too personal when asking questions during the verbal assessment. Gather pertinent information about the client's musculoskeletal and health issues without delving into their private lives (Price and Bratcher 2010).

- Belittling the past efforts of clients who have used the services of professionals whose methods you disagree with, or who have had unnecessary surgeries, will only make them feel foolish (Price and Bratcher 2010). Always applaud their efforts to find solutions.

- If a prospective client highlights a specific place on his body that is painful and wants you to examine it during the verbal consultation, stay on track with the verbal assessment process, but use that opportunity to inform him of what will take place in the visual and hands-on assessments to follow.

- The verbal assessment is only one part of the assessment process. Complete the entire assessment process (including the visual and hands-on portions), gathering all the necessary clues before making a decision about a client's musculoskeletal issues.

STRESS AND MUSCLE TENSION

Since mental pressures often manifest as muscular tension, stress is another matter that should factor into your verbal assessment conversation. While it is not necessary (or appropriate) for you to inquire about the specific cause of a client's stress, it is your job to educate people about how stress can affect their musculoskeletal health. To stay within your scope of practice, simply ask prospective clients if they find aspects of their work, relationships, or home life to be stressful. If the answer is yes, you can talk about some exercise strategies, such as self-massage techniques, to help negate the physical effects of stress (Price 2015).

VISUAL AND HANDS-ON ASSESSMENT PROCESS

Once you have completed the verbal assessment, you will commence the visual and hands-on assessment process. As with the verbal assessment, we will examine two perspectives on this experience—the client's and your own.

CLIENT'S PERSPECTIVE

Upon completion of the verbal assessment, most prospective clients believe that their mental involvement in the assessment process is over. This impression may result from past consultation experiences when they answered some initial health questions and then relaxed and waited for the professional to examine them, diagnose the problem, and offer up the recommended treatment. Although common, this approach to assessment reinforces clients' lack of self-confidence by making them think their involvement is not important. As you now know, in order for your clients to succeed, they need to take responsibility for the desired outcome (Reeve 2015). Therefore, the visual and hands-on assessment process requires as much, if not more, client participation than the verbal assessment.

Once clients realize that they will be actively involved in the visual and hands-on evaluation, they will likely feel a rush of self-consciousness. You can minimize their anxiety by

- keeping them focused on the process,
- avoiding comments about their aesthetic appearance or apparel, and
- limiting remarks about any physical abnormalities you observe.

It is also important to bear in mind that if a client does have a physical deviation, he may try to brush over that area of his body when it is being assessed. This is particularly common when it comes to physical characteristics such as bunions or calluses. For example, when you note a person's bunions during the visual and hands-on assessment for the feet and begin to ask questions, many clients will casually remark that the bunions have been there for a long time and do not really hurt at all. In fact, they may be excruciating or extremely embarrassing. The only way to gauge how clients truly feel about an unusual physical trait is to pay attention to their body language in addition to what they say during the assessment (Griffin 2006).

YOUR PERSPECTIVE

The visual and hands-on assessment process enables you to uncover the cause of a client's pain or dysfunction, and it gives you an opportunity to demonstrate your skills. However, this part of the assessment process is also where your anxieties may take over as you try to show the person how much you know. Remember that extraneous information will only detract from the effectiveness of the assessments. Focus on conducting the assessments and conveying the findings in a practical way that makes sense to the client.

PRACTICAL CONSIDERATIONS

To ensure a smooth and productive experience at this stage of the consultation, bear in mind the following points.

MAKE CONNECTIONS

Before commencing the visual and hands-on assessments, explain to the prospective client what you will be doing. People will feel more comfortable when they know what to expect (Shah and Gardner 2008). Refer to the Client Assessment Diagram for guidance until you are completely familiar with the visual and hands-on assessments you need to perform and in what order.

Talk the client through each assessment as you perform it, and link each assessment to the next area of the body. For example, if you have assessed a person's feet and ankles and found that they overpronate, explain how overpronation affects the function of her knees. Although this kind of information may seem simple to you, it may be the first time she has ever been made aware of the functional relationship between her feet and her knees. Helping clients to understand these links reassures them that their bodies are not broken—they are simply reacting to imbalances elsewhere (Price and Bratcher 2010).

USE APPROPRIATE LANGUAGE

For clients to meaningfully participate in the assessment process with you, you must convey crucial technical information so a layperson can understand it (Donaldson 2007). Here are suggestions on how to phrase technical assessment information in client-friendly ways:

Technical term	Client-friendly term
Overpronation	Flattening of the foot
Excessive lumbar lordosis	Too much arch in the-lower back
Excessive thoracic kyphosis	Rounded shoulders
Excessive cervical lordosis	Too much arch in the neck
Valgus knee	Moved toward the middle
Anterior rotation	Front of pelvis has tipped down
Tibia and fibula	Lower leg
Femur	Upper leg or thigh bone
Acetabulum	Hip socket
Lumbar spine	Lower back
Thoracic spine	Mid- to upper back
Cervical spine	Neck
Glenohumeral joint	Shoulder joint
Scapula	Shoulder blade

ACCOMMODATING LEARNING STYLES

In addition to the language you use, another part of engaging someone in the assessment process is to integrate their style of learning into the proceedings. Once the visual and hands-on assessment is underway, tune in to whether the prospective client learns most effectively by watching (visual learning style), listening (verbal learning style), or doing (kinesthetic learning style) (Winnick and Porretta 2017). Some people might learn using a combination of all three styles. Generally, a person will use descriptive words that match his learning style.

- A verbal learner might respond to your explanations with statements such as, "I *hear* what you are saying" or "That doesn't *sound* good!" Verbal learners benefit from detailed and clear instructions that enable them to focus on the words being used versus the actions being performed (Winnick and Porretta 2017).

- Visual learners might respond to your instructions with statements such as, "I *see* what you're saying" or "That didn't *look* good!" This type of learner would benefit most from observing the assessments as you conduct them (e.g., watching you perform them in a mirror so they can see the results for themselves) (Winnick and Porretta 2017).

- Kinesthetic learners might respond to something you have said with a statement such as, "I really *feel* that when my foot collapses," or "I can also *sense* what happens to my knee when my foot flattens." Kinesthetic learners need to physically experience what their particular imbalances feel like. You can help them achieve this by coaching them to place their own hands on parts of their bodies as you perform each assessment (Winnick and Porretta 2017).

MAXIMIZING ASSESSMENT IMPACT

Teaching prospective clients how to perform some of the structural assessments you use is a great way to maximize their participation in the process (Price and Bratcher 2010). Also, if they know how to perform assessments on their own, then they will be able to monitor their own progress after their programs begin. Furthermore, if prospective clients learn to perform some of the assessments during the consultation, they may try them on friends or family members. This can spark interest in your corrective exercise services from other people and lead to promising referrals (Price and Bratcher 2010).

While you might mention one or two exercise solutions as you perform the assessments, do not provide too much exercise information during the assessment process. A good rule of thumb is that once you get an indication that the prospective client is buying into the program (and excited about the exercises he will learn), do not discuss any more sample solutions. Leave clients feeling eager for more at the end of the assessment process because this will prompt them to sign up for the program (Price 2012).

CONCLUDING THE ASSESSMENT PROCESS

When you are ready to bring the consultation to a close, return to a quiet place and summarize your findings from the structural assessment. Ending the consultation in a private area enables you to hold the client's attention while you explain your findings. It also gives you a much more appropriate place to discuss the issue of money (Griffin 2006). Following is an example of how to summarize the assessment process:

Mr. Stone, based on the assessment findings, we discovered that both of your feet flatten out more than they should. This is probably caused by the fact that your shoulders are rounded forward, which is causing your body to fall forward of its center of gravity and to place more stress on your feet. The rounding of your shoulders forward also makes you have to arch the back of your neck excessively to keep your eyes aligned with the horizon. This musculo-skeletal imbalance in your upper back is what is making both your neck and your feet hurt.

CLOSING THE DEAL

The last part of the consultation process involves providing program information that will lead to the person signing up for your services (Crane 2013). This section will discuss each party's perspective with regard to closing the deal and will cover practical considerations and tips for success during this final stage.

CLIENT'S PERSPECTIVE

When the assessment process is over, the prospective client will typically want to know:

- How much do your corrective exercise services cost?
- How many sessions will it take to reach my goals?
- How often do I need to see you?

People may also have special circumstances that are of concern to them. For example, prospective clients who travel often will want to know if they will be able to move forward with their corrective exercise programs when they are away from home. Others may have to travel a long way to see you and, therefore, may find it difficult to attend sessions on a regular basis. In special circumstances such as these, be prepared to provide alternate program suggestions and to help these people set realistic goals about what to expect from a modified program (Price and Bratcher 2010).

While some of the questions asked during the consultation wrap-up are legitimate, often they are indications of last-minute pangs of insecurity. This is natural behavior for anyone who is deciding to pledge substantial time and money to a new course of action. However, if you listen to the prospective clients' concerns and address each question in a logical and empathetic manner, their fears will be lessened, and they will feel more confident about deciding to use your services (Bandura 1986).

YOUR PERSPECTIVE

By now you should be more self-assured when it comes to your structural assessment and corrective exercise skills. However, you may be less confident, or even intimidated, by the act of selling your products and services. While this is a common challenge for many personal service providers, you must work on strengthening your sales abilities. If you appear nervous when discussing program variables, duration, or costs, prospective clients may misinterpret this as dishonesty, weakening their confidence in you and your programs. Therefore, it is important for you to navigate this final portion of the consultation process confidently (Bly 1991). Remember that

---

Visual and Hands-On Assessment: Keys to Success

- Nervous clients may try to divert your attention during the assessment process by talking about different topics or showing you exercises they have done in the past. Note their anxieties and listen to their concerns, but stick to the step-by-step nature of the assessment process (Price and Bratcher 2010).

- Some clients will make flattering comments during the assessment process that classify you as an authority figure. Always bring the tone of the assessment back to you as a facilitator, not the authority (Schwarz 2017).

- The assessment process is psychologically taxing for clients. Keep the consultation to an hour or less by sticking to your assessment plan and following the assessment protocols.

- Never diagnose a medical condition or provide an opinion about a medical issue. This is completely beyond the scope of practice of most health and fitness professionals (Bryant and Green 2010).

selling the program to a potential client is no different from any other part of the consultation process. You simply follow a structured and well-practiced routine to ensure that you cover all the important sales and transaction details.

PRACTICAL CONSIDERATIONS FOR CLOSING THE CONSULTATION

Following are some vital elements for bringing your consultation wrap-up to a successful close.

OUTLINING THE PROPOSED PROGRAM

Once you have summarized your assessment findings and plan of action, explain that The BioMechanics Method corrective exercise programs are comprised of three phases that are designed to help the body adapt to the musculoskeletal changes you will be making together: self-myofascial release (or self-massage), stretching, and strengthening exercises. Explain that these phases will be introduced in that order, and then briefly describe each one so the client understands the rationale (Price and Bratcher 2010).

Self-myofascial release and self-massage could be explained as follows:

Self-massage is akin to chewing gum before you blow a bubble. You have to work the gum first in order to make it soft and flexible, otherwise it will tear when you try to blow the bubble. Think of your muscles the same way. Your imbalances have created some inflexible areas in your muscles and soft tissues. If we start off with exercises that try to move your body into increased ranges of motion without first loosening up the tissues, we might hurt something. That's why I will teach you the self-massage component first so your body loosens up before we begin asking it to perform greater ranges of movement like stretching.

The stretching component could then be summarized as follows:

Once you have loosened up your muscles and soft tissues with the self-massage exercises, we can focus on moving those muscles and joints that have not been working correctly. This is done through various types of stretching.

Finally, explain the strengthening component of the program:

When your muscles and joints can move more effectively, we will start adding exercises that will help your body get stronger so you can eliminate your imbalances and maintain better alignment. As you progress with the strengthening exercises, they will become more integrated, meaning that your whole body will be working together like what happens in real life. For example, I'll be teaching you exercises that will help you to walk without pain or to play tennis or golf better (if these are two sports that clients have indicated that they enjoy).

Providing a succinct overview of the proposed program also helps a client understand that corrective exercise is a process that requires time and perseverance (Simpson 2011).

GIVING SPECIFIC EXAMPLES

After the program overview, give one specific example of a corrective exercise and illustrate how this particular strategy will address the person's current musculoskeletal issue(s) if needed. For example, you might explain what a foam roller is and how you will teach the client to use it to massage the muscles of her upper back to address her rounded shoulder posture and alleviate her shoulder and neck pain. If appropriate, also share one or two nonexercise-related tactics, such as changing shoe types or adjusting sleeping posture, that will be included as part of the corrective exercise program. Highlighting small, nonexercise-related changes will make the corrective exercise process appear easy to implement and will build the client's confidence (Price 2012).

DESCRIBING A TYPICAL SESSION

Once a prospective client has learned about the general components of the program, describe what may happen during a typical session.

- State how long each session will last and, if you are integrating corrective strategies into other exercise programs like sport-specific training, how much time you will spend per session learning, progressing, and regressing the corrective exercises.

- Advise clients that they will be required to perform homework exercises outside of the times you meet together. Further explain that you will take a picture of each exercise you recommend and provide written instructions for how to perform it (Simpson 2011). More information on how to present a client's homework in a professional format is provided in chapter 25.

- Explain that each session will begin with a review of the exercises the client has been working on and then adjusted based on his progress.

ESTIMATING PROGRAM DURATION AND FREQUENCY

Most people want to know how long they will need to perform the corrective exercises and how long their corrective exercise program will last. The answers to these questions will depend largely on how much time and effort they are willing to commit. The importance of getting clients to tell you how much time they have available, rather than you telling them how much time they must commit, cannot be understated.

To help clients determine how long it will take to reach their corrective exercise goals, ask them how much time they are prepared to commit to their homework exercises. If they tell you they can spend 20 minutes a day, then the homework program you design should be no longer than 20 minutes. Getting clients to identify their desired homework session length gets them involved in the process and makes them responsible for finding the time each day to do the work. If instead you tell them how much time they must commit, they will blame you if they cannot set aside the necessary time (Price and Bratcher 2010).

The subject of how many corrective exercise sessions you think clients will need should be addressed in conjunction with the discussion of how much time they can commit to the homework exercises. If they say they can only commit 5 to 10 minutes a day, explain that it might take longer than average for them to reach their goals. If they can spend more time each day on their homework exercises, they will reach their objectives more quickly.

DISCUSSING PROGRAM COSTS

The assessment and consultation process is carefully designed to make a prospective client recognize your specialty skills. Consequently, most people will expect that your program rates reflect the expert services you offer (Bly 1991). Whether you offer single sessions, session packages, or a combination of sessions and packages, confidently convey what your prices are for each possibility and inform clients of their payment options. It is advantageous to provide several payment choices, including cash, checks, direct deposit, and credit cards. This will give clients more flexibility to invest in their programs and will ensure that you have the opportunity to help them realize their goals (Price and Bratcher 2010).

Closing the Deal: Keys to Success

- Extraneous talk or additional information about other products or services you offer will hinder your ability to sell your corrective exercise programs. Aim to retain the positive feelings about the assessment and consultation to close the deal (Swain and Brawner 2014).

- A prospective client's enthusiasm can be contagious, but avoid going into too much program detail during the consultation close. Offer only a couple of examples of what the program entails, and keep those examples brief.

- If clients are not prepared to put in the necessary work to achieve their goals, help them to develop realistic expectations about your programs or services.

- Although it can sometimes be beneficial for you to allow a bit of flexibility with regard to program costs or duration when closing the consultation, do not let a potential client regulate your fees or your area of expertise (Price 2012).

- Trying to get an eager client to sign up for as many sessions as possible in order to boost your income can be tempting. However, it is your responsibility to help every client to succeed in the most efficient manner possible.

Review of Key Points

The assessment and consultation process is used to sell your corrective exercise services and to set up the right kind of relationship with prospective clients. When performed well, it can alleviate client anxieties, increase potential adherence, and accurately shape expectations about the program.

- Whenever possible, speak with prospective clients on the telephone (as opposed to communicating via text or email) before meeting them in person.

- Ask open-ended questions at the beginning of the in-person consultation to enable the client to guide the initial stages of the conversation. As the consultation progresses, ask closed-ended questions, such as those detailed on the Client Assessment Diagram (CAD), to gather specific information about the client's health history and musculoskeletal condition.

- As you conduct the visual and hands-on assessments, use jargon-free language, and employ verbal, visual, and kinesthetic teaching methodologies to ensure that potential clients can follow along and participate.

- Summarize your results at the end of the assessment process, answer any questions the prospective client may have about their musculoskeletal health, and briefly discuss the general components of The BioMechanics Method corrective exercise programs.

- Always ask potential clients how much time they are prepared to dedicate to their homework each day rather than telling them how much you expect of them.

- Be direct and confident when discussing money and providing information on estimated program costs and payment options.

Self Check 1

It is important to practice the visual and hands-on assessment portion of the initial consultation often. Ask a friend or family member to allow you to perform the visual and hands-on assessment process, and record your results on a copy of the CAD provided in the appendix. When you are finished, use the following questions to elicit feedback on the person's consultation experience.

1. What would you like to have known to help you feel more comfortable before we began the visual and hands-on assessments?
2. Did you understand each of the assessments as we went through them and the explanations of how your imbalances might be causing your aches and pains? If not, what was confusing?
3. What could I have done better during the assessment process from a teaching standpoint?
4. Did you feel like you were contributing to the assessment process? If so, how?
5. If not, are you referring to the whole process or a specific part?
6. Is there anything I could have done differently to help you feel more comfortable during the assessment process?

Self-Check 2

In order to practice your consultation wrap-up and sales skills, ask your subject from Self-Check 1 to give you 10 minutes to try to sell him on the program of corrective exercise you propose. Use the following chart to guide you through this process. After completing the items in the left column, ask him for specific feedback on how you did and what you could have done differently to improve the experience. Record his responses in the right column.

Points to cover	Client feedback
Summarize the results of the assessment.	
Describe how the program is structured.	
Give one or two examples of exercises or techniques you plan to incorporate into his program to help him alleviate his issues.	
Describe how a session is structured.	
Ask whether the person is prepared to do homework and how often.	
Outline the number of sessions recommended and the frequency of visits.	
Discuss the program cost and payment options.	

CHAPTER 24

Structuring Sessions and Programs

After you sign a client up for your services, you will begin the process of developing a comprehensive corrective exercise program to address his underlying musculoskeletal imbalances. Just as you and your client would have experienced the consultation process differently, each of you will also have different psychological needs and practical requirements with regard to the design and application of his program. Understanding these needs (and the best way to satisfy them) will ensure that individual exercise sessions, and the program as a whole, progress smoothly and successfully.

BEGINNING AND BUILDING PROGRAMS

To create and deliver exercise sessions and complete programs, you must understand the process from a typical client's perspective as well as from your own. The following section will explore these different points of view. It will also cover practical considerations and tips for beginning and building a successful program.

CLIENT'S PERSPECTIVE

Your new client will now feel much more comfortable working with you as a result of her positive consultation experience. However, she will still have concerns when she arrives for her first appointment about whether the program will be effective. To help your client overcome these lingering fears, begin the first session by

- reminding her of the step-by-step nature of the program,
- emphasizing the importance of regular adherence to her homework, and
- restating the realistic expectations you set up together during the consultation process (Shah and Gardner 2008).

Continue by starting the self-myofascial exercise portion of your session as planned, but refrain from discussing the more complex exercises that will be introduced later. As the client progresses with her first session and begins to feel results, her confidence in her ability to perform more challenging activities will grow (Caissy 1998). Later sessions will become more motivating as her musculoskeletal health improves, and then you can begin sharing your plans for advancing her program.

Although it may seem counterintuitive, sometimes clients who have been unsuccessful at resolving their musculoskeletal problems in the past will unconsciously set themselves up to fail with your program. This is because humans are creatures of habit—we tend to repeat the same behaviors rather than make necessary (and sometimes difficult) changes to reach our goals (Berdik 2012). These clients may not be aware that they are sabotaging their own efforts. For example, consider a new client with severe hip pain who has tried other pain reduction programs such as physical therapy, chiropractic, and acupuncture. Although the other professionals offered treatments that should have brought relief, the client continued to experience pain and dysfunction. When you ask him why the other programs did not work, he tells you that he has no idea why. When you probe further, you learn that he was not willing to adjust or stop doing those activities that caused pain (e.g., running five miles a day). Based on this new information, you now understand that his frequent running was partly to blame for the failure of his previous treatments, and it may also sidetrack your program. In such a case, it is your job not only to provide appropriate corrective exercises, but also to help the client to identify behavioral and lifestyle changes he needs to make to ensure that his program succeeds (Bandura 1986).

YOUR PERSPECTIVE

Your main objective at this initial stage of the program is to address clients' problems as rapidly as possible. You want them to start to experience noticeable improvements, which will deepen their commitment and trust in you, your services, and the program. However, you may be anxious about performing well during this crucial meeting, and it can have adverse effects (Skovholt and Trotter-Mathison 2016).

The way you behave during your first corrective exercise session with a new client sets the tone for how you will continue to work together. At this stage, you both know the initial consultation went well, and you left that meeting feeling optimistic. Now you may feel an enormous amount of pressure to make sure your client stays happy and also quickly sees results. So you might talk a lot, or you might try to do too much in the initial session. This can be overwhelming for the client, and it may create unrealistic expectations about what a single session should look like. Therefore, in the first session and in all later sessions, it is vital to

- remain calm,
- use communication strategies that reduce the client's anxieties, such as avoiding technical jargon, and
- follow The BioMechanics Method structured exercise selection and design process (Price and Bratcher 2010).

PRACTICAL CONSIDERATIONS FOR BEGINNING AND BUILDING PROGRAMS

As you build corrective exercise programs and structure the sessions, there are many things to take into account to ensure a productive series of meetings and promote mutually beneficial relationships with your clients.

ESTABLISHING INITIAL PROGRAM VARIABLES

During the initial consultation wrap-up, you will have given your prospective client an overview of a general corrective exercise program. You will have explained that it progresses from self-myofascial release techniques to stretching and then to strengthening. This does not mean, however, that you need to use all of these modalities in every session. If someone has chronic or long-standing myofascial restrictions, for instance, then you may spend the first two to five sessions doing only self-myofascial release exercises before you move on to any stretching (Price and Bratcher 2010).

Once you start working with a client, you will be able to evaluate his ability to perform certain movements. With this information, you can determine which corrective exercises are most appropriate and how long you will need to concentrate on each modality before progressing to the next technique.

After you have evaluated the client's abilities and established your plan of action for a session, share your plan with the client. Toward the end of that session, assign appropriate corrective exercise homework, and outline your plan for the following session. Letting your clients know what to expect at each stage of the program will keep them motivated to perform their homework activities so they can make progress (Shah and Gardner 2008).

TIMEKEEPING

Regardless of what you do during a session, you must work within the time frame designated for each appointment. Predetermined session time frames are crucial for two reasons:

1. When clients know how long a session will last, they can better manage their time for the appointment itself and their other commitments.

2. Keeping an appointment to its specified time gives you clear parameters for managing the session content.

If you do not stick to your predetermined time frames, clients can become dissatisfied (Salvo 2016). Imagine you are working with a client and the session is going very well. Since you are making great progress, you decide to extend the session by 20 minutes because you do not have anyone scheduled during the next appointment block. You think you are doing the client a favor by giving her extra time and attention. In actuality, you are creating the expectation that she will receive extra time whenever you do not have someone booked immediately after her. Then when you cannot or choose not to give her extra time in the future, she will feel cheated.

PROVIDING CLEAR INSTRUCTIONS

Clients must learn to do their exercises correctly so they can do them well both in your presence and for homework. Following are some important points about giving exercise instructions.

- Always address clients' learning styles when you present new exercises, and link the benefits of each exercise back to the reason they came to see you (Winnick and Porretta 2017). For example, if a client wants to be able to bend down and pick up a child without his back hurting, link the benefits of doing the exercise you have chosen to that activity.

- Once a client understands an exercise and can do it correctly, have her perform it again and explain to you what movements she is making. For instance, a client performing the Butt Lift exercise may cue herself to keep her pelvis neutral and lift up using her butt muscles. As she describes her movements, make a mental note of the words she uses (or write them down), and use them in her homework instructions. Using the client's own wording allows you to incorporate her learning style into the instructions and verify that she understands what is required (Dempsey and Sales 1993).

- If a client forgets how to perform or fails to describe an exercise correctly, remind him of the technique and tell him you will add those instructions to his homework to help him remember. That way he can focus on learning the exercise now without worrying about whether he will forget it later.

- As the client performs each exercise, use a phone or digital camera to take a picture (or video if needed) of him performing it to include with his homework instructions.

- Once clients are confident they can do an exercise correctly on their own, discuss performance frequency and duration. Consider how much time they said during the initial consultation that they could spend on homework exercises. Make sure the number of exercises, sets, and reps fits into that time frame. A homework program that is outside the client's level of commitment will only result in nonadherence (Price 2016).

- Toward the end of each session, write down the mutually agreed-upon homework exercise instructions with the client present. Using session time to devise homework plans gives your clients every opportunity to understand what they need to do to reach their goals (Gallahue and Donnelly 2003).

- Print the photos you took during the session to accompany the instructions, or text or email them to the client the same day.

- Even though you will ask clients for input and feedback, it is your responsibility to make sure the homework instructions are clear and accurate (Bosworth 2010). For detailed information on how to teach each corrective exercise modality correctly, refer to chapters 15, 16, and 17.

- The use of customized client program workbooks can help clients to manage their homework instructions and consolidate program information. For more information on creating client program workbooks, refer to chapter 25.

> Go to the online video and watch video 24.1, where Justin talks about strategies for successful cueing.

EXERCISE REGRESSIONS, PROGRESSIONS, AND ALTERNATIVES

Occasionally, you and a client may disagree on whether they are ready to perform an exercise on their own. If clients are confident they can do the exercise, encourage them to do it, as long as they are not in danger of hurting themselves. But offer them a regression or an alternative movement in case they have problems. This will help build their self-confidence (Price and Bratcher 2010). Similarly, if you think someone will master his homework exercise quickly, offer a progression he can move on to before his next session with you. He will feel like an enormous success when you review his achievements and discuss further progressions.

When choosing exercises and designing programs, consider any obstacles that may prevent clients from doing the exercises on their own regularly. Some clients will have demanding work or travel days, for example. On those days, they will not be able to commit the normal amount of time to their homework. For these people, create a shorter program for those busier days. Alternatives like these will enable clients to continue to make progress even when other commitments compete for their time (Price and Bratcher 2010). For more information on how to progress, regress, and find alternatives for different types of corrective exercises, see chapters 15, 16, and 17.

MONITORING AND PROGRESSING PROGRAMS

Assigning homework is a vital part of achieving results and keeping corrective exercise programs moving forward. Therefore, beginning with the second session, always review the homework exercises you have given your clients, even if they tell you they have been doing their homework consistently and have no questions. Take as long as you need to do this at the start of each session, and make sure the exercises are being performed correctly. There are three reasons that this is important:

1. It enables you to observe their technique and give positive feedback on their progress.
2. It provides you with an opportunity to build their confidence.
3. You can highlight those behaviors and decisions you want the client to adapt as their own (Hale and Crisfield 2004).

Beginning and Building Programs: Keys to Success

- If a client arrives on time for an appointment, never start the session late. If you have trouble with time management, stagger your appointments so you have enough time at the end of each session to wrap up properly, but still enough wiggle room to begin the following session on time (Lynch 1992).

- If unavoidable circumstances result in you running a couple of minutes late, tell your next client that you will begin her session shortly. This helps waiting clients to know what to expect and helps the session to begin on a positive note.

- Do not conduct any part of a corrective exercise session in a busy place where people typically gather, such as near a drinking fountain, or where other activities occur at the same time (Griffin 2006). Corrective exercises require a lot of concentration, and clients need to be able to focus.

- Give clients exercises that they can feel confident performing, and move forward with small steps to ensure success at each stage (Price 2016).

- Do not assume or take a client's word that homework exercises have been done correctly. If a client has been doing them incorrectly, they may be doing more harm than good (Roberts 1992). Therefore, it is essential to always review homework.

- Running sessions to the last minute will not give you enough time to prepare your client's homework, so be sure to leave time for this. If you finish the homework planning before the session is due to end, spend the remaining time reviewing what the client has done during that session or what to expect in the next one (Price and Bratcher 2010).

- Do not be vague when scripting homework. Even if they say they can remember everything, people often forget details when they later try to replicate an exercise. Incorrectly completed homework exercises can slow program progress (Gallahue and Donnelly 2003).

For example, if during the review process a client says they discovered another tight spot toward the front of the thigh while performing the Foam Roller IT Band exercise for homework, you could commend him on his discovery. Then you could suggest he target that area by adding the Foam Roller Quadriceps to his program, and you could explain why this additional exercise would help. Reviewing homework also helps you to determine whether new exercises should be added based on the client's progress.

At the end of every session, schedule the next appointment and tell clients what you would like them to do between meetings. If you book the next appointment in a week, for example, you might suggest that the client do the homework at least five to six times before then (assuming the client has communicated to you that they are willing to do their homework almost every day). Scheduling a future appointment at the end of a current session also helps to reinforce the client's commitment to the program.

Review of Key Points

You will probably spend a lot of time working with each client throughout the course of a corrective exercise program, so it is important to create working relationships that foster trust and mutual respect. You must also pay close attention to your client's mental and physical needs, and facilitate their programs accordingly.

- Creating productive corrective exercise programs requires you to approach each client differently and focus on individual needs. It also requires appropriate teaching strategies so they understand exactly what they must do to reach their goals.

- You can alleviate clients' initial anxieties by taking things slowly, keeping things simple, and implementing program variables they can achieve.

- Provide a clear picture of what to expect in each exercise session, and structure your time accordingly. Follow The BioMechanics Method exercise progression protocol from self-myofascial release techniques to stretches and then to strengthening.

- Always link your exercise recommendations to your clients' goals. For example, if a client's ultimate goal is to be able to play tennis again, explain how each exercise relates to movements he will need on the tennis court.

- Progress a program when you feel a client is ready. Appropriate progressions keep clients motivated about moving forward.

- If a client is having difficulty mastering an exercise, it is your job to notice this before she becomes frustrated or hurts herself. Whenever necessary, regress the exercise to help maintain the client's confidence in herself and in the program.

- All information about a client's homework (whether exercise-related or not) should be recorded in a personalized workbook. Pictures (and videos if appropriate) should be taken of all homework exercises, and clear instructions should be provided so the client knows exactly what is expected.

Self-Check

The following table contains four sample exercises from the exercise library (chapters 19, 20, and 21). For each exercise, identify different cueing strategies you could use to teach the exercise based on your evaluation of whether a client is predominantly a visual, verbal, or kinesthetic learner. Then identify two ways to progress, two ways to regress, and two alternatives for each exercise. A sample has been provided.

Name of exercise	Visual cues	Verbal cues	Kinesthetic cues	Progressions	Regressions	Alternatives
Lunge With Knee Pull	"Watch how I pull my knee toward the midline."	"The key is to rotate the hip of your front leg around toward your back foot."	"Do you feel when you rotate your hip back that the glute works harder?"	1. Lunge With Knee Pull (with rotation) 2. Perform in bare feet on unstable surface	1. Glute Stretch 2. Foam Roller on Gluteal Complex	1. The Pivot 2. Lunge With Side Reach
Foam Roller Thoracic Spine						
Door Frame Stretch						
Butt Lift						
Hip Flexor Stretch (Sagittal)						

CHAPTER 25

Sample Sessions and Program

In this chapter you will learn how your program design skills can be applied in a comprehensive case study. You will meet a client who enrolled in a program of corrective exercise with The BioMechanics Method to help her overcome chronic back pain and recurring shoulder pain so she could return to the activities she enjoys.

This case study includes a summary of the information that was gathered during the client's initial consultation, her completed Client Assessment Diagram, and the homework exercises given during her first five sessions. After the description of each session, there is a detailed explanation for why each technique was included.

CLIENT BACKGROUND INFORMATION

Marion Hurst (name changed) is 60 years old and has experienced chronic lower back pain for the last three years. Her back pain is at its worst when she first gets out of bed in the morning and has to bend over to pick up the bowls to feed her dogs. As the morning progresses and she gets ready for work, her back loosens up. Marion has a sedentary job as an executive in an office. When she stands up at work after sitting for long periods of time, her back tightens up again. This causes her to become tired during the day, and she always feels exhausted when she gets home in the evening. As part of her job, Marion also has to attend many social functions where she must stand for long

periods of time. This prolonged standing also irritates her lower back. Marion finds the pain frustrating and sometimes creates excuses to get out of these social functions. Marion believes that she should wear high-heeled shoes to work and to all social gatherings to maintain a professional appearance.

During her free time, Marion likes to play golf two to three times a week. Her back pain is always worse in the evening after playing golf, and she also experiences more aches and pains the following morning. She also likes to go for long walks with her husband on weekends. However, typically after a couple of miles her back tightens up so much that she has to stop the walk. She finds this very frustrating because the pain is interfering with this fun activity that she and her husband have enjoyed together for years. In recent months her husband has been walking without her, while she stays at home watching television or reading. Because of this decrease in physical activity, Marion has gained 10 pounds and is feeling her energy levels lessen and her self-confidence diminish.

Marion has five grandchildren who come to visit every couple of weeks and who love to play in her large backyard. She has always relished playing with the grandkids, but in the last year or so her back has gotten so bad that she can no longer join in the fun and games. More recently, she has had to sit in a patio chair and just watch the kids. Not being able to participate in these physical activities with her grandchildren is quite depressing for Marion.

In addition to her back pain issues, Marion also experiences right-side shoulder pain and a little right knee pain after playing a lot of golf. She has noticed that if she plays golf on two consecutive days, her right shoulder is very uncomfortable for many days after. Consequently, Marion cannot play golf on both Saturday and Sunday when she has the most time to enjoy her favorite sport.

CLIENT GOALS

Marion identified five goals that she hopes participation in a corrective exercise program will help her achieve:

1. Get through her workday (and associated obligations) without back pain.
2. Return to walking with her husband.
3. Play golf without pain and discomfort in her lower back and shoulder.
4. Actively play with her grandchildren when they come to visit.
5. Feel better when she gets out of bed in the morning so that she doesn't feel so "old."

Marion indicated in her initial consultation that she can commit to 25 to 35 minutes a day for her corrective exercise homework.

STRUCTURAL ASSESSMENT RESULTS

The completed Client Assessment Diagram (figure 25.1) contains additional information about Marion's musculoskeletal condition that was gathered during her initial consultation and assessment.

EXERCISE PROGRAMMING AND RECOMMENDATIONS

This section contains an overview of the first five sessions of the corrective exercise program that was designed to help Marion successfully alleviate her chronic back pain. The details of each session and the rationale for choosing each exercise are provided. This will help you to better understand the strategic nature of The BioMechanics Method approach to corrective exercise program design, and it will help you to apply your skills when working with real clients. All of the exercises included in Marion's program are contained in chapters 19, 20, and 21.

SESSION 1

Duration: 1 hour

EXERCISE SELECTION INFORMATION

The exercises that were chosen for Marion's first session and subsequent homework were designed to address her underlying musculoskeletal issues, but they were also intended to help reduce her symptoms as quickly as possible. This would show her the value of the program and would motivate her to complete her homework while preparing for her next session.

Daily Homework Exercises and Instructions

The following exercises were chosen for Marion's first session based on her assessment results and stated goals. The wording of all instructions in this and later sessions were created together by Marion and her corrective exercise specialist (certified in The BioMechanics Method) at the conclusion of each session in an effort to increase her adherence and motivation. A photograph of Marion performing each exercise was also taken to accompany the written homework instructions, and these were added to her client program workbook.

1. Foam Roller Gluteal Complex: Place ankle on opposite knee. Lean on elbow or balance on hand while you pull knee toward chest. Roll all sore spots on butt for 1 to 2 minutes on each side.
2. Foam Roller IT Band: Roll all sore spots you find from side of hip down to knee. Pause on the worst areas for 10 to 20 seconds to help them release. Roll both sides for 1 to 2 minutes on each leg.
3. Two Tennis Balls on Upper Back: Begin with balls on middle of upper back at about bra height. "Scoot" body down to move balls up. Tilt pelvis to increase pressure. Use pillow to keep line of sight perpendicular to floor. To decrease pressure, increase pillow height. Spend 2 to 3 minutes finding all sore spots.
4. Calf Massage (with baseball): Massage calf muscles with baseball placed on hard-covered book. Find as many sore spots as possible, and spend 1 to 2 minutes on each calf.

5. Calf Stretch: Keep back foot straight and raise arch. Stretch both sides for 20 to 30 seconds.

6. Glute Stretch: Pull knee to chest as you drop hip down and away from knee to keep butt bone on floor. Rotate torso gently to increase stretch if needed. Do both sides for 20 to 30 seconds.

After Marion was asked at the beginning of her session if she was prepared to purchase a foam roller for use at home, it was agreed that her program (and homework) would commence with these initial exercises.

RATIONALE FOR EXERCISE SELECTION

The reasoning behind each exercise choice for Marion's first corrective exercise session and homework assignments follows.

Session 1: Exercise 1

Name of Exercise: Foam Roller Gluteal Complex

Selection Rationale: This exercise was chosen first for several reasons. Marion's structural assessment results revealed that she has an anterior pelvic tilt and excessive lumbar lordosis. As a result, the muscles that originate on the back and sides of the pelvis, sacrum, and fascia of the lower back are restricted and tight. This exercise would help release some of the tension in this area of her body to reduce her lower back pain.

This exercise was also chosen to rejuvenate the muscles and tissues of this area in preparation for stretching and strengthening exercises that will be introduced later. These progressions will be designed to help improve function when Marion is walking and playing golf.

Finally, this exercise was selected as the opening exercise for the program because it is fairly easy to do, and there is direct kinesthetic feedback when a person is doing it correctly—she can feel when she is on the right spot. The use of this simple, yet effective, exercise enables Marion to feel confident that she can replicate the exercise at home.

Session 1: Exercise 2

Name of Exercise: Foam Roller IT Band

Selection Rationale: This exercise was selected for a similar reason to the Foam Roller Gluteal Complex. The IT band is the connective tissue that helps continue the attachment of the gluteus maximus muscle to just below the knee. Therefore, the IT band has a direct impact on the function of both the lower back and the knee. During the assessment, Marion stated that she sometimes also experiences knee pain, so rolling the IT band will help this issue as well as her lower back.

Session 1: Exercise 3

Name of Exercise: Two Tennis Balls on Upper Back

Selection Rationale: This exercise was chosen next because Marion's structural assessment indicated that she has excessive thoracic kyphosis and spends much of her day in a rounded shoulder position hunched over a desk. This exercise will rejuvenate and regenerate the muscles of this area in preparation for strengthening exercises that will be added later in the program to help pull her thoracic spine back into extension (i.e., more upright). Training the thoracic extensors to work correctly will also help reduce stress on the lower back since it will not have to arch so much to help keep the spine upright. Lastly, this exercise is included in her program early on because it will target the underlying cause of Marion's lower back pain (excessive thoracic kyphosis as identified in her CAD).

Session 1: Exercise 4

Name of Exercise: Calf Massage (with baseball)

Selection Rationale: This exercise was chosen partly because of Marion's typical choice of footwear: high-heeled shoes. Marion's assessment results indicate that she overpronates, and this imbalance (and her choice of footwear) has caused her calf muscles to become tight and restricted. Consequently, these muscles are always irritated and prevent her from being able to dorsiflex at the ankle correctly. This lack of dorsiflexion prevents her from being able to move her pelvis and lower back into a more neutral position when standing or walking. The baseball on a book variation of the calf massage was chosen so that Marion would not have to round her shoulders forward to reach down to massage her calves. Instead, she can release her calf muscles while sitting upright.

CLIENT ASSESSMENT DIAGRAM

NAME
DATE 9/22/17

'X' for "Quick Check"

ANTERIOR VIEW

CHECKLIST	✓	DETAILS
Feet and Ankles:		
Pain?	✓	both after walking
Arthritis/Conditions?	✓	none reported
Function?	✓	affects walking
What makes better/worse?	✓	heels/golf shoes
Causal links?	✓	feet sore = back
Visual irregularities?	✓	swelling R side
Pronated?	✓	both R worse
Ab/Adducted?	✓	both R worse
Condition of toes?	✓	bunions (both)
Condition of plantar fascia?	✓	both sore R worse
Condition of calf muscles?	✓	both tight
Client knows neutral?	✓	yes
Knee:		
Pain?	✓	R after golf
Arthritis/Conditions?	✓	none reported
Function?	✓	not affected
What makes better/worse?	✓	golf
Causal links?	✓	feet/knee/back
Visual irregularities?	✓	none
Single leg squat?	✓	R knee moves in
Patella tracking?	✓	R side bad/pops
Client knows neutral?	✓	yes
Lumbo-Pelvic Hip:		
Pain?	✓	lower back
Arthritis/Conditions?	✓	none reported
Function?	✓	always bad/hurts

'X' for "Quick Check"

POSTERIOR VIEW

CHECKLIST	✓	DETAILS
What makes better/worse?	✓	shoes, sitting, standing
Causal links?	✓	feet & knees
Visual irregularities?	✓	arch in low back
Excessive lordosis?	✓	YES
Anterior rotation?	✓	YES
Client knows neutral?	✓	yes
Thoracic Spine/Shoulder:		
Pain?	✓	front R shoulder
Arthritis/Conditions?	✓	none reported
Function?	✓	raising arms
What makes better/worse?	✓	golf & typing
Causal links?	✓	R knee
Excessive kyphosis?	✓	YES - A LOT
Protracted/Elevated scapula?	✓	yes - R worse
Internally rotated arms?	✓	yes - R more
Muscle tension?	✓	yes - R more
Client knows neutral?	✓	yes
Head and Neck:		
Pain?	✓	R trag a bit
Arthritis/Conditions?	✓	none reported
Function?	✓	none reported
What makes better/worse?	✓	work & golf
Causal links?	✓	R shoulder
Visual irregularities?	✓	none
Forward head?	✓	2½" forward
Excessive neck curvature?	✓	yes
Client knows neutral?	✓	yes

ADDITIONAL NOTES

Occupation/Activities	8-10 hrs per day seated & then has to stand a lot in bad shoes. Loves golf & walking w/ spouse
Injuries/Surgeries	none reported
Footwear Considerations	need to address shoes - pronated feet placing stress on lower back by ant. rot. pelvis → ex. lum. lordosis
Major Deviation(s)	extremely bad ex. thor. kyphosis made worse by job - sits a lot - strengthen thor. erectors & glutes keep torso mobile

Figure 25.1 Completed CAD from case study client.

Session 1: Exercise 5

Name of Exercise: Calf Stretch

Selection Rationale: This exercise was selected next because it is a natural progression from the Calf Massage (with baseball). Increasing the flexibility of Marion's calf muscles will help her to reduce her anterior pelvic tilt and the associated lower back pain.

Session 1: Exercise 6

Name of Exercise: Glute Stretch

Selection Rationale: The Foam Roller Gluteal Complex exercise performed earlier in the session was in preparation for this stretching exercise. It was selected at this point because it follows the recommended order of progression from self-myofascial release exercise to stretching. This exercise also helps release tension from her lower back and sets her up for a further progression to glute strengthening exercises later in the program.

In addition, Marion's overpronation causes her knee to move toward the midline and her leg to internally rotate. The gluteus maximus muscle, which originates on the lower back and the back of the pelvis and attaches to the lower leg, is negatively affected by this movement dysfunction. Every time Marion overpronates, the insertion of the gluteus maximus is pulled away from its origin on her lower back. If she can gain some flexibility in her gluteus maximus by performing this stretch, her overpronation issues will not affect the position of her lower back (and her pain) to the same degree.

SESSION 2

Duration: 1 hour

EXERCISE SELECTION INFORMATION

At the start of Marion's second session, the exercises she had been performing for homework were reviewed. It was determined that she had been doing her exercises regularly and correctly. Therefore, some of the exercises were ready to be progressed (the Foam Roller Gluteal Complex) and some new exercises were added (the Foam Roller Hip Flexors and Hip Flexor Stretch [Sagittal]). Some of the original exercises remained the same because they were still providing a benefit for Marion.

Only those exercises that were progressed, regressed, or newly added to the program required new written instructions and photographs. Clients who need to refer back to instructions or pictures for previous exercises will have easy access to this information in their client program workbooks.

Daily Homework Exercises and Instructions

The following exercises were chosen for Marion's second session based on her homework review, progress, and stated goals.

1. Baseball on Gluteal Complex*: Place baseball on 3 to 4 sore spots across top of buttocks and hold for 20 to 30 seconds on each spot. Place ankle on knee of opposite leg. Do both sides.
2. Foam Roller IT Band
3. Two Tennis Balls on Upper Back
4. Calf Massage
5. Foam Roller Hip Flexors*: Place roller perpendicular to leg and roll or hold on sore spots at top of leg, just below hip bone. Roll for about 1 minute each side.
6. Hip Flexor Stretch (Sagittal)*: Tuck hip under on side that is kneeling. Contract butt to help push hip forward. Raise arm slowly, ensuring that butt muscle does not let go. Hold for about 15 seconds on each side and repeat.
7. Glute Stretch
8. Calf Stretch

Note: * indicates progression or regression from previous session or newly added exercise.

RATIONALE FOR EXERCISE SELECTION AND PROGRAM CHANGES

The reasoning behind each new exercise choice for Marion's second corrective exercise session and new homework assignments follow.

Session 2: Exercise 1

Name of Exercise: Baseball on Gluteal Complex

Selection Rationale: While reviewing the Foam Roller Gluteal Complex exercise, Marion indicated that there were still several sore spots on her buttocks. She also said she felt like releasing the tension in her glutes was really helping her lower back feel better. However, she also noted that if she did the Foam Roller Gluteal Complex exercise for too long on her right side, then her right shoulder would start to hurt from balancing herself on the roller. As a result of this feedback, the decision was made to continue with self-massaging her glutes, but to use a baseball instead of the roller. The smaller surface area of the baseball would target the muscle specifically to continue releasing tension; however, using a baseball instead of the roller would allow her to lie down while releasing her glutes so her shoulder would not hurt while performing this exercise.

Session 2: Exercise 5

Name of Exercise: Foam Roller Hip Flexors

Selection Rationale: This exercise was included in Marion's program to address one of the major environmental causes of her musculoskeletal issues and back pain: namely, the fact that she sits for many hours a day in hip flexion. Marion's hip flexors have become chronically shortened as a result of her desk job. This is problematic because the major hip flexor muscle, the psoas major, originates from the lumbar spine and inserts at the top of the femur. Hence, chronically shortened hip flexor muscles pull the lumbar spine forward toward the legs. This pulling motion increases Marion's lumbar lordosis and resultant back pain. The Foam Roller Hip Flexors exercise will release tension and help restore flexibility to this muscle group, thereby reducing unnecessary stress to her lumbar spine.

Session 2: Exercise 6

Name of Exercise: Hip Flexor Stretch (Sagittal)

Selection Rationale: This exercise was chosen as a progression from the Foam Roller Hip Flexors exercise. It is important to work on the mobility of Marion's hip flexors because in her next session, the plan is to integrate an exercise to strengthen her glutes. The hip flexors are the antagonist muscles of the gluteus maximus. If they are tight, they will restrict hip extension and the ability of the glutes to contract concentrically to push the hips forward. Therefore, both the self-myofascial release and stretching exercises for Marion's hip flexors were taught during this session so she can perform them as additional homework exercises in preparation for the next session. If Marion performs these exercises regularly and correctly, her hip flexors will release, allowing her program to progress effectively with the introduction of the glute strengthening exercise earmarked for Session 3.

SESSION 3

Duration: 1 hour

EXERCISE SELECTION INFORMATION

Marion has shown real dedication to performing her homework exercises and has completed them every day. She reports that her lower back pain symptoms are decreasing and that she is finding it easier to both sit and stand for longer periods of time without pain. As with previous sessions, Marion's homework exercises were reviewed, and she feels confident that she can perform all of her exercises correctly. Based on her feedback and commitment, adjustments were made to her program, including the addition of some new stretches and a strengthening exercise.

Since Marion's muscles and soft tissue structures are becoming looser and more flexible due to her continued performance of her self-myofascial release exercises, she can spend less time on those exercises and still receive the same benefits. This gives her more time to add new exercises to her program without going over the 25- to 35-minute time frame she has committed for her homework.

Daily Homework Exercises and Instructions

The following exercises were chosen for Marion's third session based on her homework review, feedback, and progress.

1. All roller and ball exercises: as shown previously

2. Foam Roller Quadriceps*: Roll on the front of thighs from the hip down to the knee, pausing on all sore spots. Pay special attention to the area on the side/front of the thigh near the top. Roll each side for 1 to 2 minutes.

3. Hip Flexor Stretch (Sagittal)

4. Glute Stretch

5. Calf Stretch

6. Quadriceps Stretch (standing)*: Place foot on armrest of couch. Keep hips aligned left to right as you tuck pelvis under. Keep torso erect without arching lower back. Use balance aid like back of a chair if needed. Hold stretch on both sides for 20 to 30 seconds.

7. Door Frame Stretch*: Stand between door frame and reach outside arm up and over head to grab one side of door frame.

Place other hand on door frame at hip level. Place foot that is farthest away from your hands behind other foot. Keep both feet planted on floor as you push outside hip away from door frame. Stretch both sides for about 15 seconds and repeat.

8. Butt Lift (on ball)*: Balance mid- to upper back on ball with feet on floor. Keep the hips tucked under as you lift and lower the hips. Lift only as far as you can without letting go of a neutral pelvic position. Touch your hands to the ground if you need help balancing. Do 6 to 10 repetitions or less if your technique falters.

Note: * indicates progression or regression from previous session or newly added exercise.

RATIONALE FOR EXERCISE SELECTION AND PROGRAM CHANGES

The reasoning behind each new exercise choice for Marion's third corrective exercise session and new homework assignments follow.

Session 3: Exercise 2

Name of Exercise: Foam Roller Quadriceps

Selection Rationale: Marion's center of gravity is positioned slightly forward (due to her excessive thoracic kyphosis and anterior pelvic tilt), so her quadriceps muscles are tight and overworked from trying to stop her body from falling forward. The rectus femoris muscle (one of the quadriceps) originates from the front of the pelvis and attaches to the kneecap. When this quadriceps muscle is restricted and irritated, it can pull the front of the pelvis down toward the kneecap, making her anterior pelvic tilt and resultant back pain worse. This foam roller exercise will rejuvenate and regenerate Marion's quadriceps and prepare them for the exercise that follows.

Session 3: Exercise 6

Name of Exercise: Quadriceps Stretch (standing)

Selection Rationale: This exercise is a natural progression from the Foam Roller Quadriceps exercise. As mentioned previously, releasing tension in the quadriceps will help lessen Marion's anterior pelvic tilt (and accompanying

excessive lumbar lordosis), thereby alleviating her back pain. Stretching the quadriceps (especially the rectus femoris) will also enable Marion's hips to extend more easily, which will enable her to shift her center of gravity over her pelvis, her base of support. This combination of factors means that Marion will experience much less stress in her feet, knees, lower back, and neck when she is standing and walking.

Session 3: Exercise 7

Name of Exercise: Door Frame Stretch

Selection Rationale: Marion has been doing the Two Tennis Balls on Upper Back exercise consistently since the beginning of her program. Her thoracic extensors are now suppler, and the structures of her thoracic spine and rib cage should be ready for the introduction of some integrated movement. The Door Frame Stretch was added to Marion's program for the purpose of moving and loosening up her thoracic spine in the frontal plane (i.e., bending from side to side).

The overall goal of her program will be to increase the range of motion in Marion's thoracic spine in all three planes of movement so the lower back will not have to work overtime to generate most of her torso motions. This stretch was added to promote side-to-side motion in her thoracic spine. Subsequent exercises will be added later in the program to increase mobility in the transverse and sagittal planes, that is, in rotation and forward and backward.

Session 3: Exercise 8

Name of Exercise: Butt Lift (on ball)

Selection Rationale: Throughout her program, Marion has progressed through the appropriate self-myofascial and stretching progressions for her glutes. She is now ready to begin strengthening the gluteus maximus muscle concentrically to enable her hips to extend fully, thereby taking stress off the structures of her lumbar spine and knees. Since Marion sometimes has pain in her right shoulder, this exercise was adapted with Marion supporting her torso on a stability ball to avoid placing undue stress on her shoulder. Marion already had a stability ball at home, so this alternative version of the Butt Lift exercise was an easy solution.

SESSION 4

Duration: 1 hour

EXERCISE SELECTION INFORMATION

Marion has continued to perform all of her homework exercises regularly and correctly. She was happy to report at the beginning of this session that she attended a work function several days ago and was able to stand for three hours without pain. She had also gone for a walk with her husband on the weekend and said it was the longest walk they had enjoyed together for years. She still finds that her back is quite sore after golf, but she is pleased with her other improvements. Based on her feedback, adjustments were made to her program, including exercises designed to target Marion's torso and upper back.

Daily Homework Exercises and Instructions

The following exercises were chosen for Marion's fourth session based on her homework review, feedback, and continued progress.

1. All rollers and balls: as previously shown
2. Foam Roller Quadratus Lumborum*: Roll between top of pelvis and bottom of ribs. Do not place direct pressure on ribs. Keep knees bent, and roll each side for 30 seconds to 1 minute.
3. Tennis Ball Around Shoulder Blade*: Place ball on all sore spots between shoulder blade and spine. Hug opposite shoulder to move shoulder blade away from spine. Bend knees and use pillow to support head if needed. Spend 2 to 3 minutes on each side.
4. Hip Flexor Stretch (Sagittal)
5. Glute Stretch
6. Calf Stretch
7. Quadriceps Stretch (standing)
8. Door Frame Stretch
9. Butt Lift (on ball)
10. Wave Goodbye (Lying)*: Support both elbows and head with small pillow or rolled-up towel. Rotate backs of hands onto larger pillows placed to side of head. Keep shoulders back and down and pelvis tucked under to make sure you don't cheat with lower back. Hold each contraction for about 20 seconds and do 2 to 3 repetitions.

Note: * indicates progression or regression from previous session or newly added exercise.

RATIONALE FOR EXERCISE SELECTION AND PROGRAM CHANGES

The reasoning behind each new exercise choice for Marion's fourth corrective exercise session and new homework assignments follow.

Session 4: Exercise 2

Name of Exercise: Foam Roller Quadratus Lumborum

Selection Rationale: During the review of Marion's homework from the previous session, she indicated that she felt a large degree of stretch on the sides of her lower back when she performed the Door Frame Stretch. The Foam Roller Quadratus Lumborum self-myofascial release exercise was added to her program to help loosen up the sides of her lower back and torso to gain more benefit from the Door Frame Stretch. Loosening her quadratus lumborum will also help improve the flexibility of the soft tissues that lie between the back of her pelvis, the lumbar spine, and the bottom of her rib cage. This will enable her entire spine, pelvis, and rib cage to move more freely and will increase Marion's torso mobility. This will be especially helpful both for improving her golf swing and for reducing her pain after walking and playing golf.

Session 4: Exercise 3

Name of Exercise: Tennis Ball Around Shoulder Blade

Selection Rationale: Marion now has a number of exercises to reduce her back pain and strengthen the muscles of her lumbo-pelvic hip region while also mobilizing her thoracic spine. Therefore, attention can now turn to addressing the imbalances around her shoulder girdle to help alleviate her shoulder pain. The Tennis Ball Around Shoulder Blade exercise will loosen up her rhomboids and trapezius muscles in preparation for later strengthening exercises to move her scapula, thoracic spine, and shoulder into better alignment. This exercise was chosen because it is one that Marion can easily add to her program while performing her other floor-based exercises.

Session 4: Exercise 10

Name of Exercise: Wave Goodbye (Lying)

Selection Rationale: The Wave Goodbye (Lying) is a progression from the Tennis Ball Around Shoulder Blade exercise. The Wave Goodbye (Lying) exercise will strengthen Marion's scapula depressors, retractors, and the muscles that externally rotate her arms. Strengthening these muscles will help correct the imbalances in her thoracic spine and shoulder girdle. Correcting these imbalances will alleviate her shoulder pain and will enable her to extend her upper back, thereby reducing her lower back pain as well.

SESSION 5

Duration: 1 hour

EXERCISE SELECTION INFORMATION

Marion has been diligent with her corrective exercise program, and she is seeing much improvement in the reduction of her painful symptoms. She continues to be virtually pain-free when standing, and she has been able to take increasingly longer walks with her husband. She rarely experiences tightness in her lower back when she wakes up, and this has made a noticeable difference in her disposition. She is looking forward to an upcoming visit from the grandkids, and she thinks she will be able to participate in many of the activities they have planned. Although her thoracic spine mobility has improved, her excessive thoracic kyphosis remains the biggest obstacle to the complete eradication of her symptoms. Based on her feedback, adjustments were made to Marion's program to continue focusing on the torso and upper back, and an integrated eccentric strengthening exercise (Lunge With Knee Pull) was added.

Daily Homework Exercises and Instructions

The following exercises were chosen for Marion's fifth session based on her homework review, feedback, and the need to progress her program to more directly address her excessive thoracic kyphosis.

1. All rollers and balls: as previously shown
2. Tennis Ball Around Shoulder Blade
3. Hip Flexor Stretch (Sagittal)
4. Glute Stretch
5. Calf Stretch
6. Quadriceps Stretch (standing)
7. Door Frame Stretch
8. Wall Rotation Stretch*: Keep feet straight and hips level. Rotate sternum toward wall without rotating hips. Keep head looking forward and spine erect. Do not let hips shift left or right or spine bend to the side. Hold stretch for about 20 seconds on both sides.
9. Straight Arm Raise (Lying)*: Bend knees, and keep pelvis tilted. Pull shoulders back and down as you try to pull straight arms down toward a large pillow or a foam roller placed above your head. Use additional smaller pillow to support head if needed. Hold each contraction for about 20 seconds and do 2 to 3 repetitions.
10. Wave Goodbye (Standing)*: Lean back against the wall with your knees slightly bent and pelvis tucked under to flatten your lower back to the wall. Keep elbows forward and shoulders back and down as you rotate backs of hands to wall. Hold contraction for about 20 seconds. Do 2 to 3 repetitions.
11. Lunge With Knee Pull (with rotation)*: In lunge position, pull knee toward midline as you rotate hip back and away from knee toward back foot. Don't round shoulders; keep head looking down and forward. Use opposite arm to help rotate torso back. Hold each repetition for a few seconds. Try 3 to 4 repetitions total or less if technique falters.

Note: * indicates progression or regression from previous session or newly added exercise.

RATIONALE FOR EXERCISE SELECTION AND PROGRAM CHANGES

The reasoning behind each new exercise choice for Marion's fifth corrective exercise session and new homework assignments follow.

Session 5: Exercise 8

Name of Exercise: Wall Rotation Stretch

Selection Rationale: Marion's thoracic spine has started to gain mobility in the frontal plane (that is, from side to side) from performing the Door Frame Stretch. The Wall Rotation Stretch was added to help increase her mobility in this area in the transverse plane. Increasing her ability to rotate her thoracic spine will help decrease stress on her lower back when she is walking and playing golf. Both of these activities require the torso to rotate to swing the arms. If the torso cannot rotate, then the lumbar spine and hips typically compensate by overrotating.

Session 5: Exercise 9

Name of Exercise: Straight Arm Raise (Lying)

Selection Rationale: Several exercises have already been incorporated into Marion's program to improve the mobility of her thoracic spine. The Two Tennis Balls on Upper Back exercise has helped her gain more thoracic extension, the Door Frame Stretch has helped her improve lateral movement, and the Wall Rotation Stretch will help increase her ability to rotate this area. The addition of the Straight Arm Raise (Lying) exercise will strengthen her thoracic extensors with the goal of retraining this area so that she can maintain a better posture during the day when seated at work.

This variation of the exercise was chosen because Marion can perform this exercise on the floor. She can control her lower back by tilting her pelvis instead of arching her lower back, and she can keep her shoulders from shrugging. Control over these movements will ensure that she strengthens the right muscles without further stressing those areas that are already irritated or overworked.

Session 5: Exercise 10

Name of Exercise: Wave Goodbye (Standing)

Selection Rationale: Marion was previously given the Wave Goodbye (Lying) exercise for homework, and she was able to do it proficiently. Marion appeared ready to progress to the standing version of this exercise to increase its benefit. Progressing to the standing version will result in the continued strengthening of her thoracic extensors, scapula depressors, retractors, and external rotators of the arm. It will also ensure that Marion continues to improve the position (and condition) of her torso. This will relieve stress on her knees, lower back, and shoulders. Marion will perform this exercise with her feet slightly away from the wall so she can tilt her pelvis more easily and avoid any tendency to cheat by using her lower back.

Session 5: Exercise 11

Name of Exercise: Lunge With Knee Pull (with rotation)

Selection Rationale: This exercise replaces the Butt Lift, and is the first in Marion's program where she will be trying to coordinate a fairly complex movement against the force of gravity. After careful consideration, the decision to add the Lunge With Knee Pull (with rotation) exercise was made based on her significant reduction in symptoms, her dedication to accurate technique, and her regular performance of her homework exercises.

The fact that Marion is ready for this complex exercise is very exciting from a program design standpoint. She will now be learning to control her lower and upper body simultaneously to coordinate movements that resemble many of the activities she enjoys. The Lunge With Knee Pull (with rotation) exercise is designed to strengthen the gluteal muscles eccentrically as they slow down hip flexion and internal rotation of the leg. To achieve this, the torso must rotate correctly away from the front leg to pull the origin of the gluteus maximus away from its insertion just below the knee. This replicates the movements Marion makes when she walks and plays golf, and it will bring her closer to her goal of participating in those activities without pain.

CASE STUDY CONCLUSION

The session just described marked the completion of Marion's fifth corrective exercise session and homework, but not the end of her corrective exercise program. Marion continued to participate fully in the program and was dedicated to completing her homework exercises. After 10 sessions, Marion was pain free during daily activities and was able to golf, walk, and play with her grandkids regularly without pain. Based on her progress, Marion was also able to return to a program of regular exercise. She continued to integrate corrective exercise techniques into her workouts to maintain and to keep improving her musculoskeletal health.

Revisit this case study regularly as you continue to practice, refine, and apply your consultation skills, your assessment skills, your anatomy knowledge, and your corrective exercise program design abilities.

DOCUMENTING YOUR OWN CLIENTS' HOMEWORK

In addition to Marion's hard work and dedication, an important part of her success was organizing and tracking her homework exercises in her client program workbook. Documenting your client's homework is imperative to keeping programs on track and ensuring progression. While client program workbooks are ideal for helping clients to maintain, organize, and easily refer to their homework exercises, emailing homework instructions (and pictures or video), or copying the files to a flash drive or to accessible online storage, can also be used effectively to manage your client's homework assignments.

Following are some guidelines for creating a client's homework instructions and visual aids.

- When recording assessment information and homework exercise information, write legibly (or print in large, clear type) so the client can easily read what you have written.
- If clients prefer, you can allow them to write out their own instructions. Some clients may need more written instructions and key points than others, so provide as many pages as they need.
- When taking still pictures or video of clients, pay attention to what they are wearing because the color of their clothing may affect the quality of the images. Clothing that blends in with the background may produce unclear images. Find a way to contrast the client with the background before taking pictures.
- Some clients may need their pictures printed in a larger size so they can see what they are doing in each exercise. Sending pictures via email, or saving them onto a portable storage device, will enable them to make their pictures as large as they need.
- Exercises that are more complex or require many coordinated movements may require more than one picture. Take several pictures of the exercise from different angles, or use video.
- For ease of reference, number or name each picture or video so it corresponds to the number or name of each written instruction for an exercise.
- Include the date on each set of homework instructions. This is for ease of reference, and it helps you review information from previous sessions.
- Include the date and time of your next appointment as part of the homework instructions. Including this information acts as a tangible reminder for the client and can prevent aggravation and possible arguments if a client misses a scheduled appointment time.

Self-Check

As you know, Marion needed additional sessions to ensure that all her needs and program goals were met. Based on this case study about her program aims and current progress, consider what exercises might be of benefit to Marion for her next two sessions. Write your exercise selection choices and rationales in the tables that follow.

Note: While the tables include all three types of exercise modalities (self-myofascial release, stretching, and strengthening) and up to three exercises for each, it is not necessary to fill every cell in each table because this would be too many exercises to add to Marion's program. Choose only exercises that you think are appropriate for Marion's next two sessions.

Session 6	Exercise	Exercise	Exercise
Self-myofascial			
Stretching			
Strengthening			
Rationale for selected exercises			

Session 7	Exercise	Exercise	Exercise
Self-myofascial			
Stretching			
Strengthening			
Rationale for selected exercises			

Part VI

Business of Corrective Exercise

In part VI, you will learn to enhance your professional image by perfecting the procedures and protocols you learned in parts I through V and marketing your skills appropriately. The consistent application of your knowledge and skills to help clients will also enable you to promote your expertise in ways that attract more clients. Your investment of time to learn and use the techniques contained in this final part will prove invaluable to your growth as a fitness professional.

Part VI will teach you how to position yourself, your corrective exercise services, and your place of business in a manner that not only attracts new customers but also improves patronage from your current clients. You will learn to work within your scope of practice; polish your professional appearance; and update your business name, logo, website, facility, equipment, procedures, practices, and programming to effectively showcase your corrective exercise talents.

Detailed marketing strategies that will help to highlight your business strengths, build up areas of weaknesses, identify potential opportunities, and thwart potential obstacles to success are also discussed in part VI. Marketing tactics for defining your competitive edge, beating out the competition, and providing noticeable value to current and potential customers are included as well. You will also learn how to create and distribute successful marketing materials and build valuable networks with other health care professionals.

CHAPTER 26

Enhancing Your Professional Image

Throughout this text, at the conclusion of each chapter, there have been a series of Self-Checks designed to build your confidence surrounding the use of corrective exercise skills in real-life settings. Polishing your skills will enhance your ability to help people with musculoskeletal imbalances and begin to bolster your professional image.

As your practical corrective exercise knowledge improves, it is time to focus on developing a professional image that will reflect your abilities. You want to position yourself as a knowledgeable professional in the field of corrective exercise and attract people to use your services. This will require integrating structural assessments and corrective exercise into your business offerings (Price and Bratcher 2010).

Adding corrective exercise services to your existing fitness business, or beginning a new service dedicated to corrective exercise, is a great way to help people with musculoskeletal limitations and muscle and joint pain. It also gives you an opportunity to profit from this rapidly growing service area. To do this, you must

1. cultivate an image of yourself as a knowledgeable and successful professional proficient in corrective exercise, and
2. consistently use specific, systemized, and effective corrective exercise procedures when working with clients.

When you consistently use your assessment and corrective exercise skills, you strengthen your image as a trusted professional. Making the effort to shape your professional image will enable you to more easily attract new clients and introduce corrective exercise services to your current clients.

PERFECTING YOUR PROTOCOLS AND PROCEDURES

When you first begin to integrate The BioMechanics Method protocols, assessments, and exercises into your service offerings, it will be natural to experiment to see what works best for your business. However, avoid making it appear that you are applying the procedures in a random fashion; it will only diminish your effectiveness and damage your image. Instead, refer back to this textbook as often as needed to remind you of the step-by-step nature of the assessments and exercise protocols. You should also regularly practice the communication and teaching techniques as they are presented in this text, and create procedures for their implementation. The routine application of these methods will help refine your skills and establish you as an experienced professional (Gerber 2001).

Following is a summary of important points about presenting corrective exercise procedures to clients.

■ Be straightforward and concise about what potential clients should expect during their initial consultation. Providing clear instructions will help to reduce their anxiety about their first meeting with you (Price and Bratcher 2010).

- Make people feel comfortable and confident about consulting with you by having protocols in place for welcoming all new or potential clients (Norman 1999).

- Conduct each initial consultation in a similar fashion using The BioMechanics Method format for verbal, visual, and hands-on assessment (Price and Bratcher 2010).

- Once you have completed your assessments, summarize the findings for clients in a jargon-free manner, and answer any questions they may have about their results.

- Explain the corrective exercise strategies you intend to teach to help them resolve their musculoskeletal issues. Base your recommendations on the assessment results, and link your strategies directly to ways they can improve a client's condition.

- Conclude the initial consultation with an explanation of your use of client workbooks, the number of sessions the client may require, and your rates.

- Whether working with a new corrective exercise client or integrating corrective exercise into a current client's program, the procedures are exactly same. All sessions should include:

  1. A review of all homework exercises at the start of each session.
  2. Exercise recommendations based on findings from the review process and the client's primary fitness goals.
  3. Continual use of assessments during exercise sessions to provide feedback for both you and the client. Performing assessments after your client has successfully adhered to his corrective exercise program for a few weeks will help to reinforce his efforts; it will also produce information you may need for program adjustments (O'Donohue and Levensky 2006).

IMPROVING YOUR IMAGE TO ATTRACT NEW CLIENTS

Perfecting your assessment and exercise procedures is an ongoing process. As you work on this aspect of your professional identity, you will find it necessary to expand the number and variety of people with whom you interact. Whether you are an existing fitness business owner or starting a new enterprise, you will need to attract new clients to your services.

"You only get one chance to make a first impression" is a saying that is particularly relevant in terms of developing your professional image. Potential clients will make judgments and assumptions about your credibility and skills based on their first encounter with you (Galai, Hillel, and Wiener 2016; Sobel and Sheth 2000). It is vital to convey to any prospective client that you know exactly what you are doing. There are many ways to instill feelings of confidence about your services. Following are some suggestions.

BUSINESS NAME AND LOGO

Your business name (and logo, if you have one) is the first thing people see when they consider using your services. Therefore, your business name and logo should reflect your commitment to helping people with corrective exercise needs. Many fitness professionals choose business names that they think will be motivational for clients, such as John's Buff Bodies or Lean and Trim with LeAnn. However, names like these may intimidate prospective corrective exercise clients because these people often do not feel confident in their physical abilities and appearance. More appropriate names would include references to improved function and movement—for example, Movement Matters, or Functional Fitness. Similarly, logos can easily send the wrong message (Price 2003). When thinking about your business name and logo, be prepared to revise them a few times to ensure that you are communicating your services and business image as intended.

PERSONAL APPEARANCE

Another crucial aspect of portraying yourself in a professional manner is your appearance, which includes your clothing, grooming, and demeanor. While fitness environments are more tolerant of casual dress standards, avoid dressing in shorts and tank tops or in revealing fitness outfits. Choose clothing that gives the impression you are a professional who provides services to like-minded professionals and people who are serious about reaching their goals. You may even want to consider branding your apparel or investing in a style makeover that reflects your professionalism and service offerings. Looking the part goes a long way toward convincing people that you have the skills and expertise that go along with your appearance (Price 2003). Portraying a professional image will also boost your confidence when dealing with clients. This will come across to prospective clients and will help you to turn more initial consultations into sales. Furthermore, if you give the impression that you are a knowledgeable and successful professional, clients who seek you out will expect to pay a premium for your services.

LOCATION, FACILITY, AND EQUIPMENT

The appearance of your place of business should also convey your professional status. People should know from looking around your premises that you regularly integrate corrective exercise techniques into your business offerings. While it is easier to create this type of atmosphere if you own the facility, you need not own the place if you are savvy in the use of props. The inclusion of some or all of the following items will help create the impression of a well-qualified professional:

1. *Textbooks.* Several books relating to musculoskeletal health, corrective exercise, or biomechanics should be visible to potential customers. If you do not have a regular workplace where you can easily display these items, bring a few books with you to meetings and consultations for use as visual aids.

2. *Anatomy props.* If at all possible, have a small anatomy skeleton in your office or consultation space. It is a very handy prop that creates a good impression for clients. It can also be used during your structural assessment procedures to help explain results.

3. *Equipment.* Foam rollers and other self-myofascial release tools are great conversation starters that can pique the interest of a prospective client. Keep these types of equipment in view so that your place of business becomes recognizable as a facility that offers corrective exercise procedures.

WEBSITE

The Internet and social media have forever changed the way people seek out goods and services. In today's consumer world, 80 percent of people research a company online before making a purchasing decision (Lamb, Hair, and McDaniel 2017). The creation (or redesign) and promotion of a well-thought-out and professionally constructed website is absolutely necessary for helping potential clients find out more about your services. A website, particularly one with links to your company's social media platforms, may also facilitate referrals from current clients and other professionals who may want to endorse your services.

In chapter 27, you will learn how to further develop your website, expand your corrective exercise offerings, and drive traffic to your site. However, during the initial business development stages (before you invest substantial time and money in an expensive website), there are a number of low-cost strategies you can use on your site that will enhance your professional image and help to reflect your commitment to providing specialty skills in corrective exercise (Price and Bratcher 2012).

DETAIL YOUR AVAILABLE SERVICES

Research has found that more than 47 percent of potential customers look at a company's products and services before checking out any other section of their website (Huff, Edmond, and Gillette 2015). Make it easy for customers with musculoskeletal pain and dysfunction to determine if at least some of your services appeal to them. For example, you may want to include a section in the menu bar or list of services titled Muscle and Joint Pain, or Injury Prevention—anything that potential clients can identify with when they look up your available services.

LINK TO BLOGS AND ARTICLES

Include links on your website to articles and blogs about corrective exercise, the causes and cures for various injuries, or biomechanics. This is another way to establish yourself as an authoritative source of information. If you are confident in your writing skills, consider posting your own articles and blogs on your website to make potential customers aware of your specialty knowledge. However, it is not necessary to create articles and blogs yourself. It is always better to link and give credit to a well-written, professionally created piece than to display work that may harm, rather than enhance, your credibility.

HIGHLIGHT YOUR QUALIFICATIONS

Obtaining and maintaining specialty certifications in corrective exercise is an essential part of crafting a professional appearance. Highlighting these qualifications on your website or mentioning them on your About Us page will help reassure prospective clients about your skills and knowledge.

CONNECT TO SOCIAL MEDIA

Social media platforms such as Facebook and Twitter are used by three billion people around the world (Lamb, Hair, and McDaniel 2017). That's nearly half of the population on Earth! You can effectively use these platforms to publicize your corrective exercise talents and link them back to your website. If you are short on content for your social media platforms, link to posts from other sites that offer corrective exercise strategies and solutions for musculoskeletal problems.

OFFER NEWSLETTERS

The addition of a weekly, monthly, or quarterly newsletter dedicated to corrective exercise that customers can sign up for on your site is another way to bolster your image while gathering contact information for future marketing purposes. Smart topics could include sample exercises that demonstrate how to alleviate certain aches and pains. Current clients can benefit from the information, but more importantly, they may forward the newsletter to their friends and family. This can help increase your exposure and strengthen your reputation.

HIGHLIGHT SUCCESS STORIES

Potential clients like to see that a business has a proven track record helping people like themselves. Include an area on your website that highlights testimonials and success stories from people you are currently helping or have assisted in the past.

INTEGRATING CORRECTIVE EXERCISE PROTOCOLS WITH CURRENT CLIENTS

If you already run a successful fitness business, you may be somewhat less focused on attracting new clients because you already have an established client base. While this is an advantage from an income standpoint, it can make it hard to change your existing practices and services. Clients who are used to a particular exercise routine may not feel comfortable if you decide to incorporate different features into their programs. However, almost 90 percent of all fitness clients will experience musculoskeletal limitations at one time or another. So your continued success depends on finding ways to begin integrating musculoskeletal assessment and corrective exercise strategies (Schroeder and Donlin 2013). The following strategies can help you to do this.

CREATE AWARENESS OF YOUR NEW SKILLS

Integrating corrective exercise into your current programs is much easier to do if you arouse your clients' curiosity about it (Conrad 1998). Tell them about books you are currently reading, talk with them about courses you are taking on the subject, and share insights from any conferences you attend that may be pertinent to their circumstances. This will make them aware of your interests in this area. Moreover, when you start discussing corrective exercise and biomechanics with clients, many will start telling you about their own aches, pains, and movement issues. They may also tell you about all the people they know who have similar issues, and they may ask whether corrective exercise can help. Starting a dialogue about corrective exercise provides the perfect segue to introducing it into your current clients' programs.

BEGIN PROGRAM CHANGES

Once you have started a conversation about corrective exercise and its benefits, take every opportunity to demonstrate how it can be included in people's exercise programs. Following are several ways to familiarize current clients with your newfound talents while enhancing your professional image in the process.

OFFER FREE TRIALS

A free offer or trial of your corrective exercise services is an excellent way to enable current clients to experience your new skills and to earn their trust (Kumar and Meenakshi 2011). Simply suggest that they arrive 10 minutes early for their regular sessions so that you can show them a new assessment or exercise. This gives you the opportunity to pique their interest without taking time away from their normal appointments. You can either perform an assessment on a body part or teach them one or two self-myofascial release warm-up techniques to help them prepare for their scheduled workouts. As they express further interest in corrective exercise, you can show them some stretches or corrective strengthening techniques.

ASSESS IMBALANCES DURING WORKOUTS

Integrate corrective exercise into clients' fitness programs by using musculoskeletal assessments during their normal workouts. For example, if a client doing a squat complains that the front of her ankle is hurting, stop the exercise and perform a quick visual or hands-on assessment of her foot and ankle to see if she is overpronating (see chapter 2). You can use assessment procedures to demonstrate your knowledge of the musculoskeletal system, help your client to understand the possible cause of the ankle problem, and offer some solutions.

FOLLOW UP AFTER SESSIONS

Whenever you teach clients to perform a corrective exercise, follow up with them later to review their technique. This review gives clients an opportunity to ask questions. It also gives you the opportunity to give them positive feedback about the gains they have made by using corrective exercise techniques. This will increase their acceptance of corrective exercise as part of a regular exercise program (Price and Bratcher 2010).

PROVIDE REMINDERS OF YOUR CORRECTIVE EXERCISE TALENTS

Seize opportunities as they arise to remind clients of your corrective exercise skills. While this may take time, there are many tactics you can use.

- Each time you teach a current client a new corrective exercise, take a picture of him performing the exercise. This will make him feel involved in the process and convey that you are choosing exercises that address his specific condition. Email or text these pictures to him after his session, or print them out so he can take the images with him.

- Cooperate with clients to write the directions for their exercise homework. Include written instructions with accompanying photographs whenever possible. Not only are pictures and instructions a great way to give clients a physical reminder of their positive experience with your corrective exercise services, but it will also help them feel they have provided valuable input into their programs.

- Create personalized program workbooks for current clients, the same as you would for new clients, so they can track and record their progress. This tangible evidence of their efforts and achievements provides valuable positive feedback that will also enhance their perception of you as a corrective exercise specialist.

RUN AN OPEN HOUSE

Introducing clients to your corrective exercise skills individually is a very effective way to bolster their esteem for your professional capabilities. But you can also reach a wider audience of both existing and potential clients by holding an open house. An open house is an event that showcases your corrective exercise services. You don't need to own your own facility to host one; you can simply hold it at your gym, club, or current work location. Here are some tips to ensure open house success:

- Choose a corrective exercise–related topic you feel comfortable talking about.

- Devise a name for the open house related to that topic, such as Get Your Feet in Shape or Great Exercises to Alleviate Back Pain, so that people know what to expect by attending.

- Choose a date for the open house, and advertise it by sending out invitations to all of your contacts and current clients, posting it in your social media platforms, and placing notices around the location where the event is being held.

- Send out a press release to local newspapers and other community organizations to inform them of the event (Price and Bratcher 2012). (Information on how to write a press release can be found in chapter 27.)

- On the day of the open house, give a 10- to 15-minute talk for attendees about your chosen topic, use your new skeleton, textbooks, and charts to help illustrate your knowledge, and include demonstrations on how to perform a couple of exercises to help alleviate musculoskeletal issues related to the topic being discussed.

- Conclude the presentation by inviting those who are interested to attend a subsequent talk or to schedule an appointment with you for an assessment.

In addition to your own presentation at the open house, you could invite other like-minded health professionals to give a short talk or demonstration about their businesses. For example, a massage therapist could talk and then perform brief 10-minute massages on some of the attendees. This will serve not only to help attendees feel physically better when they leave your event, but it also enables you to begin developing your network of professional referrals (Price and Bratcher 2012). (For more on networking and referrals, see chapter 28.)

Go to the online video and watch video 26.1, where Justin talks about how to enhance your professional image.

KEYS TO SUCCESS

Enhancing your professional image involves two interconnected concepts: (1) applying your skills consistently and successfully and (2) looking the part of a knowledgeable and proficient practitioner. As you begin publicizing or expanding your services, however, be careful in the claims you make. Clients with long-standing and recurring musculoskeletal issues may doubt that a health and fitness professional can improve their musculoskeletal conditions because they may have had previous negative experiences. Therefore, when crafting your professional image, you must use descriptions and examples that are unambiguous, grounded in reality, and supported by results. You also want them to instill a sense of hope, confidence, and optimism in the people seeking out your services.

Review of Key Points

- Professionals in any industry have methods to ensure that no part of their process or service is overlooked. You can integrate corrective exercise into your business by consistently applying The BioMechanics Method procedures and practices.

- As you gain competence and confidence in your skills, it is important to enhance your professional image so that you can attract new clients and expand your services to existing clients.

- First impressions count. Giving the impression that you are a knowledgeable and professional specialist in the field of corrective exercise will reassure prospective clients.

- You can enhance your professional image by creating an appropriate business name and website, wearing professional attire, and making sure your place of business conveys that image.

- Part of honing your skills involves integrating assessment and corrective exercise procedures into your services to current clients. Doing so will elevate your status as a professional in their eyes, and it will also improve your chances of success with their current fitness programs.

Self-Check

Dedicating time and attention to specific aspects of your business will enable you to convey the right message to potential and current clients. Consider the business topics in the following chart, and identify one or two improvements you can make in each area.

Business topic	Areas for improvement
Business name	
Logo	
Personal appearance	
Website	
Your current qualifications	
Client testimonials/success stories	
Business location	
Initial consultations	
Conducting client sessions	

CHAPTER 27

Marketing Your Corrective Exercise Services

As your corrective exercise skills and professional reputation develop, you must start considering marketing strategies to effectively promote your business. Marketing a business is not just about launching a website, handing out brochures, and offering everyone you meet a business card. It is a thoughtful process designed to educate potential clients in a manner that encourages them to purchase what you have to sell, make current clients feel better about patronizing your business, and increase potential referrals (Hayes 2012; Silk 2006).

UNDERSTANDING HOW MARKETING WORKS

Successful marketing takes time and effort, and it can also cost a lot of money. Therefore, your marketing efforts should be deliberate, well-prepared, and focused on a specific audience. Developing an effective marketing strategy requires an in-depth appreciation of the things that make your business unique. This includes your business processes, your current customer base, your competition, your current services and products, any services you plan to add, and the needs and wants of potential clients. The particulars of these elements of your business will have a direct impact on the way you market it.

This chapter presents some simple assessments and activities you need to conduct in order to gather this information about your business so that you can develop an effective marketing strategy. They are as follows:

- Conducting a SWOT analysis
- Considering your competitive edge
- Defining your service features and benefits
- Surveying your current clients
- Developing a value proposition statement

Gathering this valuable information will help you to understand your current business position and to identify those aspects of your business that should be highlighted with your marketing efforts. It will also help you to identify any weaknesses in your operations that need improving, as well as opportunities that you can capitalize on (Hall 2003).

CONDUCTING A SWOT ANALYSIS

A SWOT analysis is a simple but effective tool commonly used in the development of marketing plans. It is used to assess your business *strengths* and *weaknesses* and to determine the *opportunities* and *threats* you may encounter as you try to attract clients to your corrective exercise services. Conducting this type of business assessment can help you focus your marketing activities on areas where you can derive the most benefit. This type of analysis is also an effective way to determine what parts of your business are helping you to move forward and what parts may be holding you back. It can also help you to predict potential problems so you can attend to them before they disrupt your business (Hall 2003).

The best way to complete a SWOT analysis is by answering the following questions and recording your responses. The more thought you put into this assessment of your business, the more it will help you in developing your marketing plan.

IDENTIFY YOUR BUSINESS STRENGTHS

- What advantages do you have over peers in your community or industry?
- What do you do well?
- What do others see as your strengths?
- What relevant resources do you have access to?

Consider these questions as they pertain both to you and to your competitors. For example, if all of your competitors offer corrective exercise programs, then the provision of corrective exercise services is not considered a strength; it is a market expectation. However, if you are one of only a few professionals in your business area with a corrective exercise background or qualification, then you should consider that a strength.

IDENTIFY YOUR BUSINESS WEAKNESSES

- What can you do to improve your business skills, communication techniques, or networking abilities?
- How strong are your qualifications or certifications?
- What things do you do badly?
- What do you (or should you) avoid doing?
- What makes your business vulnerable?

Consider your responses carefully and from every perspective. For example, what do your competitors do better than you? What would your clients say you need to improve? An honest assessment of your weaknesses will help you to target areas for growth and development.

IDENTIFY YOUR BUSINESS OPPORTUNITIES

- What are the industry trends in corrective exercise at the moment?

- What networking opportunities are you aware of or can you create?
- Does the use of technology factor into your business?
- What kinds of local events are happening in your area?
- Whom do you know who can be a resource or an asset (and do they owe you favors)?

Think carefully about whether your identified strengths can open up any additional opportunities for your business. For example, if you have contacts in the hotel and hospitality industry, you could discuss with these people the possibility of creating in-room, spa-like bundles in order to provide guests with corrective exercise self-massage treatments. You should also ask yourself if opportunities might present themselves by eliminating your previously identified weaknesses. If you are not very well versed in the nuances of social media, could you open up new marketing opportunities by educating yourself on the topic, or hiring someone part-time to help you set up and manage your social media platforms?

IDENTIFY THREATS TO YOUR BUSINESS

- What is your competition doing?
- What is your cash flow situation like?
- What business obstacles do you face?
- Can any of your weaknesses threaten the success of your business?

Identifying those things that could negatively affect your business can enable you to sidestep adversity. For example, if all of your competitors offer free consultations but you do not, you should investigate whether your decision not to do so is perceived positively or negatively by potential customers. If your target customers expect free consultations, your decision not to offer them may prove to be a threat to your livelihood.

DEFINING YOUR COMPETITIVE EDGE

A competitive edge refers to the characteristics of your business that make you stand out over the competition (Hall 2003). Pinpointing your competitive edge is a valuable exercise because once you determine what your business has that others do not, you can highlight that in your marketing materials to attract potential customers and even entice them away from the competition.

To determine your competitive edge, consider how you and your business differ from others in your area. An obvious example is that you might be the only person in your community who offers corrective exercise services. While this is certainly an advantage, it would be helpful from a marketing standpoint to clarify this point in more detail. For example, in addition to being the only corrective exercise service provider, you may have documented success helping clients specifically overcome lower back pain so they

---

SWOT Example

The following SWOT analysis is for a self-employed personal trainer who currently sees regular personal training clients and runs a few boot camps per week. She also intends to add dedicated corrective exercise services as one of her offerings.

Strengths

- As a sole proprietor (and my own boss), I can adjust my services as needed to meet the needs of my clients.
- My current workload enables me to devote time to clients and provide exceptional customer service.
- I have a good reputation in the gym where I am an independent contractor.
- I am mobile, so I can travel to clients' homes if necessary.
- My overhead costs are low, so I can offer value to my clients and have money to spend on quality marketing materials.
- I am one of the only personal trainers in my community who has a structured approach to corrective exercise.

Weaknesses

- Outside of my current clients, I have very little market presence in the community.
- When I am sick or out of town, I do not get paid (and my clients also suffer).
- My cash flow is unreliable due to fluctuations in my client load.
- The gym I work out of is noisy and is not conducive to helping clients who have corrective exercise needs.
- I do not market myself as a trainer with specialty skills.

Opportunities

- The field of corrective exercise is greatly expanding, and there are many opportunities for success.
- My competitors are slow to realize this expanding market opportunity.
- People are discouraged with the traditional approaches to helping to alleviate musculoskeletal pain and dysfunction.
- Boot camp classes are popular, but people do not want to get injured.

Threats

- People are using the Internet to find exercises for their musculoskeletal problems.
- People tend to use physical therapy instead of corrective exercise because it is covered by insurance.
- Routine prescription of pain medication may lessen the demand for corrective exercise.

The results of this trainer's SWOT analysis enable her to understand her strengths and where she can capitalize on her opportunities. This may prompt her to create a market presence in her community by promoting her corrective exercise services and "injury-free" boot-camp classes at the gym where she sees clients. If it is not feasible for her to see additional clients or run specialty classes in her current workspace, her independence, schedule flexibility, and access to a vehicle would allow her to provide mobile corrective exercise services and classes. As her corrective exercise clientele and service roster grows, she may consider opening her own facility to create an optimal teaching and training environment.

In reviewing her weaknesses and threats, she may realize the advantage of advertising her services as personalized, unlike the cookie-cutter approach of Internet-based program suggestions. She may also come to realize that rather than viewing physical therapists as a business threat, she can network with them to act as a referral source once a client has been discharged from physical therapy. (For more on networking, see chapter 28.)

can return to working out regularly. Alternatively, you may have strong relationships in place with the medical community. Or, if you are not the only professional in your business area with corrective exercise expertise, you might be the only one who has a recognized certification or the only one who specializes in helping professional athletes.

Being aware of your competitive edge is obviously helpful for making marketing decisions. However, it is also a valuable way to determine where your time and resources should be spent on further developing those skills you need to make sure you always stay ahead of the competition (Hall 2003).

IDENTIFYING FEATURES AND BENEFITS

All of the services you now offer (or plan to offer in the future) have features and benefits. The *features* of your corrective exercise services are the characteristics that describe your offerings (e.g., you use self-myofascial release [SMR] exercises). The *benefits* of your service are the positive value that the features bring to your customers (e.g., the benefits of SMR exercises include increased range of motion and decreased pain). Understanding the difference between features and benefits, and knowing which of these to highlight in your marketing messages, will prove helpful when the time comes to create your promotional pieces (Kuzmeski 2010).

Creating a list of features and benefits for your service offerings is useful for two reasons:

1. It compels you to take stock of the types of services you offer.
2. You can use the information from this assessment to develop compelling marketing and advertising messages.

The best way to discern the benefits of your corrective exercise services is to think about and list their unique features. Once you have identified what the features are, you can extract all the possible benefits of those features to describe how they will appeal to customers. Figure 27.1 provides an example of some features and benefits of corrective exercise services in general.

Effective marketing typically emphasizes the benefits of a service rather than the features because these benefits are what customers really want (Kuzmeski 2010). For example, consider a yoga instructor who plans to offer a corrective exercise stretching class along with her traditional yoga classes. A feature of the special class is static and dynamic stretching exercises based on the concepts of functional anatomy. However, potential clients probably will not be interested in the stretching exercises themselves or their scientific justification; they are more interested in the benefits (pain relief and increased mobility) that the stretches can bring them. Therefore, although this instructor may mention the features of her stretching class in her advertising materials, the focus should be primarily on the benefits clients will receive from attending the class.

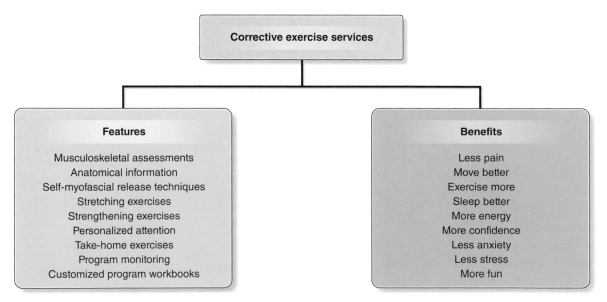

Corrective exercise services

Features

Musculoskeletal assessments
Anatomical information
Self-myofascial release techniques
Stretching exercises
Strengthening exercises
Personalized attention
Take-home exercises
Program monitoring
Customized program workbooks

Benefits

Less pain
Move better
Exercise more
Sleep better
More energy
More confidence
Less anxiety
Less stress
More fun

Figure 27.1 Sample list of corrective exercise features and benefits.

EXAMINING YOUR CURRENT CLIENT BASE

If you already have a strong client base, you may wonder why you need to assess your business to develop a marketing strategy at all. This may be a valid point if you are never interested in expanding your services, increasing your revenue, or knowing for certain that your client base will not shrink. However, if you want to raise your rates, grow your business, and improve your reputation as a corrective exercise service provider, you must continue to improve your understanding of your target market. Asking clients directly for input, either in person or in a survey, about what they want, what they would like to have available, and why they choose to work with you will give you the answers you need to satisfy both current and future customers.

The following questions can be used to help you gather information from your existing client base:

- Do you have any musculoskeletal or movement limitations that are affecting your ability to exercise or enjoy daily activities? If so, what kind(s) of problems do you experience, and what do you currently do about it?

- Do you seek professional help for these problems? If so, who do you see?

- Are you satisfied with the service you receive from these other professionals? If so, what do you like about their service?

- If you are not satisfied with the services you receive, what could the service provider do differently to make you more satisfied?

- How important is it that you address your musculoskeletal imbalances and get rid of your aches and pains?

- What could I do to help you with these problems?

- What could I do differently to help you in general?

- What are you prepared to do to help alleviate your musculoskeletal problems?

Assessing your existing client base will help you to appreciate what your current (and potential) clientele want and need from a corrective exercise provider. It also keys you in to what may be currently missing from your business in terms of corrective exercise services so you can tailor your future offerings and marketing strategies accordingly (Humbatov 2015).

CREATING A VALUE PROPOSITION STATEMENT

The final assessment activity to help you focus your marketing strategy is to state the aims and objectives of your business in terms of the unique value you offer to clients (e.g., injury prevention, injury recovery, pain relief, performance enhancement, maintenance). This statement is called a value proposition. Creating a value proposition statement helps direct your marketing strategies by assessing and defining your target market group, the benefits you offer, and the relative pricing of your services in relation to your competitors (Schultz and Doerr 2011).

Here is an example of how a personal trainer with the business name Advantage Fitness could phrase a value proposition statement to include corrective exercise services:

Advantage Fitness offers busy executives convenient, mobile exercise services that help alleviate muscle and joint pain and improve fitness at an exclusive price point.

In this example, the target market is clearly defined (i.e., executives pressed for time). The benefits of the services are also identified (i.e., mobile services that save the customer time by not having to travel, exercise programs that improve fitness as well as alleviate muscle and joint pain), and there is a clear indication that the cost for the services is going to be high (i.e., exclusive) compared to other providers.

When using your value proposition statement to develop and implement your marketing strategy, it is important that your marketing messages accurately reflect the stated elements of your business. Every part of your value proposition—target market, benefits, and pricing—should be communicated through your advertising, promotions, positioning, public relations, customer service policies, networking, and day-to-day operations (Schultz and Doerr 2011). For example, the value proposition statement for Advantage Fitness would direct them to use high-quality, professionally created advertising and promotional materials that reflect their exclusive price point and exceptionally high levels of customer service. It would also require that they use name-brand equipment, have recognized and respected qualifications in corrective exercise, drive a nice vehicle (since it is a mobile business), have excellent punctuality and time-keeping skills, be able to accept credit card payments, and other such considerations that would echo the message promised in their value proposition statement.

Developing a value proposition statement can be challenging, but it is one of the most important assessment activities because it requires you to have a precise understanding of your business objectives. Identifying your business aims and stating them in terms of what you will deliver (and to whom and at what price) is an excellent way to direct marketing decisions (Schultz and Doerr 2011).

CREATING MARKETING MESSAGES

Once you have completed the assessment of all the unique qualities of your business and know the image you want to present to consumers, it is time to begin creating content and selecting methods for distributing your marketing messages. This will include the content itself and the vehicles you will use to inform and attract your target market, such as your website, brochures, or word-of-mouth advertising (Price and Bratcher 2010).

Marketing messages are the verbal, nonverbal, and written communications used to attract potential customers and keep current customers satisfied (Kuzmeski 2010). While everyone's message will be unique, the process by which the marketing content is produced is similar for everyone. Use the information from your SWOT analysis, your features and benefits chart, your competitive advantage summary, your current client analysis, and your value proposition statement to develop the core content for your marketing materials. Focus on the following aspects:

1. Emphasize the positive traits of your business.
2. Identify the specific yields your services can provide for both current and prospective clients.
3. Capitalize on elements that differentiate your business from the competition.
4. Maintain continuity of content across all your messages.

EVALUATING DELIVERY METHODS

As you create your marketing messages, you must decide how you will get this information to your intended audience. There are many distribution channels you can use, ranging from inexpensive options such as social media to very costly options like running your own infomercials on television.

Most delivery methods fall at various points along the cost spectrum. Websites, email marketing campaigns, brochures, newspaper and magazine ads, flyers, and press releases are all delivery methods that can vary in price. Before putting energy and money into developing and distributing your messages, revisit the research you have already done on your business and potential market to help you to narrow your options. Also consider the following questions when choosing what delivery methods to use:

- *How does your target market spend their time?* Thinking about the ways in which your potential customers spend their time will help you to figure out the smartest ways to get your marketing messages in front of them. For example, if your target market consists of retired professionals who mostly stay at home, consider how they might spend a typical day. If they read magazines, check the mail, and occasionally go to health-related appointments, then the use of direct mail postcards or newsletters, circulars or flyers, or advertisements in relevant magazines or local newspapers might be good distribution options for your business. You might also consider networking with other health professionals who serve your target market or make brochures available at their offices (Cynthia 2012; Urquhart-Brown 2008).

- *What distribution methods will emphasize your skills and services?* When considering ways to persuade customers to buy your services, choose distribution methods that will present your business and your skills in the best possible light. For instance, if you have a knack for developing warm relationships with people as you help them with personal matters related to their musculoskeletal health, this would be something you would want to highlight in your marketing materials. Pictures or videos that show you working with relaxed and satisfied clients would likely help potential customers with similar issues feel comfortable about approaching you (Cynthia 2012).

- *What kind of message do you want to send potential customers?* Your target market's opinions and attitudes will greatly influence their perception of your marketing pieces, so take that into account when determining which distribution methods to use. For example, if you plan on marketing private corrective exercise sessions to very successful business professionals (who have a lot of discretionary income), then the marketing and distribution channels you choose must give the impression that your services are exceptional and worth the amount of money you intend to charge. Flyers taped to car windshields or brochures delivered to receptionists are not going to convey that message. In fact, such distribution choices may have the opposite effect, so you must evaluate whether these choices are congruent with your marketing messages (Cynthia 2012).

- *How much money do you have to spend?* The most vital aspect of deciding what distribution method(s) to use for your marketing messages is how much you can reasonably afford to spend. It does not matter how appealing a distribution method may appear, or how many potential customers may be exposed to it. If you spend more than you can afford, your business might go bankrupt before you can see any return on your marketing efforts (Price and Bratcher 2012).

IMPLEMENTING YOUR MARKETING STRATEGY

Creating the content for your marketing strategy and choosing the best delivery methods for your marketing messages is an extensive, but invaluable process. To help you evaluate the best distribution techniques for you and your business, and the most effective way to use them, some of the most popular methods are described next.

WEBSITES

In chapter 26, you learned about the importance of having an online presence in today's marketplace and some basic website tactics for informing both potential and current clients about your new skills. As you further expand and distribute your marketing messages, you will need to revisit your website to update the content, redesign its structure (if necessary), and employ strategies to maximize your website's search engine exposure (Rieva 2001).

When you begin the process of refining or building your site, first determine what the main purpose of the site will be. Decide whether you want to use your website to

- be a first point of contact for interested prospects,
- sell corrective exercise products and services,

- interact with customers (e.g., through the use of a forum or members-only area), or
- serve mainly as a virtual information display.

Understanding the primary marketing function of your site will make it easier to develop or adjust the content (Rieva 2001). Once you have decided what type of site to build (or rebuild), seek out a reputable web design company to help you. If you want to be able to make changes and updates to your website yourself once it is complete, ask your designer to include a content management system or administrative portal in conjunction with the site (Rieva 2001).

The use of relevant keywords that correspond to your site content is what enables well-designed websites to appear higher in search engine results than others. This is important because sites that appear higher in search engine results are more likely to be seen and visited by potential customers (Shepherd and Augenti 2012). If you decide to submit your site for paid inclusion to search engines like Google or Yahoo!, you will need to generate a list of relevant keywords or phrases that describe your business so search engine robots can find and rank your site. When you create your list of keywords, do not just use words or phrases that include your name, professional label, credentials, or the processes you use to help clients. Remember that potential customers are more interested in their own musculoskeletal problems than in your resumé, and they will search for services using keywords that relate to their problems. The keyword search engine optimization site Semrush.com, for example, reported that on March 31, 2017, the term "lower back pain" was searched on the Internet 330 times more often than "corrective exercise specialist." (Keyword Magic Tool, *Semrush*, accessed March 31, 2017, https://www.semrush.com/features/keyword-magic-tool/) You can generate a list of useful keywords or phrases for your website by identifying words that focus on your prospects' problems. Once you have exhausted that list, think of words that describe the solution to their problems (i.e., the benefits of your services). There are several online tools that can help you find words and phrases that your prospects are interested in. You can also use these services to test phrases and words to find out which ones are most often used by people for Internet searches (Neuman 2007).

In additional to optimizing your site's keywords and content, linking (and backlinking) your website to the most popular social media platforms (i.e.,

Facebook, Twitter, Instagram) will also raise your search engine visibility (Shepherd and Augenti 2012). Potential customers often use social media when searching for services, and you can use this to your advantage. Furthermore, linking to social media platforms will enable you to easily update your customers about developments with your business, provide them with useful information, or generally keep you and your business in the forefront of their minds. Encouraging current clients to share your social media feeds with their friends, families, and colleagues is also a terrific way to encourage new referrals (Price and Bratcher 2012). If you are unsure how to set up or create quality social media platforms, ask your website designer to include this as part of the website development service.

PRESS RELEASES

Another excellent way to inform people of your new or expanding corrective exercise services is to send out press releases to local television stations, community magazines, and newspapers (Hiam 2014). The submission of press releases to media outlets is a free distribution method you can use to build potential hype around you and your business. There are also online press release companies that provide press release services for a fee. Regardless of whether your choose paid or free release services, bear in mind that media outlets typically receive press releases in abundance, so make sure the content of your release is unique and interesting from a news and marketing perspective. A press release should contain the following elements:

- The date of your release and the words "For Immediate Release"

- A catchy headline that sums up the contents of the release

- Information about you and your business that is newsworthy from a particular media outlet's perspective (e.g., notify local TV and newspapers that your business won a national corrective exercise award)

- A summary of the who, what, where, when, and why of your announcement in the first paragraph and a brief expansion of the details in the following paragraph(s)

- Concise and easy-to-read content with no grammatical or punctuation errors

- Information and details on the person to contact for further information

- A separate section in the release that summarizes your company background information and contact details

MASS MARKETING CAMPAIGNS

If you plan to offer generalized services such as weight loss in association with your corrective exercise services, and you intend to appeal to a broad market of clients with similar needs, you might want to consider implementing a mass marketing campaign (Frazer-Robinson 2003). Mass marketing promotion is designed to get your name out to as many potential customers as possible through the use of distribution channels such as television, radio, flyers, direct mail, print ads, email campaigns, and Internet-based ad promotions through sites like Facebook and YouTube. While it can potentially be an effective way to distribute your marketing message, the outlay for these channels can be costly. It is also important to remember that although mass marketing campaign messages may be received by many people, it does not mean that the leads generated by such campaigns will translate into paying customers (Frazer-Robinson 2003). If you choose to deploy a mass marketing campaign, it is critical to ensure that all the elements of that campaign match the image you wish to convey due to the vast numbers of people who will be exposed to it.

WORD-OF-MOUTH ADVERTISING

The most valuable distribution method for your marketing messages is word-of-mouth marketing. It is, by far, the most effective way of getting and keeping business referrals—and it is virtually free! The best way to generate word-of-mouth marketing is to provide clients with program success, exceptional customer service, and positive experiences every time you interact with them (Friedmann 2009). You can then draw on the positive experiences of those clients (or family members or friends you have helped with their musculoskeletal issues) to establish new business. Many of your clients, friends, family members, and colleagues love to talk about their involvement with you, so give them an excuse to do so. Here are some ways to do this:

- Encourage clients to invite friends, family members, spouses, or work colleagues to attend sessions with them so these potential customers can witness your expertise in person.

- Use client workbooks to inspire word-of-mouth marketing for your business to potential customers who might see these materials in use by one of your clients. Consider branding each page of the workbook with your business name and logo, or including informational pages about The BioMechanics Method process, because this is an excellent way to add value to your services and promote your business.

- Offer incentives for referrals such as free T-shirts, free sessions, or discounted rates to clients who refer their friends. Similarly, developing professional networking relationships with the medical community is a great way to cultivate word-of-mouth referrals (see chapter 28).

Many small businesses pay lip service to the importance of marketing, but they do not spend the required time or invest the necessary capital to create the right type of exposure for their businesses. However, just as you need to practice your corrective exercise assessment, anatomy, and program design skills, you must continually improve your marketing know-how to ensure a steady stream of customers. By frequently reexamining your service offerings, communicating with clients to understand their needs, predicting future requirements, paying attention to what your competition is doing, and adapting to evolving trends in the industry, you can tailor your marketing messages and the way you deliver them to constantly improve your marketing skills and promotional efforts.

 Go to the online video and watch video 27.1, where Justin talks about how to market your corrective exercise skills.

TRANSITIONING TO A FULL-TIME CORRECTIVE EXERCISE SPECIALIST

As you continue to experience success by applying your expertise and marketing yourself effectively, the demand for your services will grow. Eventually, there may come a time when you need to make a decision about the direction you would like your business to take. If you are enjoying your standing as a specialist in corrective exercise, it may be advantageous to become a full-time corrective exercise service provider. Narrowing your business focus to specialize exclusively in corrective exercise has many benefits:

- You can target your marketing specifically to people who have chronic musculoskeletal issues, thereby reducing marketing costs and achieving a better return on your efforts.

- You can charge higher fees that reflect your specialty services.

- You can focus your education efforts purely on corrective exercise and biomechanics to improve your skills and streamline your continuing education requirements, both of which will lead to increased client success and increased revenue for your business.

- You will have a platform from which to be recognized as an industry expert, and you will be able to develop secondary revenue streams by presenting, writing, and educating others about corrective exercise.

- You can work less and have more time to pursue leisure activities and interests as your rates increase with your elevated status.

Making the decision to transition to a full-time corrective exercise specialty business can be a very profitable one. However, in order to realize your full business potential as a specialist provider in corrective exercise, you must continue to take a calculated approach to developing your image as an expert in the field and positioning your business as a leader in the industry.

OBTAIN THE NECESSARY QUALIFICATIONS

As with any type of specialist, clients want to know that the people they are working with are indeed qualified to do what they are doing. Obtaining a corrective exercise specialty certification from a reputable education provider in the fitness industry (and keeping your certifications current) is an absolute must if you plan to be a full-time corrective exercise provider. You will also need to update your qualifications on a regular basis.

CONCENTRATE YOUR BUSINESS AIMS

In order for consumers to instantly recognize you as a successful corrective exercise provider, every component of your business will need to reflect your commitment to corrective exercise. This includes your marketing materials, website, newsletters, social media efforts, continuing education courses, speaking engagements, and media opportunities.

Restricting your business focus to your area of expertise will help concentrate your operations as well as increase your perceived value as a specialist practitioner of corrective exercise.

RESTRUCTURE YOUR CLIENT PROFILE

If you have operated a successful health and fitness business for quite some time, you will likely have established clientele on your appointment rosters who are not corrective exercise service clients. If you intend to become a full-time corrective exercise specialist, begin the process of transitioning or reducing the number of sessions "traditional" clients come to see you for non–corrective exercise services. It is also important that you reshape the programs of these clients so that you help them primarily with corrective exercise needs and raise their rates progressively to meet your current fees. While this may be a difficult and uncomfortable challenge for you, this restructuring of your business will cement your reputation as a corrective exercise specialist, allow you to attract quality referrals, and enable you to increase your rates accordingly. You can refer your non–corrective exercise clients to other professionals (such as a personal trainer, nutritionist, or weight loss specialist) as you restrict your services to corrective exercise. You will likely find that these colleagues will, in turn, begin referring clients with musculoskeletal limitations to you for specialty corrective exercise services.

OPEN YOUR OWN FACILITY

When you have enough revenue and a solid roster of clients, you might consider opening your own corrective exercise facility. This will give you the opportunity to design your workspace to fully accommodate corrective exercise clients and brand your business to reflect the specialty services you offer. Operating your own facility can be more costly than other workplace arrangements, but it can also help you to create an unmistakable professional image as a specialist and open up many possibilities for additional revenue streams (Rieva 2001).

Review of Key Points

Marketing your corrective exercise services effectively requires you to take an in-depth look at your business, your current offerings, your competition, and the needs of your client base. Once you have completed this assessment of your business, use that information to develop attention-grabbing and persuasive marketing messages, and implement them in ways that will attract customers and support your business growth.

- Completing a SWOT analysis will help you to evaluate your strengths and weaknesses and any threats or opportunities you may have in the market.

- The creation of a value proposition statement will help you to be clear about the image you want to project for your services and to whom you will offer them.

- Assessing your business rivals enables you to pinpoint the competitive advantage you have over them in order to cultivate a unique image for your corrective exercise business.

- All services have features and benefits. Potential clients are typically more interested in benefits than in features, so emphasize those in your marketing messages.

- Researching current and potential customers enables you to evaluate precisely how your business can satisfy their needs, and it helps determine what specific niche your services fill in the marketplace.

- The distribution options you choose for your marketing messages will vary depending on your target market and the goals of your marketing campaign. Choose options that accurately reflect your business image and that fall within your budget.

- The most productive of all marketing channels is word of mouth. You can generate this type of marketing by providing exceptional customer service, concrete results, and positive experiences every time you interact with clients and potential customers.

Self-Check

Effectively marketing your corrective exercise services requires that you understand not only your own business but also your potential clients' needs and wants so that you can create convincing and persuasive marketing messages. To help you hone your marketing message skills, use the space that follows to create marketing copy (i.e., the words you would use) for a 100-word promotional message about one of your corrective exercise offerings. An example is provided here:

The BioMechanics Method Corrective Exercise Specialist course (TBMM-CES) is the health and fitness industry's highest-rated corrective exercise education program, with qualified professionals in more than 60 countries. To earn a TBMM-CES credential, students complete a comprehensive course designed to enhance their skills in musculoskeletal assessment, anatomy, corrective exercise selection, and program design. Professionals who have earned The BioMechanics Method corrective exercise specialist credential are sought-after the world over for their unique ability to help people address the underlying musculoskeletal causes of muscle and joint pain so they can regain or continue a program of regular exercise and an active lifestyle.

Your Marketing Copy

CHAPTER **28**

Scope of Practice, Networks, and Referrals

As you begin to integrate corrective exercise techniques into your exercise programs, it is extremely important that the services you offer remain firmly within your scope of practice as a fitness professional (Bryant and Green 2010). Working within a clearly delineated role is beneficial for you and your clients because it enables you to practice and promote your specialty skills. It also enables you to build strong networking relationships with other businesses and to increase your ability to generate quality client referrals.

MAINTAINING YOUR SCOPE OF PRACTICE

While the laws differ among states and countries, it is universally accepted that professionals must not work outside the bounds of their experience, education, training, and demonstrated competencies (Howley and Thompson 2016). As a fitness professional, your expertise lies in understanding the musculoskeletal system and how it is influenced by posture and movement. This specialized knowledge helps you to recognize clients' physical limitations and enables you to design exercise programs to help them reach their health, movement, and fitness goals. The integration of corrective exercise into fitness programming and personal training is a key to your success and that of your clients (Price and Bratcher 2010).

As you work, however, it is important not to confuse your role with that of a licensed medical professional. It is never appropriate for you to diagnose, prescribe for, or treat a specific medical condition (Bryant and Green 2010). While it is not your job to be an authority figure on diagnosed conditions or medical care, it is within your scope of practice to work with clients to take actions that will improve their musculoskeletal health (Price and Bratcher 2010).

Maintaining your occupational boundaries can also benefit your business by enhancing your reputation as a reliable professional (Price and Bratcher 2012). Doctors often require qualified fitness professionals to whom they can refer patients who need guidance with exercise (DiNubile and Patrick 2005). Unfortunately, they can be reluctant to refer patients with musculoskeletal conditions out of a concern that their clients' problems might be made worse by a fitness professional or personal trainer. When you have specialty qualifications in musculoskeletal assessment and corrective exercise, and when you work within your scope of practice, medical professionals will feel confident in sending clients your way (DiNubile and Patrick 2005).

As you advance in your use of corrective exercise procedures, it is highly recommended that you obtain The BioMechanics Method Corrective Exercise Specialist (TBMM-CES) credential. Not only will this strengthen your skills, but it can also result in more referrals from medical professionals. This internationally recognized CES qualification can lend credibility to your networking efforts. As your network grows, you will also find it easier to refer clients to other specialists when their condition lies beyond your scope of practice.

 Go to the online video and watch video 28.1, where Justin talks about the benefits of working within your scope of practice.

DEVELOPING PROFESSIONAL NETWORKS AND REFERRALS

Networking is the creation of strategic business relationships with licensed medical professionals and other health and fitness practitioners. When done well, it can produce a mutually beneficial referral system of clients and patients (Levinson and Mann 2007). Networking is one of the least expensive and most effective ways to market your business and build your client base. However, successful networking involves more than handing out business cards or getting others to hand them out for you. It requires time to cultivate relationships with selected professionals you trust and who, in turn, have confidence in you and your business. While successful networking takes time and energy, the referrals generated through your network are likely to be genuine prospects who may become clients (Price and Bratcher 2012).

Before you begin networking, ask yourself what you want to get out of your business relationships. Is your primary goal to connect with other professionals so they will refer clients to you? Or is it to build a network of professionals to whom you can refer your own clients for other specialty services? Perhaps it is a combination of both. Once you have defined your objectives, you must then identify appropriate opportunities and partners (Price and Bratcher 2012).

IDENTIFYING GOOD NETWORKING OPPORTUNITIES

There are many ways to meet people with whom you can network: conversations with current clients, dinner parties for clients, lunch meetings with other professionals, community gatherings, social media sites, and conversations with work colleagues. Some of these opportunities give you the chance to meet face-to-face with others to create lasting and productive networking relationships; other, less-structured meetings are more likely to result in sporadic client referrals. You must determine which types of networking opportunities are most likely to help you achieve your objectives. You also must understand that the key to building networking relationships lies in the quality, not the quantity, of the events you attend (Price and Bratcher 2012).

APPROACHING POTENTIAL NETWORKING PARTNERS

Once you have identified potential referral sources or networking partners, approach them in a professional manner (Ciletti 2011). You should send a letter introducing yourself, your business, the types of services you offer, and how you envision working together to help their customers or those clients you share. As with everything else you do in your business, your letter of introduction and accompanying materials should present the high-quality, expert image you want to portray. Once you have sent the letter, follow it up immediately with a telephone call or email to let the prospective networking partners know it is coming and that you will follow up soon to answer any questions. Do not make the mistake of simply contacting people by email. Many business owners are used to being solicited this way, and they will often ignore this type of introduction.

Once the potential networking partners have received your letter, follow up as promised, gauge their interest in collaborating, and try to set up a meeting to introduce yourself in person (Brocato 2010). Do not be discouraged if they do not have time to meet with you. If they are successful medical practitioners, they are likely very busy. Your efforts to make contact and follow up in a timely manner will still demonstrate your desire to help clients to reach their goals and they may produce referrals in the future.

If you can set up a meeting with your target partner, be ready to make the most of that opportunity by preparing a brief summary about you and your business. This is crucial for piquing someone's interest, and it is the first step in developing successful networking relationships (Knoote-Parke 2009; Price and Bratcher 2012).

FORMING YOUR SALES PITCH FOR PROSPECTS

The more you prepare and rehearse your business summary, the more confident and interesting you and your business will appear to a networking prospect. While the details of your presentation will vary according to your audience, the core content will be the same.

- *Your business basics:* Clearly describe the primary purpose of your business in one or two sentences. If the person you are speaking to is interested and wants to know more, she will indicate this, and you can expand from there (Knoote-Parke 2009). Here is an example of the business basics for a person who owns a personal training studio that specializes in corrective exercise for amateur athletes:

  "I specialize in helping people overcome musculoskelctal problems and movement limitations so they can excel in the sporting endeavors they love."

  A concise, yet descriptive statement such as this will prompt an interested party to ask more questions, such as, "Do you have your own facility?" or, "What types of athletes do you help?" Once they begin asking questions, you will be able to tell what types of services they want to hear about, and you can tailor the rest of the conversation to meet their interests (Price and Bratcher 2012).

- *Benefits your business provides:* A wise speaker knows that people are typically more interested in themselves than in what the speaker has to say. If you can find out a little bit about networking prospects before talking with them, you can tie that into your presentation (Thomas 2014; Bryant, Green, and Newton-Merrill 2013).

- *Add credibility:* Always frame your business in a positive manner to add credibility to your undertakings, but be careful about making false claims. Exaggerating your successes may prompt listeners to end the conversation (Knoote-Parke 2009). On the other hand, selling yourself short with statements like, "We only have…" or "I've just started…" can have the same negative effect (Price and Bratcher 2012).

- *Associated fees:* Unless it works to your benefit, or is part of your strategy with a particular person, avoid discussing prices or costs for your services when initially meeting potential networking partners. The aim of the pitch is to get them interested enough in your services that the price is not a determining factor in their decision to refer to you.

DISTINGUISHING YOURSELF AS A NETWORKING PARTNER

Once you have made headway with your networking pitch, capitalize on your progress. Following are some strategies that can increase the chances that targeted professionals will refer clients your way.

- *Skill demonstration:* When you meet with prospective networking or referral sources, have a strategy to help them remember your unique skills. When appropriate, demonstrating any of The BioMechanics Method visual or hands-on procedures will enable you to showcase your talents. If it is inappropriate to demonstrate your skills at that time, give them a certificate for a complimentary session with you for use at a future date (Price and Bratcher 2012).

- *Session swap:* If you are networking with professionals who also provide services for alleviating musculoskeletal conditions—such as chiropractors, acupuncturists, or massage therapists—offer to exchange sessions. Swapping sessions with potential partners enables you to see each other in action, and that can boost your confidence about having them in your referral network (Phillips 2014).

- *Offer discounts:* Extending a small discount to a potential networking partner's clients or patients may encourage professionals to remember and refer to you. Their ability to arrange discounts for your services makes the referring professionals appear to be doing clients a favor, and it also helps motivate the potential client to book an appointment with you (Price and Bratcher 2012).

- *Commissions:* While the custom of offering discounts for a network partner's clients is recommended, offering commissions to the referring professional is not. This type of arrangement creates relationships based on monetary gains instead of mutual respect, and it can affect the long-term success of the networking arrangement (Price and Bratcher 2012).

- *Web referral page and links:* Once you have established a networking partnership, consider setting up a Referral Page on your website dedicated exclusively to affiliated health care, medical, and fitness professionals you recommend. Advertising reputable networking partners can enhance your own credibility.

- *Maintenance:* After you have developed a networking source, reach out to that person periodically to keep lines of communication open and referrals forthcoming (Thomas 2014). If it appears that someone is no longer interested in working with you, thank them for their valuable time, and let them know that you are always available if they need your help in the future.

SOCIAL MEDIA AND NETWORKING GROUPS

Face-to-face networking is the strongest way to build your referral streams and business partnerships. There are, however, a number of business-related social networking sites, such as LinkedIn, Viadeo, PartnerUp, and Xing that are designed for building professional networks online. These sites enable users to invite and endorse other professionals (Phillips 2014). However, these sites lack the individual touch that is vital to developing successful professional networks; they should only be used as an adjunct to more personal networking strategies. While social media sites such as Facebook and Twitter are valuable for advertising and marketing your business, they are not recommended for developing reliable referral networks.

Similar to online networking, opportunities exist to join professional networking groups set up by a third party or networking organization. This type of networking alliance consists of professionals from different areas who agree to refer to each other so that the members of the group can mutually benefit (Thomas 2014). This type of prearranged referral system can work well for some people. However, these types of networking groups are open to virtually anyone, and the caliber of professionals in them can vary greatly. In rare cases, joining such a group where certain members have a poor standing in the community may actually harm your own business reputation.

NETWORKING WITH YOUR CLIENTS

Professional networking relationships are needed in order to generate quality referrals from outside of your business. If your company is established and you have a solid client base, one of the best ways to increase referrals is to solicit them from satisfied clients (Blakemore 2011). Following are some strategies for networking with existing customers.

- *Use gift certificates:* All of your clients will know someone with aches and pains, and your skills will be in high demand if you can get in front of those people. Encourage current clients to make these referrals by providing them with a gift certificate for a complimentary assessment or session to pass on to someone they think might like to see you (Fisher 2001). Asking clients to pass on the certificate is an easy way to motivate them to refer business to you, but be careful not to give away too many gift certificates because this will devalue your services.

- *Homework for a client's friend, family, or colleague:* Giving clients an opportunity to use the knowledge they are gaining about corrective exercise to help their friends, family members, or colleagues is another great way to generate

---

Creating Professional Networks and Referrals: Keys to Success

- Some people think the best salespeople are also the best talkers. On the contrary, the best salespeople are the best listeners. The more you listen to potential networking partners, the more you will learn about them, and the better you will be able to tailor your networking spiel to appeal to their interests.

- Every networking opportunity is different. People respond differently to different approaches, so be prepared to be flexible in your networking pitch.

- Building a solid professional networking and referral platform takes a lot of time and effort. It may require many hours of work, and it may take months before you start to see developments in terms of referrals. Be patient, and continually work on fostering constructive networking relationships.

- There is a common tenet in the business world about networking and referrals: People refer to people they know and trust. Keeping the lines of communication open with your networking partners is the best way to generate solid referrals and build trusted business relationships.

referrals (Burg 2006). Imagine, for instance, that you are teaching your client a stretch she can do for her calf muscles to help alleviate soreness after running. As you are teaching her the exercise, she mentions that her husband also gets the same pain after he plays a round of golf. When you review the client's corrective exercise homework at the end of the session, ask if she thinks her husband would be interested in doing a couple of exercises to help eliminate his calf pain. If she is agreeable, provide a couple of general exercises, like a calf massage and stretch, that she could show her husband to perform before and after he plays golf. Write the information for the husband on a piece of letterhead paper (or other professional-looking materials that you have developed for this purpose), and tell your client her husband can give you a call if he has any questions about the exercises.

- *Invite people to observe:* You can also generate new referrals through your current clients by inviting their friends, family members, medical professionals, and other associates to observe their sessions with you (Aluise 1980). Often,

these people will want to see what the client is doing that is working so well.

- *Network with your client's health care providers:* You can expand and strengthen your professional networks by including a client's health care providers in your dealings with that client. For example, if a client returns after a period of absence due to illness or injury, ask who his doctor is, and ask whether you can contact that person to see if there is any additional input that can help you to provide better service for your client. Your client will appreciate the extra effort, and you will benefit from the knowledge you gain from speaking to the doctor (as well as developing a potential referral source). You can use this strategy for any type of health professional your clients use. Building networks with other health and medical professionals is a lot easier if you both share a customer to act as the point of reference (Price and Bratcher 2012).

> **Go to the online video and watch video 28.2, where Justin talks about how to network with the medical profession.**

Review of Key Points

Creating referrals through professional networks and client-generated leads is necessary to ensure a steady stream of customers. Staying within your scope of practice and developing strategic networking relationships can help boost your professional standing in the industry and can enhance your reputation for helping people with musculoskeletal dysfunctions.

- Before you begin networking or cultivating referral sources, develop a concise presentation that highlights your business. Once you have developed the basic presentation, tailor it to particular audiences as needed.

- There are many strategies for setting up an initial meeting or encouraging a potential networking source to refer business, such as exchanging services and offering discounts or gift certificates for their clients.

- Providing current clients with gift certificates for their friends, family members, or colleagues, encouraging them to invite guests to attend their sessions, and suggesting corrective exercise homework for people they know may encourage new client referrals.

- Keeping in contact with other health professionals and following up on networking or referral opportunities can help you to develop successful professional networks.

- Productive networking takes time and effort. Treat networking as an ongoing business requirement, and devote time to it regularly.

Self-Check

It is important to introduce yourself to potential networking partners in a professional way. Use the following prompts to draft a letter you can send to other practitioners to acquaint them with you and your services, with the goal of setting up a mutually beneficial referral network.

Your business name/logo
Your business address

Recipient's name and address

Dear _____,

This first paragraph should pique your readers' attention so they continue to read the letter. For example:

How many of your patients complain of recurring muscle and joint pain? Are these problems affecting their daily lives, thwarting their ability to exercise regularly, or preventing the achievement of their health and fitness goals? Who do you turn to for assistance in helping patients with these problems?

Use the second paragraph to introduce yourself, and explain how your services meet the needs you have identified.

The third paragraph should briefly describe in more detail what you do specifically to meet these needs (*e.g., use a methodical approach to identify musculoskeletal imbalances that are either causing or contributing to movement and muscle dysfunction; the strategic application of individualized corrective exercise programs; the appropriate referral of clients to like-minded professionals when a condition is encountered that might require additional assistance*).

The final paragraph should thank recipients for their time and let them know that you will be contacting them soon to discuss their needs further and to explore potential networking opportunities.

Appendix: Blank Client Assessment Diagram

The reproducible Client Assessment Diagram on the following page may be used to record information gathered during client consultation and assessment. An example of a completed version of this form can be found in chapter 25.

CLIENT ASSESSMENT DIAGRAM

NAME
DATE

'X' for "Quick Check"

CHECKLIST	✓	DETAILS
Feet and Ankles:		
Pain?		
Arthritis/Conditions?		
Function?		
What makes better/worse?		
Causal links?		
Visual irregularities?		
Pronated?		
Ab./Adducted?		
Condition of toes?		
Condition of plantar fascia?		
Condition of calf muscles?		
Client knows neutral?		
Knee:		
Pain?		
Arthritis/Conditions?		
Function?		
What makes better/worse?		
Causal links?		
Visual irregularities?		
Single leg squat?		
Patella tracking?		
Client knows neutral?		
Lumbo–Pelvic Hip:		
Pain?		
Arthritis/Conditions?		
Function?		

ANTERIOR VIEW

'X' for "Quick Check"

CHECKLIST	✓	DETAILS
What makes better/worse?		
Causal links?		
Visual irregularities?		
Excessive lordosis?		
Anterior rotation?		
Client knows neutral?		
Thoracic Spine/Shoulder:		
Pain?		
Arthritis/Conditions?		
Function?		
What makes better/worse?		
Causal links?		
Excessive kyphosis?		
Protracted/Elevated scapula?		
Internally rotated arms?		
Muscle tension?		
Client knows neutral?		
Head and Neck:		
Pain?		
Arthritis/Conditions?		
Function?		
What makes better/worse?		
Causal links?		
Visual irregularities?		
Forward head?		
Excessive neck curvature?		
Client knows neutral?		

POSTERIOR VIEW

ADDITIONAL NOTES

Occupation/Activities	
Injuries/Surgeries	
Footwear Considerations	
Major Deviations(s)	

From J. Price, *The BioMechanics Method for Corrective Exercise* (Champaign, IL: Human Kinetics, 2019).

Glossary

abducted—The position of a digit or limb that has moved away from the midline of the body.

acetabulum—A deep socket in the pelvis where the head of the femur articulates with the pelvis to form the hip.

Achilles tendon—A soft tissue structure in the lower leg that connects the calf muscles to the calcaneus (i.e., heel bone).

acromion—The part of the scapula (i.e., shoulder blade) that extends over the top of the humerus (i.e., upper arm) forming the upper border of the shoulder girdle.

active stretching—An exercise technique that requires the target muscle to be maintained in a stretched position while simultaneously contracting the opposing muscle.

adducted—The position of a digit or limb that has moved toward the midline of the body.

anterior pelvic tilt—A common musculoskeletal imbalance of the lumbo-pelvic hip girdle characterized by an excessive downward tilted position of the front of the pelvis.

atlas bone—The first vertebra of the cervical spine (i.e., C1).

bones—Hard structures made of fibrous collagen and calcium that provide the internal framework for the body.

calcaneus—The heel bone.

cervical spine—The uppermost part of the spine comprised of seven small vertebrae that form the neck.

clavicle—A bone that extends outward from either side of the sternum and across to the acromion to help form the front of the shoulder girdle. Also referred to as the collarbone.

Client Assessment Diagram (CAD)—A form unique to The BioMechanics Method that lists all the questions a client should be asked during the verbal consultation as well as the musculoskeletal assessments that should be conducted during the visual and hands-on assessment process.

competitive edge—The skills, characteristics, or positive aspects of a business that make it stand out over the competition.

concentric contraction or movement—A contraction resulting in the shortening of a muscle to produce movement.

consultation—The process of meeting with a prospective client for the purpose of conducting a structural assessment and getting him interested in corrective exercise programming.

corrective exercise—A specialty area of the fitness industry that focuses on identifying and remedying musculoskeletal imbalances through the strategic application of self-myofascial release, stretching, and strengthening exercises.

cranium—The immobile, rounded part of the skull formed by several bones held together by sutures or fibrous joints. Bones in the cranium include the occipital, frontal, sphenoid, and ethmoid bone, two parietal bones, and two temporal bones.

cruciate ligaments—Connective tissue inside the knee joint that attaches the bone of the upper leg (i.e., femur) to the lower leg (i.e., tibia) in a diagonal fashion to minimize rotational stress across the knee joint. These ligaments—the anterior cruciate ligament and the posterior cruciate ligament—also prevent excessive forward or backward movement of the tibia in relation to the femur.

diaphragm—A dome-shaped muscle that extends across the bottom of the rib cage that separates the thoracic cavity of the torso from the abdominal cavity. It is the main muscle used for breathing.

dynamic stretching—An exercise technique used to mimic everyday movements and functional activities.

eccentric contraction or movement—A contraction against resistance that results in elongation of a muscle. Used to decelerate a body part or slow movement.

elevated scapula—A common musculoskeletal imbalance of the thoracic spine and shoulder girdle characterized by an atypical, upward position of the scapula upon the rib cage.

excessive cervical lordosis—A common musculoskeletal imbalance of the neck and head characterized by an increased curvature (or overarching) of the neck that accompanies a forward head position.

excessive lumbar lordosis—A common musculoskeletal imbalance of the lumbo-pelvic hip girdle characterized by an excessive curvature (or overarching) of the lumbar spine.

excessive thoracic kyphosis—A common musculoskeletal imbalance of the thoracic spine and shoulder girdle characterized by an excessive rounding forward of the thoracic spine.

exercise alternative—An exercise or technique that will enable a client to achieve a desired program objective when an initial exercise recommendation is deemed not suitable or possible.

fascia—A three-dimensional web of pliable connective tissue that intertwines and binds every muscle, organ, and soft tissue structure throughout the body to enable it to move as an integrated system of functional parts.

femur—The long bone in the upper leg.

fibula—The bone located beside the tibia on the lateral side of the lower leg.

forefoot—Forward most area of the foot, which includes the toes and serves to increase the surface area of the foot to aid with balance.

forward position of the head—A common musculo-skeletal imbalance of the neck and head characterized by a projection of the head forward of the body's center plumb line.

glenohumeral joint—The main joint of the shoulder where the humerus (i.e., upper arm) articulates with the glenoid (i.e., part of the shoulder blade).

gravity—A natural force of attraction put out by the earth that pulls objects toward the core of the planet.

ground reaction forces—A concept in physics that states when force is applied by one object to another object, the same amount of force is returned in the opposite direction. Also referred to as impact.

hindfoot—Area of the foot directly below the ankle that helps absorb shock and displace forces.

humerus—The long bone in the upper arm.

iliotibial band (IT band)—A dense strip of connective tissue that runs along the lateral side of the thigh that connects the fibers of the gluteus maximus and tensor fasciae latae muscles to the lower leg.

intercostals—A group of muscles between the ribs used to facilitate breathing.

internally rotated arms—A common musculoskeletal imbalance of the thoracic spine and shoulder girdle characterized by an inwardly rotated position of the upper arms.

ischial tuberosity—The bottom portion of the rounded bone at the bottom of the pelvis. Also called the sit bone.

isometric strengthening—A strengthening technique that results in a muscle becoming activated by holding a desired body position in a static contracted position.

kinetic chain exercises—A type of strengthening exercise comprised of a sequential series of motions, actions, and body parts that rely on each other to produce a desired movement or create a chain of motion.

labrum—A ring of cartilage on the edge of the scapula that gives the end of the upper arm (i.e., the humerus) a cup-shaped socket in which to sit to help form the glenohumeral joint.

lack of dorsiflexion—A common musculoskeletal imbalance of the feet and ankles characterized by a diminished ability to bring the lower leg over the foot (or vice versa).

lateral collateral ligament—Connective tissue that acts as a guide rope between the fibula and the femur to give side-to-side stability to the knee.

lateral longitudinal arch—The arch on the outside of the foot.

learning style—An individual's preferred method of learning. The most common learning styles are visual, verbal, and kinesthetic.

ligament—A tough band of connective tissue that links bones together at a joint.

lumbar spine—The lower portion of the spine that contains the five largest vertebrae. The lumbar spine is responsible for helping flex, side-bend, extend, and rotate the spine.

lumbo-pelvic hip girdle—The area of the body where the lumbar spine, pelvis, and top of the legs come together.

mandible—The bone at the bottom of the skull that forms the jaw, chin, and lower mouth. Also known as the jawbone, the mandible is connected to the cranium via the temporomandibular joint.

marketing—A deliberate process for educating potential clients about a business's products and services in a manner that encourages them to purchase what the business has to sell.

marketing messages—The verbal, nonverbal, and written marketing communications a business uses to attract potential customers and maximize client retention.

medial collateral ligament—Connective tissue that acts as a guide rope between the tibia and femur to give side-to-side stability to the knee.

medial longitudinal arch—The prominent arch that runs along the inside (i.e., medial border) of the foot.

menisci—Discs of cartilage in the knee that act as shock absorbers between the bones of the upper and lower leg.

midfoot—Area in the middle of the foot designed to absorb shock that encompasses the highest part of the arches of the foot.

multijoint strengthening—A type of exercise involving the movement of multiple joints (and simultaneous strengthening of all the muscles that affect those joints) at once.

multiplanar/multidimensional exercises—Types of strengthening exercises designed to move the body in different directions or planes of motion.

muscles—Specialized soft tissues made up from bundles of cells responsible for controlling movement in the body.

musculoskeletal imbalance—An area(s) of the body where muscles, bones, or joints are out of balance or have assumed a nonneutral position as a result of pain, injury, chronic muscle tension, activity choice, habit, fascial restrictions, or ineffective movement patterns.

musculoskeletal system—System of the body comprised of the skeleton, muscles, tendons, ligaments, and fascia.

myofascial systems—Arrangements of fascia that follow the paths of muscles, bones, ligaments, and tendons as they travel up, down, and around the body. Myofascial systems enable coordinated movement in all three planes of motion.

networking—The process of creating strategic business relationships with clients, licensed medical professionals, and other health and fitness practitioners, usually for the purpose of initiating or facilitating client referrals.

nuchal ligament—A band of connective tissue that extends from the base of the skull to the seventh cervical vertebra (i.e., C7).

overpronation—A common musculoskeletal imbalance of the feet and ankles characterized by excessive collapsing of the feet and ankles toward the midline of the body.

passive stretching—An exercise technique that involves holding a fixed position for a predetermined amount of time with the goal of increasing range of movement around a joint or number of joints. Also called static stretching.

patella—A small bone in the center of the knee. Also referred to as the kneecap.

patellar ligament—Connective tissue that attaches the patella to the tibia in the lower leg.

pelvis—A ringlike structure comprised of three fused bones (ilium, ischium, and pubis) located at the base of the spine. These sets of fused bones form each side of the pelvis.

plantar fascia—A broad, dense, fairly rigid connective tissue that runs the length of the underside of the foot and helps give the arches of the feet their shape and structure.

progression—An advancement to a more challenging exercise or moving forward to more dynamic types of movements or techniques.

protracted shoulder girdle—A common musculoskeletal imbalance of the thoracic spine and shoulder girdle characterized by the shoulder blades moving forward on the back of the rib cage, resulting in the vertebral border of the scapula (the edge closest to the spine) moving away from the spine.

Q angle—The position of the thigh bone in relation to the center of the knee.

quadriceps tendon—Connective tissue that attaches the quadriceps muscles of the upper leg to the patella.

rationale—The reason for recommending the inclusion of an exercise or strategy in a client's corrective exercise program based on her assessment results, needs, and goals.

referral—A client or potential client who is obtained as a direct result of a recommendation or endorsement by another party.

regression—A return to an earlier exercise or technique that is easier for a client to perform.

rib cage—The rib cage is formed by 24 bones (12 on each side of the thoracic spine) that attach to the sternum at the front of the chest and to the sides of each thoracic vertebra at the back (the bottom two sets of ribs do not attach to the sternum). These bones form a ringlike structure that protects the organs in the mid- and upper torso and increase the size of the torso, providing a greater surface area for muscles and other soft tissues to attach.

sacroiliac joint—A main joint of the lumbo-pelvic hip girdle where the sacrum meets the ilium of the pelvis. There is a left and a right sacroiliac joint.

sacrotuberous ligament—A band of connective tissue that spans from the base of the sacrum to the ischial tuberosity of the pelvis. Often found to be a direct continuation of the tendon of the biceps femoris (a hamstring muscle) and consequently helps link structures of the lower body to the upper body.

sacrum—A triangular series of fused vertebrae at the base of the spine between the lumbar spine and the coccyx (tailbone).

scapula—A broad, flat bone that sits on the back of the upper rib cage, forming the back of the shoulder girdle. Also referred to as the shoulder blade.

scope of practice—The boundaries of a professional's experience, education, training, and demonstrated competencies.

self-myofascial release—A form of self-massage used to restore and rejuvenate soft tissues that have become adversely affected by chronic musculoskeletal imbalances.

shoulder joint—The part of the shoulder girdle where the humerus articulates with the scapula via the glenoid. Also called the glenohumeral joint. The three other joints that make up the shoulder girdle are the acromioclavicular, scapulothoracic and sternoclavicular joints.

side-to-side alignment— Alignment of the femur and tibia and the movement and position of these bones in relation to the centerline of the body.

single-joint strengthening—A type of exercise used to strengthen muscles that move one joint at a time.

skull—The bony structure consisting of the cranium and the mandible that provides the general framework for the head.

sternum—A T-shaped bone at the top and center of the front of the rib cage to which the clavicles and rib bones attach.

strengthening—A type of exercise used to fortify specific soft tissue structures (e.g., muscles) and reeducate the body so it can move more effectively and efficiently.

stretching—A type of exercise used to increase the flexibility of the muscles and fascia and to increase the range of motion of the joints.

structural assessment—A verbal, visual, and hands-on evaluation process used to gain insight into a person's musculoskeletal condition before creating a program of corrective exercise.

subtalar joint—A joint in the ankle located beneath the talus bone that transfers forces forward and across the foot.

SWOT analysis—A tool commonly used in the development of marketing plans to assess a business's potential strengths, weaknesses, opportunities, and threats.

talus bone—A bone near the bottom of the ankle that helps connect the lower leg to the foot.

temporomandibular joint (TMJ)—One of the most important joints in the neck and head area, formed where the mandible (i.e., jawbone) articulates with the temporal bone of the cranium.

tendon—A flexible, yet tough connective tissue that attaches muscle to bone.

thoracic spine—The part of the spine between the lumbar and cervical segments consisting of 12 vertebrae in the middle and upper torso area.

thoracolumbar fascia—Layers of fascia on the back of the torso that connect many of the ligaments and big muscles of the lower back, pelvis, and rib cage. Also referred to as the lumbodorsal fascia.

tibia—The wide shin bone on the medial side of the lower leg.

tibiofibular joint—The joint where the tibia and fibula come together at the ankle.

tracking problems of the knee—A common musculoskeletal imbalance of the knee characterized by an inability of the patella to glide smoothly over the end of the femur during knee flexion and extension.

tragus—The fleshy piece of skin that covers part of the opening at the front of the ear.

transverse arches—A series of small dome-shaped arches that run from side to side across the foot just behind the toes.

true ankle joint—The joint below the lower leg bones and above the talus bone that helps the lower leg to interact with the foot and ankle and helps displace stress to the heel.

valgus knee position or displacement—A common musculoskeletal imbalance of the knee characterized by the knee collapsing too far in toward the midline of the body.

value proposition statement—A marketing strategy used to state the aims and objectives of a business in terms of the unique value those elements offer clients or customers.

verbal assessment—The first part of the structural assessment process used to acquire relevant health history information as it relates to a client's musculoskeletal well-being.

visual and hands-on assessment—The portion of the structural assessment process used to visually and manually inspect each major area of a client's body for the presence of musculoskeletal imbalances.

References

Preface

IHRSA. 2017. *IHRSA health club consumer report.* Boston: International Health, Racquet and Sportsclub Association.

Schroeder, J., and A. Donlin, eds. 2013. *IDEA fitness programs and equipment trends report.* San Diego, CA: IDEA Health & Fitness Association.

Chapter 1

Bryant, C.X., and D.J. Green, eds. 2010. *ACE personal trainer manual: The ultimate resource for fitness professionals,* 4th ed. San Diego, CA: American Council on Exercise.

Bryant, C.X., D.J. Green, and S. Newton-Merrill, eds. 2013. *ACE health coach manual: The ultimate guide to wellness, fitness, and lifestyle change.* San Diego, CA: American Council on Exercise.

Kendall, F.P., E.K. McCreary, and P.G. Provance. 2005. *Muscle testing and function with posture and pain,* 5th ed. Baltimore, MD: Lippincott Williams and Wilkins.

Price, J. 2012. *How to turn prospective clients into paying clients: The art of initial consultations.* PTontheNet.com. Accessed August 30, 2016. www.ptonthenet.com/articles/art-of-initial-pt-client-consultations-3580

Price, J. 2016. *How to increase client adherence.* PTontheNet.com. Accessed October 12, 2017. www.ptonthenet.com/articles/how-to-increase-client-adherence-4119

Price, J., and M. Bratcher. 2010. *The fundamentals of structural assessment. Module 1: The BioMechanics Method corrective exercise specialist certification program.* San Diego, CA: The BioMechanics Press.

Whitworth, L., H. Kimsey-House, K. Kimsey-House, and P. Sandahl. 2007. *Co-active coaching: New skills for coaching people toward success in work and life,* 2nd ed. Palo Alto, CA: Davies-Black Publishing.

Chapter 2

Arnot, B. 2003. *Wear and tear: Stop and put the spring back in your body.* New York: Simon & Schuster.

Barnes, J.F. 1999. Myofascial release. In *Functional soft tissue examination and treatment by manual methods.* 2nd ed., edited by W.I. Hammer. Gaithersburg, MD: Aspen Publishers.

Cook, G. 2010. *Movement: Functional movement systems. Screening, assessment, corrective exercise strategies.* Santa Cruz, CA: On Target Publications.

Davis, M., P. Davis, and D. Ross. 2005. *Expert guide to sports medicine.* Philadelphia: American College of Physicians.

Frowen, P., et al. 2010. *Neale's disorders of the foot,* 8th ed. St. Louis: Elsevier.

Gray, H. 1995. *Gray's anatomy.* New York: Barnes & Noble Books.

Hertel, J. 2002. Functional anatomy, pathomechanics, and pathophysiology of lateral ankle instability. *Journal of Athletic Training* 37(4): 364-375.

Hobrough, P. 2016. *Running free of injuries: From pain to personal best.* New York: Bloomsbury.

Hyde, T., and M. Gegenbach. 2007. *Conservative management of sports injuries.* Sudbury, MA: Jones & Bartlett.

Johnson, D., and R. Pedowitz. 2007. *Practical orthopedic sports medicine and arthroscopy.* Philadelphia: Lippincott Williams & Wilkins.

Kelikian, A. 2011. *Sarrafian's anatomy of the foot and ankle: Descriptive, topographic, functional.* Philadelphia: Lippincott Williams & Wilkins.

Kendall, F., E. McCreary, and P. Provance. 2005. *Muscles: Testing and function with posture and pain.* 5th ed. Philadelphia. Lippincott Williams & Wilkins.

Lowe, W. 2009. *Orthopedic massage: Theory and technique.* 2nd ed. St. Louis: Mosby Elsevier.

Magee, D., and D. Sueki. 2011. *Orthopedic physical assessment atlas and video: Selected special tests and movements.* St. Louis: Elsevier Sanders.

Miller, P. 1995. *Fitness programming and physical disability.* Champaign, IL: Human Kinetics.

Muscolino, J. 2009. *The muscle and bone palpation manual with trigger points, referral patterns and stretching.* St. Louis: Mosby Elsevier.

Petty, N., and A.P. Moore. 2002. *Neuromusculoskeletal examination and assessment: A handbook for therapists.* Edinburgh: Churchill Livingstone.

Price, J., and M. Bratcher. 2010. *The fundamentals of structural assessment. Module 1: The BioMechanics Method corrective exercise specialist certification program.* San Diego, CA: The BioMechanics Press.

Schamberger, W. 2002. *The malalignment syndrome: Implications for medicine and sport.* Edinburgh: Churchill Livingstone.

Snell, R. 2008. *Clinical anatomy by regions.* Philadelphia: Lippincott Williams & Wilkins.

Chapter 3

Clippinger, K. 2016. *Dance anatomy and kinesiology.* Champaign, IL: Human Kinetics.

Dimon, T., and M. Day. 2008. *Anatomy of the moving body: A basic course in bones, muscles, and joints.* 2nd ed. Berkeley, CA: North Atlantic Books.

Fernandez des-la-Penas, C., J. Cleland, and J. Dommerholt, eds. 2016. *Manual therapy for musculoskeletal pain syndromes: An evidence and clinical-informed approach.* St. Louis: Elsevier.

Frisch, H. 1994. *Systematic musculoskeletal examination: Including manual medicine diagnostic techniques*. Berlin: Springer Verlag.

Hamel, J., and K.M. Knutzen. 2003. *Biomechanical basis of human movement*. 2nd ed. Philadelphia: Lippincott Williams & Wilkins.

Hyde, T., and M. Gengenbach. 2007. *Conservative management of sports injuries*. Sudbury, MA: Jones & Bartlett.

Kendall, F., E. McCreary, and P. Provance. 2005. *Muscles: Testing and function with posture and pain*. 5th ed. Philadelphia: Lippincott Williams & Wilkins.

McLester, J., and P. St. Pierre. 2008. *Applied biomechanics: Concepts and connections*. Belmont, CA: Thomson Wadsworth.

Magee, D., J. Zachazewski, and W. Quillen. 2009. *Pathology and intervention in musculoskeletal rehabilitation*. St. Louis: Saunders Elsevier.

Petty, N., and A.P. Moore. 2002. *Neuromusculoskeletal examination and assessment: A handbook for therapists*. Edinburgh: Churchill Livingstone.

Price, J., and M. Bratcher. 2010. *The BioMechanics Method corrective exercise specialist certification program*. San Diego, CA: The BioMechanics Press.

Chapter 4

Boos, N., and M. Aebi, eds. 2008. *Spinal disorders: Fundamentals of diagnosis and treatment*. New York: Springer.

Cramer, G., and S. Darby. 2014. *Clinical anatomy of the spine, spinal cord, and ANS*. 3rd ed. St. Louis: Mosby.

Dimon, T., and M. Day. 2008. *Anatomy of the moving body: A basic course in bones, muscles, and joints*. 2nd ed. Berkeley, CA: North Atlantic Books.

Gajdosik, R., R. Simpson, R. Smith, and R.L. DonTigny. 1985. Pelvic tilt intratester reliability of measuring the standing position and range of motion. *Physical Therapy* 65(2): 169-174.

Heino, J.G., J.J. Godges, and C.L. Carter. 1990. Relationship between hip extension range of motion and postural alignment. *Journal of Orthopaedic and Sports Physical Therapy* 12(6): 243-247.

Houglum, P. 2016. *Therapeutic exercise for musculoskeletal injuries*. 4th ed. Champaign, IL: Human Kinetics.

Kendall, F., E. McCreary, and P. Provance. 2005. *Muscles: Testing and function with posture and pain*. 5th ed. Philadelphia: Lippincott Williams & Wilkins.

McGill, S. 2016. *Low back disorders: Evidence-based prevention and rehabilitation*. 3rd ed. Champaign, IL: Human Kinetics.

Palmer, L., M. Epler, and F. Epler. 1998. *Fundamentals of musculoskeletal assessment techniques*. New York: Lippincott Williams & Wilkins.

Petty, N., and A.P. Moore. 2002. *Neuromusculoskeletal examination and assessment: A handbook for therapists*. Edinburgh: Churchill Livingstone.

Price, J., and M. Bratcher. 2010. *The BioMechanics Method corrective exercise specialist certification program*. San Diego, CA: The BioMechanics Press.

Schamberger, W. 2002. *The malalignment syndrome: Implications for medicine and sport*. Edinburgh: Churchill Livingstone.

Solberg, G. 2008. *Postural disorders and musculoskeletal dysfunction: Diagnosis, prevention and treatment*. 2nd ed. Toronto: Elsevier.

Ward, K., ed. 2016. *Routledge handbook of sports therapy, injury assessment and rehabilitation*. New York: Routledge.

Whiting, W.C., and R.F. Zernicke. 2008. *Biomechanics of musculoskeletal injury*. 2nd ed. Champaign, IL: Human Kinetics.

Chapter 5

Betts, J.G., P. Desaix, E. Johnson, J.E. Johnson, O. Korol, D. Kruse, B. Poe, J. Wise, M.D. Womble, and K.A. Young. 2013. *Anatomy & physiology*. Houston, TX: OpenStax College, Rice University.

Bontrager, K.L., and J. Lampignano. 2014. *Textbook of radiographic positioning and related anatomy*. 8th ed. New York: Elsevier.

Brumitt, J. 2010. *Core assessment and training*. Champaign, IL: Human Kinetics.

Bryant, C.X., and D.J. Green, eds. 2010. *ACE personal trainer manual: The ultimate resource for fitness professionals*. 4th ed. San Diego, CA: American Council on Exercise.

Cramer, G., and S. Darby. 2014. *Clinical anatomy of the spine, spinal cord, and ANS*. 3rd ed. St. Louis: Mosby.

Dimon, T., and M. Day. 2008. *Anatomy of the moving body: A basic course in bones, muscles, and joints*. 2nd ed. Berkeley, CA: North Atlantic Books.

Goldfinger, E. 1991. *Human anatomy for artists: The elements of form*. Oxford, England: Oxford University Press.

Hanna, T. 1988. *Somatics: Reawakening the mind's control of movement, flexibility and health*. Cambridge, MA: Perseus Books.

Imhoff, A.B., K. Beitzel, K. Stamer, E. Klein, and G. Mazzocca, eds. 2016. *Rehabilitation in orthopedic surgery*. 2nd ed. Berlin: Springer-Verlag.

Johnson, J. 2012. *Postural assessment: Hands-on guides for therapists*. Champaign, IL: Human Kinetics.

Johnson, J. 2016. *Postural correction: An illustrated guide to 30 pathologies*. Champaign, IL: Human Kinetics.

Kehr, P., and A. Weidner, eds. 1987. *Cervical spine I: Strasbourg 1985*. New York: Springer-Verlag Wien.

Kendall, F., E. McCreary, and P. Provance. 2005. *Muscles: Testing and function with posture and pain*. 5th ed. Philadelphia: Lippincott Williams & Wilkins.

McGill, S. 2016. *Low back disorders: Evidence-based prevention and rehabilitation*. 3rd ed. Champaign, IL: Human Kinetics.

McMinn, R.M.H., ed. 2005. *Last's anatomy: Regional and applied.* Hong Kong: Churchill Livingstone.

Middleditch, A., and J. Oliver. 2005. *Functional anatomy of the spine.* 2nd ed. New York: Elsevier.

Muscolino, J.E. 2011. *Kinesiology: The skeletal system and muscle function.* 2nd ed. St. Louis: Elsevier Mosby.

Palmer, L., M. Epler, and F. Epler. 1998. *Fundamentals of musculoskeletal assessment techniques.* New York: Lippincott Williams & Wilkins.

Petty, N., and A.P. Moore. 2002. *Neuromusculoskeletal examination and assessment: A handbook for therapists.* Edinburgh: Churchill Livingstone.

Price, J. 2015. Excessive thoracic kyphosis: More than just bad posture. *IDEA Mind-Body Wellness Review* 2(1): 19 paragraphs, www.ideafit.com/fitness-library/excessive-thoracic-kyphosis-much-more-than-just-bad-posture-0.

Price, J., and M. Bratcher. 2010. *The BioMechanics Method corrective exercise specialist certification program.* San Diego, CA: The BioMechanics Press.

Rolf, I.P. 1989. *Rolfing: Reestablishing the natural alignment and structural integration of the human body for vitality and well-being.* Rev. ed. Rochester, VT: Healing Arts Press.

Schenck, R.C., ed. 1999. *Athletic training and sports medicine.* 3rd ed. Rosemont, IL: American Academy of Orthopaedic Surgeons.

Solberg, G. 2008. *Postural disorders and musculoskeletal dysfunction: Diagnosis, prevention and treatment.* New York: Churchill Livingstone Elsevier.

Chapter 6

Adds, P., and S. Shahsavari, eds. 2012. *The musculoskeletal system.* Boca Raton, FL: CRC Press.

Chek, P. 2001. Primal movement patterns. Presentation at the IDEA Health and Fitness Association Conference, San Francisco, CA.

Clippinger, K. 2007. *Dance anatomy and physiology: Principles and exercises for improving technique and avoiding common injuries.* Champaign, IL: Human Kinetics.

Eriksen, K. 2004. *Upper cervical subluxation complex: A review of the chiropractic and medical literature.* Philadelphia: Lippincott Williams & Wilkins.

Griffin, J.C. 2015. *Client-centered exercise prescription.* 3rd ed. Champaign, IL: Human Kinetics.

Grimsby, O., and J. Rivard, eds. 2008. *Science, theory and clinical application in orthopaedic manual physical therapy.* Vol. 2. Taylorsville, UT: The Academy of Graduate Physical Therapy.

Johnson, J. 2016. *Postural correction: An illustrated guide to 30 pathologies.* Champaign, IL: Human Kinetics.

Jones, K.J. 2011. *Neurological assessment: A clinician's guide.* Edinburgh: Elsevier.

Kendall, F.P., E.K. McCreary, and P.G. Provance. 2005. *Muscle testing and function with posture and pain.* 5th ed. Baltimore, MD: Lippincott Williams & Wilkins.

Louw, D.A. 2007. *Human development.* 3rd ed. Cape Town, South Africa: ABC Press.

Muscolino, J.E. 2011. *Kinesiology: The skeletal system and muscle function.* St Louis, MO: Elsevier.

Palmer, L., M. Epler, and F. Epler. 1998. *Fundamentals of musculoskeletal assessment techniques.* New York: Lippincott Williams & Wilkins.

Petty N., and P. Moore. 2002. *Neuromuscular examination and assessment: A handbook for therapists.* Edinburgh: Churchill Livingstone.

Price, J., and M. Bratcher. 2010. *The BioMechanics Method corrective exercise specialist certification program.* San Diego, CA: The BioMechanics Press.

Shen, F.H., and C.I. Shaffrey, eds. 2010. *Arthritis and arthroplasty: The spine.* Philadelphia: Saunders Elsevier.

Chapter 7

Ayyappa, E. 1997. Normal human locomotion, part 2: Motion, ground reaction force and muscle activity. *Journal of Prosthetics and Orthotics* 9(2): 42-57.

Dimon, T., and M. Day. 2008. *Anatomy of the moving body: A basic course in bones, muscles, and joints.* 2nd ed. Berkeley, CA: North Atlantic Books.

Draves, D. 1986. *Anatomy of the lower extremity.* Baltimore, MD: Williams & Wilkins.

Golding, L.A., and S.M. Golding. 2003. *Fitness professionals' guide to musculoskeletal anatomy and human movement.* Monterey, CA: Healthy Learning.

Gray, H. 1995. *Gray's anatomy.* New York: Barnes and Noble Books.

Kendall, F., E. McCreary, and P. Provance. 2005. *Muscle testing and function with posture and pain.* 5th ed. Baltimore, MD: Lippincott Williams & Wilkins.

Marshall C. 2010. *Mammal anatomy: An illustrated guide.* New York: Cavandish Square Publishing.

Martini, F.H., J. Timmons, and R.B. Tallitsch. 2014. *Human anatomy.* 8th ed. San Francisco: Pearson Education.

Myers, T.W. 2008. *Anatomy trains: Myofascial meridians for manual and movement therapists.* 2nd ed. New York: Churchill Livingstone.

Price, J. 2010. Understanding muscles and movement: From theory to practice. *IDEA Fitness Journal* (7)9: 54-60.

Price, J. 2014. Build strong glutes and a pain-free lower back. *American Council on Exercise ProSource.* October. Accessed August 31, 2016: www.acefitness.org/prosourcearticle/5013/build-strong-glutes-and-a-pain-free-lower

Price, J. 2016. Swing time: Helping golfers improve scores, prevent injuries. *IDEA Fitness Journal* 13(8): 25-28.

Price, J., and M. Bratcher. 2010. *The BioMechanics Method corrective exercise specialist certification program. Module 2: Understanding muscles and movement.* San Diego, CA: The BioMechanics Press.

Rolf, I.P. 1989. *Rolfing: Reestablishing the natural alignment and structural integration of the human body for vitality and well-being.* Rev. ed. Rochester, VT: Healing Arts Press.

Siegfried, T. 2016. Einstein's gravity: One big idea forever changed how we understand the universe. In *Science news*, edited by Elizabeth Quill. New York: Diversion Books.

Chapter 8

Chinn, L., and J. Hertel. 2010. Rehabilitation of ankle and foot injuries in athletes. *Clinical Sports Medicine* 29(1): 157-167.

Clemente, C. 2011. *Clemente's anatomy dissector.* 3rd ed. Philadelphia: Lippincott Williams & Wilkins.

Clippinger, K. 2007. *Dance anatomy and physiology: Principles and exercises for improving technique and avoiding common injuries.* Champaign, IL: Human Kinetics.

Davis, M., P. Davis, and D. Ross. 2005. *Expert guide to sports medicine.* Philadelphia: American College of Physicians.

Dimon, T., and M. Day. 2008. *Anatomy of the moving body: A basic course in bones, muscles, and joints.* 2nd ed. Berkeley, CA: North Atlantic Books.

Donatelli, R., and M. Wooden. 2010. *Orthopedic physical therapy.* 4th ed. St. Louis: Elsevier.

Frowen, P., M. O'Donnell, D. Lorimer, and G. Burrow. 2010. *Neale's disorders of the foot.* 8th ed. St. Louis: Elsevier.

Golding, L.A., and S.M. Golding. 2003. *Fitness professionals' guide to musculoskeletal anatomy and human movement.* Monterey, CA: Healthy Learning.

Gray, H. 1995. *Gray's anatomy.* New York: Barnes & Noble Books.

Hyde, T., and M. Gegenbach. 2007. *Conservative management of sports injuries.* Sudbury, MA: Jones & Bartlett.

Kelikian, A. 2011. *Sarrafian's anatomy of the foot and ankle: Descriptive, topographic, functional.* Baltimore: Lippincott Williams & Wilkins.

Muscolino, J. 2010. *The muscular system manual: The skeletal muscles of the human body.* 4th ed. St. Louis: Elsevier.

Page, P., C. Frank, and R. Lardner. 2010. *Assessment and treatment of muscle imbalance: The Janda approach.* Champaign, IL: Human Kinetics.

Price, J., and M. Bratcher. 2010. *The BioMechanics Method corrective exercise specialist education program.* San Diego, CA: The BioMechanics Press.

Snell, R. 2008. *Clinical anatomy by regions.* Baltimore: Lippincott Williams & Wilkins.

Chapter 9

Agur, A., and A. Dalley. 2013. *Grant's atlas of anatomy.* 13th ed. Baltimore: Lippincott Williams & Wilkins.

Antevil, J., L. Blackbourne, and C. Moore. 2006. *Anatomy recall.* 2nd ed. Baltimore: Lippincott Williams & Wilkins.

Clippinger, K. 2007. *Dance anatomy and physiology: Principles and exercises for improving technique and avoiding common injuries.* Champaign, IL: Human Kinetics.

Dimon, T., and M. Day. 2008. *Anatomy of the moving body: A basic course in bones, muscles, and joints.* 2nd ed. Berkeley, CA: North Atlantic Books.

Gray, H. 1995. *Gray's Anatomy.* New York: Barnes & Noble Books.

Hyde, T., and M. Gengenbach. 2007. *Conservative management of sports injuries.* Sudbury, MA: Jones & Bartlett.

Kulkarni, N. 2012. *Clinical anatomy: A problem-solving approach.* London: JayPee Brothers Medical Publishers.

Price, J., and M. Bratcher. 2010. *The BioMechanics Method corrective exercise specialist certification program.* San Diego, CA: The BioMechanics Press.

Schlossberg, L., and G.D. Zuidema, eds. 1997. *The Johns Hopkins atlas of human functional anatomy.* 4th ed. Baltimore: Johns Hopkins University Press.

Chapter 10

Clark, M., and S. Lucett, eds. 2011. *NASM essentials of corrective exercise training.* Philadelphia: Lippincott Williams & Wilkins.

Clippinger, K. 2007. *Dance anatomy and physiology: Principles and exercises for improving technique and avoiding common injuries.* Champaign, IL: Human Kinetics.

Cramer, G.D., and S.A. Darby. 2014. *Clinical anatomy of the spine, spinal cord, and ANS.* 3rd ed. St. Louis: Elsevier Mosby.

DeLisa, J., B. Gans, and N. Walsh, eds. 2005. *Physical medicine and rehabilitation: Principles and practice.* Vol. 1. Philadelphia: Lippincott Williams & Wilkins.

Gamble, P. 2013. *Strength and conditioning for team sports: Sport-specific physical preparation for high performance.* 2nd ed. New York: Routledge.

Gray, H. 1995. *Gray's anatomy.* New York: Barnes & Noble Books.

Middleditch, A., and A.J. Oliver. 2005. *Functional anatomy of the spine.* 2nd ed. Edinburgh: Elsevier.

Muscolino, J.E. 2011. Kinesiology: *The skeletal system and muscle function.* 2nd ed. St. Louis: Elsevier Mosby.

Myers, T.W. 2008. *Anatomy trains: Myofascial meridians for manual and movement therapists.* 2nd ed. New York: Churchill Livingstone.

Price, J., and M. Bratcher. 2010. *The BioMechanics Method corrective exercise specialist certification program.* San Diego, CA: The BioMechanics Press.

Chapter 11

Clippinger, K. 2007. *Dance anatomy and physiology: Principles and exercises for improving technique and avoiding common injuries.* Champaign, IL: Human Kinetics.

Di Giacomo, G., N. Pouliart, A. Costantini, and A. De Vita, eds. 2008. *Atlas of functional shoulder anatomy.* Milan, Italy: Springer.

Gray, H. 1995. *Gray's anatomy.* New York: Barnes and Noble Books.

Hertling, D., and R.M. Kessler. 2006. *Management of common musculoskeletal disorders: Physical therapy principles and methods.* 4th ed. Philadelphia: Lippincott Williams & Wilkins.

Karageanes, S.J., ed. 2005. *Principles of manual sports medicine.* Philadelphia: Lippincott Williams & Wilkins.

McMinn, R.M.H., ed. 2005. *Last's anatomy: Regional and applied.* Hong Kong: Churchill Livingstone.

Maffulli, N., and J.P. Furia. 2012. *Rotator cuff disorders: Basic science and clinical medicine.* London: JP Medical.

Middleditch, A., and J. Oliver 2005. *Functional anatomy of the spine.* 2nd ed. New York: Elsevier.

Palmer, L., M. Epler, and F. Epler. 1998. *Fundamentals of musculoskeletal assessment techniques.* New York: Lippincott Williams & Wilkins.

Plotnik, R., and H. Kouyoumdjian. 2014. *Introduction to psychology.* 10th ed. Belmont, CA: Wadsworth Cengage Learning.

Price, J., and M. Bratcher. 2010. *The BioMechanics Method corrective exercise specialist certification program.* San Diego, CA: The BioMechanics Press.

Rhoades, R., and D.R. Bell, eds. 2009. *Medical physiology: Principles for clinical medicine.* 3rd ed. Philadelphia: Lippincott Williams & Wilkins.

Rockwood, C.A., and F.A. Matsen, eds. 2009. *The shoulder.* 4th ed. Vol. 1. Philadelphia: Saunders Elsevier.

Sahrmann, S. 2002. *Diagnosis and treatment of movement impairment syndromes.* St. Louis: Mosby.

Siegel, I. 2002. *All about joints: A maintenance guide.* New York: Demos Medical Publishing.

Singh, I. 2005. *Essentials of Anatomy.* 5th ed. New Delhi: Jaypee Brothers Medical Publishers.

West, J.B. 2000. *Respiratory physiology: The essentials.* 6th ed. Philadelphia: Lippincott Williams & Wilkins.

Chapter 12

Adds, P., and S. Shahsavari, eds. 2012. *The musculoskeletal system.* Boca Raton, FL: CRC Press.

Chaitow, L., and J. DeLany. 2008. *Clinical application of neuromuscular techniques: The upper body.* 2nd ed. Philadelphia: Churchill Livingstone Elsevier.

Clarkson, H.M. 2000. *Musculoskeletal assessment: Joint range of motion and manual muscle strength.* Philadelphia: Lippincott Williams & Wilkins.

Ferrari, R. 2006. *The whiplash encyclopedia: The facts and myths of whiplash.* 2nd ed. London: Jones & Bartlett.

Gray, H. 1995. *Gray's anatomy.* New York: Barnes & Noble Books.

Halim, A. 2009. *Human anatomy volume 3: Head, neck and brain.* New Delhi, India: I.K. International Publishing House.

Lee, S.W. 2017. *Musculoskeletal injuries and conditions: Assessment and management.* New York: Demos Medical.

Lieberman, D.E. 2011. *The evolution of the human head.* Cambridge, MA: Harvard University Press.

McGowan, C. 1999. *A practical guide to vertebrate mechanics.* New York: Cambridge University Press.

Palastanga, N., D. Field, and R.W. Soames. 1994. *Anatomy and human movement: Structure and function.* 2nd ed. Oxford, England: Butterworth-Heinemann.

Peterson, B.W., and F.J. Richmond. 1988. *Control of head movement.* New York: Oxford University Press.

Price, J., and M. Bratcher. 2010. *The BioMechanics Method corrective exercise specialist certification program.* San Diego, CA: The BioMechanics Press.

Salvo, S.G. 2009. *Mosby's pathology for massage therapists.* 2nd ed. St. Louis: Mosby Elsevier.

Willard, V.P., L. Zhang, and K.A. Athanasiou. 2017. Tissue engineering of the temporomandibular joint. *Comprehensive Biomaterials II* 6: 142-158.

Chapter 13

DiGiovanna, E.L., S. Schiowitz, and D.J. Dowling, eds. 2005. *An osteopathic approach to diagnosis and treatment.* 3rd ed. Philadelphia: Lippincott Williams & Wilkins.

Giangarra, C.E., and R.C. Manske. 2011. *Clinical orthopedic rehabilitation: A team approach e-book.* 4th ed. Philadelphia: Elsevier.

Houglum, P. 2016. *Therapeutic exercise for musculoskeletal injuries.* 4th ed. Champaign, IL: Human Kinetics.

Hutson, M., and A. Ward, eds. 2016. *Oxford textbook of musculoskeletal medicine.* 2nd ed. Oxford, UK: Oxford University Press.

Hyde, T.E., and M.S. Gengenbach, eds. 2007. *Conservative management of sports injuries.* 2nd ed. Sudbury, MA: Jones & Bartlett.

Karageanes, S.J., ed. 2003. *Principles of manual sports medicine.* Philadelphia: Lippincott Williams & Wilkins.

Myers, T.W. 2008. *Anatomy trains: Myofascial meridians for manual and movement therapists.* 2nd ed. New York: Churchill Livingstone.

Myers, T.W., and J. Earls. 2017. *Fascial release for structural balance.* Rev. ed. Berkeley, CA: North Atlantic Books.

Price, J., and M. Bratcher. 2010. *The BioMechanics Method corrective exercise specialist certification program.* San Diego, CA: The BioMechanics Press.

Rolf, I.P. 1989. *Rolfing: Reestablishing the natural alignment and structural integration of the human body for vitality and well-being.* Rev. ed. Rochester, VT: Healing Arts Press.

Starlanyl, D.J., and J. Sharkey. 2013. *Healing through trigger point therapy: A guide to fibromyalgia, myofascial pain and dysfunction.* Berkeley, CA: North Atlantic Books.

Swinnen, S.P., J. Massion, H. Heuer, and P. Casaer, eds. 1994. *Interlimb coordination: Neural, dynamical, and cognitive constraints.* New York: Academic Press.

Chapter 14

Bandura, A. 1986. *Social foundations of thought and action: A social cognitive theory.* Englewood Cliffs, N.J.: Prentice Hall.

Bryant, C.X., and D.J. Green, eds. 2010. *ACE personal trainer manual: The ultimate resource for fitness professionals.* 4th ed. San Diego, CA: American Council on Exercise.

Feltz, D.A. 1992. Understanding motivation in sport: A self-efficacy perspective. In *Motivation in sport and exercise,* edited by G.C. Roberts. Champaign, IL: Human Kinetics.

Fuller, C. 2004. *Thinkers, watchers, and doers: Unlocking your child's unique learning style.* Colorado Springs, CO: Pinon Press.

Myers, T.W. 2008. *Anatomy trains: Myofascial meridians for manual and movement therapists.* 2nd ed. New York: Churchill Livingstone.

Price, J., and M. Bratcher. 2010. *The BioMechanics Method corrective exercise specialist certification program.* San Diego, CA: The BioMechanics Press.

Price, J., and F. Sharpe. 2009. *The complete idiot's guide to functional training.* New York: Penguin Publishing.

Rejeski, W.J. 1992. Motivation for exercise behavior: A critique of theoretical directions. In *Motivation in sport and exercise,* edited by G.C. Roberts. Champaign, IL: Human Kinetics.

Rolf, I.P. 1989. *Rolfing: Reestablishing the natural alignment and structural integration of the human body for vitality and well-being.* Rev. ed. Rochester, VT: Healing Arts Press.

Travell, J.G. and D.G. Simons. 1992. *Myofascial pain and dysfunction: The trigger point manual. Vol. 2. The lower extremities.* Media, PA: Lippincott Williams & Wilkins.

Walker, B. 2011. *The anatomy of stretching: Your illustrated guide to flexibility and injury rehabilitation.* 2nd ed. Chichester, England: Lotus Publishing.

Whitworth, L., H. Kimsey-House, K. Kimsey-House, and P. Sandahl. 2007. *Co-active coaching: New skills for coaching people toward success in work and life.* 2nd ed. Palo Alto, CA: Davies-Black Publishing.

Chapter 15

Abelson, B., and K. Abelson 2003. *Release your pain.* Calgary: Rowan Tree Books.

Beck, M. 2010. *Theory and practice of therapeutic massage.* 6th ed. Boston: Cengage Learning.

Brummitt, J. 2008. The role of massage in sports performance and rehabilitation: Current evidence and future direction. *North American Journal of Sports Physical Therapy* 3(1): 7–21.

Calvert, R.N. 2002. *The history of massage: An illustrated survey from around the world.* Rochester, VT: Healing Arts Press.

Clark, M., and S. Lucett 2011. *NASM essentials of corrective exercise training.* Philadelphia: Lippincott Williams & Wilkins.

Feltz, D.A. 1992. Understanding motivation in sport: A self-efficacy perspective. In *Motivation in sport and exercise,* edited by G.C. Roberts. Champaign, IL: Human Kinetics.

Fritz, S. 2013. *Mosby's fundamentals of therapeutic massage.* 5th ed. St. Louis: Elsevier.

Hyde, C. 2002. *Fitness instructor training guide.* 4th ed. American Association for Active Lifestyles and Fitness. Dubuque, IA: Kendall/Hunt Publishing Company.

Inkster, K. 2015. *50 foam roller exercises for massage, injury prevention and core strength.* New York: Skyhorse Publishing.

Myers, T.W. 2008. *Anatomy trains: Myofascial meridians for manual and movement therapists.* 2nd ed. New York: Churchill Livingstone.

Price, J., and M. Bratcher. 2010. *The BioMechanics Method corrective exercise specialist certification program.* San Diego, CA: The BioMechanics Press.

Price, J. 2013. *The amazing tennis ball back pain cure.* San Diego, CA: The BioMechanics Press.

Price, J. 2016. *Increasing client adherence.* PTontheNet.com. Accessed Feb 2, 2018. http://www.ptonthenet.com/articles/how-to-increase-client-adherence-4119.

Pappaioannou, A., and D. Hackfort. 2014. *Routledge companion to sport and exercise psychology: Global perspectives and fundamental concepts.* New York: Routledge.

Rolf, I.P. 1989. *Rolfing: Reestablishing the natural alignment and structural integration of the human body for vitality and well-being.* Rev. ed. Rochester, VT: Healing Arts Press.

Scheumann, D. 2007. *The balanced body: A guide to deep tissue and neuromuscular therapy.* 3rd ed. Philadelphia: Lippincott Williams & Wilkins.

Simons, D.G., J.G. Travell, and L.S. Simons. 1998. *Myofascial pain and dysfunction: The trigger point manual, Vol. 1. Upper half of body.* 2nd ed. Media, PA: Lippincott Williams & Wilkins.

Sinah, A.G. 2001. *Principles and practices of therapeutic massage.* New Delhi: Jaypee Brothers.

Travell, J.G., and D.G. Simons 1992. *Myofascial pain and dysfunction: The trigger point manual, Vol. 2. The lower extremities.* Media, PA: Lippincott Williams & Wilkins.

Whitworth, L., H. Kimsey-House, K. Kimsey-House, and P. Sandahl. 2007. *Co-Active coaching: New skills for coaching people toward success in work and life.* 2nd ed. Palo Alto, CA: Davies-Black Publishing.

Chapter 16

Ackland,T., B. Elliott, and J. Bloomfield. 2009. *Applied anatomy and biomechanics in sport.* 2nd ed. Champaign, IL: Human Kinetics.

Alter, M. 1998. *Sports stretch: 311 stretches for 41 sports.* 2nd ed. Champaign, IL: Human Kinetics.

Bandura, A. 1986. *Social foundations of thought and action: A social cognitive theory.* Englewood Cliffs, NJ: Prentice Hall.

Bandy, W.D., J.M. Irion, and M. Briggler. 1997. The effect of time and frequency of static stretching on flexibility of the hamstring muscles. *Physical Therapy* 77(10): 1090-1096.

Bryant, C.X., and D.J. Green, eds. 2010. *ACE personal trainer manual: The ultimate resource for fitness professionals.* 4th ed. San Diego, CA: American Council on Exercise.

Calvert, R.N. 2002. *The history of massage: An illustrated survey from around the world.* Rochester, VT: Healing Arts Press.

Clark, M., and S. Lucett. 2011. *NASM essentials of corrective exercise training.* Philadelphia: Lippincott Williams & Wilkins.

Golding, L.A., and S.M. Golding. 2003. *Fitness professionals' guide to musculoskeletal anatomy and human movement.* Monterey, CA: Healthy Learning.

Gray, H. 1995. *Gray's anatomy.* New York: Barnes & Noble Books.

Hoffman, J. 2014. *Physiological aspects of sports training and performance.* 2nd ed. Champaign, IL: Human Kinetics.

Hyde, C. 2002. *Fitness instructor training guide.* 4th ed. American Association for Active Lifestyles and Fitness. Dubuque, IA: Kendall/Hunt Publishing Company.

Karageanes, S. 2005. *Principles of manual sports medicine.* Philadelphia: Lippincott Williams & Wilkins.

Kisner, C., and L.A. Colby. 2012. *Therapeutic exercise: Foundations and techniques.* Philadelphia: F.A. Davis Company.

Kovacs, M. 2015. *The stretch out strap workbook: Step-by-step techniques for maximizing your range of motion of flexibility.* Berkeley: Ulysses.

Kurz, T. 2003. *Stretching scientifically: A guide to flexibility training.* Island Pond, VT: Stadion.

Mason, J. 2004. *Believe you can: The power of the positive attitude.* Michigan: Revel.

McGill, S. 2002. *Low back disorders: Evidence based prevention and rehabilitation.* Champaign, IL: Human Kinetics.

Micheli, L. 2011. *Encyclopedia of sports medicine.* Thousand Oaks, CA: Sage Publications.

Muscolino, J. 2009. *The muscle and bone palpation manual with trigger points, referral patterns and stretching.* St. Louis: Mosby, Elsevier.

Myers, T.W. 2008. *Anatomy trains: Myofascial meridians for manual and movement therapists.* 2nd ed. New York: Churchill Livingstone.

Price, J., and M. Bratcher. 2010. *The BioMechanics Method corrective exercise specialist certification program.* San Diego, CA: The BioMechanics Press.

Rolf, I.P. 1989. *Rolfing: Reestablishing the natural alignment and structural integration of the human body for vitality and well-being.* Rev. ed. Rochester, VT: Healing Arts Press.

Taylor, D.C., J.D. Dalton, A.V. Seaber, and W.E. Garrett. 2011. Viscoelastic properties of muscle-tendon units. The biomechanical effects of stretching. *American Journal of Sports Medicine* 18(3): 300-309.

Walker, B. 2011. *The anatomy of stretching: Your illustrated guide to flexibility and injury rehabilitation.* 2nd ed. Chichester, England: Lotus Publishing.

Chapter 17

Ackland, T., B. Elliott, and J. Bloomfield. 2009. *Applied anatomy and biomechanics in sport.* 2nd ed. Champaign, IL: Human Kinetics.

Bryant, C.X., and D.J. Green, eds. 2010. *ACE personal trainer manual: The ultimate resource for fitness professionals.* 4th ed. San Diego, CA: American Council on Exercise.

Chaitow, L., and J. Delany. 2005. *Clinical application of neuromuscular techniques: Practical case study exercises.* New York: Elsevier Churchill Livingstone.

Clark, M., and S. Lucett. 2011. *NASM essentials of corrective exercise training.* Philadelphia: Lippincott Williams & Wilkins.

Coyle, D. 2009. *The talent code: Greatness isn't born. It's grown. Here's how.* New York: Random House.

Ellenbecker, T., and G. Davies. 2001. *Closed kinetic chain exercise: A comprehensive guide to multi-joint exercises.* Champaign, IL: Human Kinetics.

Fishman, S., J. Ballantyne, and J. Rathmell. 2009. *Bonica's management of pain.* Philadelphia: Lippincott Williams & Wilkins.

Fritz, S. 2013. *Mosby's fundamentals of therapeutic massage.* 5th ed. St. Louis: Elsevier.

Higgins, M. 2011. *Therapeutic exercise: From theory to practice.* Philadelphia: F.A. Davis Company.

Hoffman, J. 2014. *Physiological aspects of sports training and performance.* 2nd ed. Champaign, IL: Human Kinetics.

Houglum, P. 2016. *Therapeutic exercise for musculoskeletal injuries.* 4th ed. Champaign, IL: Human Kinetics.

Kraemer, W., and K. Häkkinen, eds. 2002. *Strength training for sport.* Malden, MA: Blackwell Science.

Magee, D.J., J.E. Zachazewski, and W.S. Quillen, eds. 2007. *Scientific foundations and principles of practice in musculoskeletal rehabilitation.* St. Louis: Saunders Elsevier.

McGill, S. 2002. *Low back disorders: Evidence based prevention and rehabilitation.* Champaign, IL: Human Kinetics.

Miller, P. 1995. *Fitness programming and physical disability.* Champaign, IL: Human Kinetics.

Price, J. 2008. Corrective exercise: Coming full circle. *IDEA Fitness Journal.* San Diego: IDEA Health and Fitness Association (January): 40-47.

Price, J., and M. Bratcher. 2010. *The BioMechanics Method corrective exercise specialist certification program.* San Diego, CA: The BioMechanics Press.

Price, J., and F. Sharpe. 2009. *The complete idiot's guide to functional training.* New York: Penguin Publishing.

Reider, B., M. Provencher, and R. Davies. 2015. *Orthopedic rehabilitation of the athlete: Getting back in the game.* Philadelphia: Elsevier Saunders.

Shumway-Cook, A., and M. Woollocott. 2007. *Motor control: Translating research into clinical practice.* 3rd ed. Philadelphia: Lippincott Williams & Wilkins.

Starkey, C., and G. Johnson, eds. 2006. *Athletic training and sports medicine.* 4th ed. Sudbury, MA: Jones & Bartlett.

Stone, M., M. Stone, and W. Sands. 2007. *Principles and practice of resistance training.* Champaign, IL: Human Kinetics.

Wrisberg, C. 2007. *Sport skill instruction for coaches.* Champaign, IL: Human Kinetics.

Chapter 18

Atkins, E., J. Kerr, and E. Goodlad. 2015. *A practical approach to musculoskeletal medicine: Assessment, diagnosis and treatment.* St. Louis: Elsevier.

Chinn, L., and J. Hertel 2010. Rehabilitation of ankle and foot injuries in athletes. *Clinical Sports Medicine* 29 (January): 157-167.

DeLisa, J., B. Gans, and N. Walsh, eds. 2005. *Physical medicine and rehabilitation: Principles and practice, Volume 1.* Philadelphia: Lippincott Williams & Wilkins.

Donatelli, R., and M. Wooden. 2010. *Orthopedic physical therapy.* 4th ed. St. Louis: Churchill Livingstone Elsevier.

Frontera, W., J. Silver, and T. Rizzo. 2015. *Essentials of physical medicine and rehabilitation: Musculoskeletal disorders, pain and rehabilitation.* 3rd ed. Philadelphia: Elsevier Saunders.

Greene, D., and S. Roberts 2017. *Kinesiology: Movement in the context of activity.* 3rd ed. St. Louis: Elsevier.

Hertling, D., and R. Kessler. 2006. *Management of common musculoskeletal disorders: Physical therapy principles and methods.* 4th ed. Philadelphia: Lippincott Williams & Wilkins.

Higgins, M. 2011. *Therapeutic exercise: From theory to practice.* Philadelphia: F.A. Davis.

Karwowski, W. 2006. *International encyclopedia of ergonomics and human factors: Volume 3.* 2nd ed. Boca Raton, FL: Taylor and Francis.

Hillstrom, K., and L.C. Hillstrom, eds. 2007. *The industrial revolution in America: Communications, agriculture and meatpacking overview/comparison.* Vols. 7-9. Santa Barbara, CA: ABC-CLIO.

McGill, S. 2016. *Low back disorders: Evidence-based prevention and rehabilitation.* 3rd ed. Champaign, IL: Human Kinetics.

Ombregt, L. 2013. *A system of orthopaedic medicine.* 3rd ed. New York: Churchill Livingstone Elsevier.

Plotnik, R., and H. Kouyoumdjian. 2014. *Introduction to psychology.* 10th ed. Belmont, CA: Wadsworth Cengage Learning.

Price, J. 2014. *How to choose the right training shoe.* Australian Fitness Network. www.fitnessnetwork.com.au.

Price, J., and M. Bratcher. 2010. *The BioMechanics Method corrective exercise specialist education program.* San Diego, CA: The BioMechanics Press.

Sahrmann, S. 2002. *Diagnosis and treatment of movement impairment syndromes.* St. Louis: Mosby.

Scheumann, D.W. 2007. *The balanced body: A guide to deep tissue and neuromuscular therapy.* 3rd ed. Philadelphia: Lippincott Williams & Wilkins.

Simons, D., J. Travell, and L. Simons. 1999. *Travell & Simons' myofascial pain and dysfunction: The trigger point manual. Volume 1: Upper half of body.* 2nd ed. Philadelphia: Lippincott Williams & Wilkins.

Weisberg, J., and H. Shink. 2015. *3 minutes to a pain-free life: The groundbreaking program for total body pain prevention and rapid relief.* New York: Atria Books.

Wilmink, J. 2010. *Lumbar spinal imaging in radicular pain and related conditions.* Netherlands: Springer.

Chapter 19

Barnes, J.F. 1999. Myofascial release. In *Functional soft tissue examination and treatment by manual methods,* 2nd ed, edited by W.I. Hammer. Gaithersburg, MD: Aspen Publishers.

Myers, T.W. 2008. *Anatomy trains: Myofascial meridians for manual and movement therapists.* 2nd ed. New York: Churchill Livingstone.

Price, J. 2013. *The amazing tennis ball back pain cure.* San Diego, CA: The BioMechanics Press.

Price, J., and M. Bratcher. 2010. *The fundamentals of corrective exercise. Module 3: The BioMechanics Method corrective exercise specialist certification program.* San Diego, CA: The BioMechanics Press.

Rolf, I.P. 1989. *Rolfing: Reestablishing the natural alignment and structural integration of the human body for vitality and well-being.* Rev. ed. Rochester, VT: Healing Arts Press.

Travell, J.G., and D.G. Simons. 1992. *Myofascial pain and dysfunction: The trigger point manual. Vol. 2. The lower extremities.* Media, PA: Lippincott Williams & Wilkins.

Chapter 20

Clark, M., and S. Lucett. 2011. *NASM essentials of corrective exercise training.* Philadelphia: Lippincott Williams & Wilkins.

Kovacs, M. 2015. *The flexible stretching strap workbook: Step-by-step techniques for maximizing your range of motion and flexibility.* Berkeley: Ulysses.

Price, J. 2013. *The amazing tennis ball back pain cure.* San Diego, CA: The BioMechanics Press.

Price, J., and M. Bratcher. 2010 *The BioMechanics Method corrective exercise specialist certification program.* San Diego, CA: The BioMechanics Press.

Chapter 21

Bryant, C.X., and D.J. Green, eds. 2010. *ACE personal trainer manual: The ultimate resource for fitness professionals.* 4th ed. San Diego, CA: American Council on Exercise.

Clark, M., and S. Lucett. 2011. *NASM essentials of corrective exercise training.* Philadelphia: Lippincott Williams & Wilkins.

Coyle, D. 2009. *The talent code: Greatness isn't born. It's grown. Here's how.* New York: Random House.

Hoffman, J. 2014. *Physiological aspects of sports training and performance.* 2nd ed. Champaign, IL: Human Kinetics.

Houglum, P. 2016. *Therapeutic exercise for musculoskeletal injuries.* 4th ed. Champaign, IL: Human Kinetics.

Magee, D.J., J.E. Zachazewski, and W.S. Quillen, eds. 2007. *Scientific foundations and principles of practice in musculoskeletal rehabilitation.* St. Louis: Saunders Elsevier.

McGill, S. 2016. *Low back disorders: Evidence-based prevention and rehabilitation.* 3rd ed. Champaign, IL: Human Kinetics.

Price, J. 2013. *The amazing tennis ball back pain cure.* San Diego, CA: The BioMechanics Press.

Price, J., and M. Bratcher. 2010. *The BioMechanics Method corrective exercise specialist certification program.* San Diego, CA: The BioMechanics Press.

Price, J., and F. Sharpe. 2009. *The complete idiot's guide to functional training.* New York: Penguin Publishing.

Wrisberg, C. 2007. *Sport skill instruction for coaches.* Champaign, IL: Human Kinetics.

Chapter 22

Altman, S., E. Valenzi, and R.M. Hodgetts. 1985. *Organizational behavior: Theory and practice.* Orlando: Academic Press.

American College of Sports Medicine. 2014. *ACSM's resources for the personal trainer.* 4th ed. Philadelphia: Lippincott Williams & Wilkins.

Bandura, A. 1986. *Social foundations of thought and action: A social cognitive theory.* Englewood Cliffs, NJ: Prentice Hall.

Brockbank, A., and I. McGill. 2006. *Facilitating reflective learning through mentoring & coaching.* Philadelphia: Kogan Page.

Bryant, C.X., D.J. Green, and S. Newton-Merrill, eds. 2013. *ACE health coach manual: The ultimate guide to wellness, fitness, and lifestyle change.* San Diego, CA: American Council on Exercise.

Caissy, G.A. 1998. *Unlock the fear: How to open yourself up to face and accept change.* Cambridge, MA: Perseus Publishing.

Price, J. 2012. How to turn prospective clients into paying clients: The art of initial consultations. *PTontheNet.com.* Accessed March 15, 2017. www.ptonthenet.com/articles/art-of-initial-pt-client-consultations-3580

Price, J., and M. Bratcher. 2010. *The BioMechanics Method corrective exercise specialist certification program.* San Diego, CA: The BioMechanics Press.

Reeve, J. 2015. *Understanding motivation and behavior.* 6th ed. Hoboken, NJ: Wiley.

Schwarz, R.M. 2017. *The skilled facilitator: A comprehensive resource for consultants, facilitators, coaches and trainers.* 3rd ed. Hoboken, NJ: Jossey-Bass.

Tyler, T.R., R.M. Kramer, and P.J. Oliver, eds. 1999. *The psychology of the social self.* New York: Psychology Press.

Williams, J. 1993. *Applied sport psychology: Personal growth to peak performance.* 2nd ed. Mountain View, CA: Mayfield Publishing.

Chapter 23

Bandura, A.1986. *Social foundations of thought and action: A social cognitive theory.* Englewood Cliffs, NJ: Prentice Hall.

Bly, R.B. 1991. *Selling your services: Proven strategies for getting clients to hire you (or your firm).* New York: Owl Books.

Boyes, A. 2015. *The anxiety toolkit: Strategies for fine-tuning your mind and moving past your stuck points.* New York: Random House.

Bryant, C.X., and D.J. Green, eds. 2010. *ACE personal trainer manual: The ultimate resource for fitness professionals.* 4th ed. San Diego, CA: American Council on Exercise.

Crane, F.G. 2013. *Marketing for entrepreneurs.* 2nd ed. Los Angeles, CA: Sage Publications.

Donaldson, M. 2007. *Negotiating for dummies*. 2nd ed. Hoboken, NJ: Wiley.

Friesen, B.K. 2010. *Designing and conducting your first interview project*. San Francisco: Wiley.

Griffin, J.C. 2006. *Client-centered exercise prescription*. 2nd ed. Champaign, IL: Human Kinetics.

Petty, N., and A.P. Moore. 2002. *Neuromusculoskeletal examination and assessment: A handbook for therapists*. Edinburgh: Churchill Livingstone.

Price, J. 2012. How to turn prospective clients into paying clients: The art of initial consultations. *PTontheNet.com*. Accessed May 22, 2017. www.ptonthenet.com/articles/art-of-initial-pt-client-consultations-3580.

Price, J. 2015. Mental aspects of chronic pain. *IDEA Fitness Journal* 12 (January): 74-78.

Price, J., and M. Bratcher. 2010. *The BioMechanics Method corrective exercise specialist certification program*. San Diego, CA: The BioMechanics Press.

Reeve, J. 2015. *Understanding motivation and behavior*. 6th ed. Hoboken, NJ: Wiley.

Schwarz, R.M. 2017. *The skilled facilitator: A comprehensive resource for consultants, facilitators, coaches and trainers*. 3rd ed. Hoboken, NJ: Jossey-Bass.

Shah, J.Y., and W.L. Gardner, eds. 2008. *Handbook of motivation science*. New York: Guilford Press.

Simpson, H.B., Y. Neria, R. Lewis-Fernández, and F. Schneier, eds. 2010. *Anxiety disorders: Theory, research and clinical perspectives*. Cambridge, UK: Cambridge University Press.

Simpson, M. 2011. *29i - Mastering your sales psyche*. Naples, FL: Xmar Publishing.

Sternberg, R.J., H.L. Roediger, and D. Halpern, eds. 2007. *Critical thinking in psychology*. New York: Cambridge University Press.

Swain, D.P., and C.A. Brawner, eds. 2014. *ACSM's resource manual for guidelines for exercise testing and prescription*. Baltimore, MD: Lippincott Williams & Wilkins.

Winnick, J., and D. Porretta. 2017. *Adapted physical education and sport*. 6th ed. Champaign, IL: Human Kinetics.

Chapter 24

Bandura, A. 1986. *Social foundations of thought and action: A social cognitive theory*. Englewood Cliffs, NJ: Prentice Hall.

Berdik, C. 2012. *Mind over mind: The surprising power of expectations*. New York: Penguin.

Bosworth, H., ed. 2010. *Improving patient treatment adherence: A clinician's guide*. New York: Springer.

Caissy, G.A. 1998. *Unlock the fear: How to open yourself up to face and accept change*. Cambridge, MA: Perseus Publishing.

Dempsey, J.V., and G.C. Sales, eds. 1993. *Interactive instruction and feedback*. Englewood Cliffs, NJ: Educational Technology Publications.

Gallahue, D.L., and F.C. Donnelly. 2003. *Developmental physical education for all children*. 4th ed. Champaign, IL: Human Kinetics.

Griffin, J.C. 2006. *Client-centered exercise prescription*. 2nd ed. Champaign, IL: Human Kinetics.

Hale, B., and P. Crisfield. 2004. *Imagery training: A guide for sports coaches and performers*. Leeds, UK: Coachwise Business Solutions.

Lynch, J. 1992. *The psychology of customer care: A revolutionary approach*. London: Macmillan.

Price, J. 2016. How to increase client adherence. *PTontheNEt.com*. Accessed May 26, 2017. www.ptonthenet.com/articles/how-to-increase-client-adherence-4119

Price, J., and M. Bratcher. 2010. *The BioMechanics Method corrective exercise specialist certification program*. San Diego, CA: The BioMechanics Press.

Roberts, G. 1992. *Motivation in sport and exercise*. Champaign, IL: Human Kinetics.

Salvo, S.G. 2016. *Massage therapy: Principles and practice*. 5th ed. St Louis, MO: Elsevier.

Shah, J.Y., and W.L. Gardner, eds. 2008. *Handbook of motivation science*. New York: Guilford Press.

Skovholt, T.M., and M. Trotter-Mathison. 2016. *The resilient practitioner: Burnout and compassion fatigue prevention and self-care strategies for the helping professions*. 2nd ed. New York: Routledge.

Winnick, J., and D. Porretta. 2017. *Adapted physical education and sport*. 6th ed. Champaign, IL: Human Kinetics.

Chapter 26

Conrad, L.J. 1998. *Guerrilla marketing: Secrets for making big profits from your small business*. Boston: Houghton Mifflin Company.

Galai, D., L. Hillel, and D. Wiener. 2016. *How to create a successful business plan: For entrepreneurs, scientists, managers and students*. Singapore: World Scientific.

Gerber, M.E. 2001. *The e-myth revisited: Why most small businesses don't work and what to do about it*. 2nd ed. New York: Harper Collins.

Huff, D., D. Edmond, and C. Gillette. 2015. 2015 B2B web usability report: What B2B buyers want from vendor websites. *Komarketing.com*. Accessed March 28, 2017. https://komarketing.com/files/b2b-web-usability-report-2015.pdf

Kumar, A., and N. Meenakshi. 2011. *Marketing management*. 2nd ed. New Delhi: Vikas Publishing.

Lamb, C.W., J.F. Hair, and C. McDaniel. 2017. *MKTG11*. Boston, MA: Cengage Learning.

Norman, J. 1999. *What no one ever tells you about starting your own business: Real life start-up advice from 101 successful entrepreneurs*. Chicago: Dearborn.

O'Donohue, W.T., and E.R. Levensky, eds. 2006. *Promoting treatment adherence: A practical handbook for health care providers*. Thousand Oaks, CA: Sage Publications.

Price, J. 2003. Blueprint of a startup (part two). *IDEA Personal Trainer* (October): 13-16.

Price, J., and M. Bratcher. 2010. *The BioMechanics Method corrective exercise specialist certification program.* San Diego, CA: The BioMechanics Press.

Price, J., and M. Bratcher. 2012. *The BioMechanics Method corrective exercise business professional educational course.* San Diego, CA: The BioMechanics Press.

Schroeder, J., and A. Donlin. 2013. *IDEA fitness programming and equipment trends report.* San Diego: IDEA Health and Fitness Association.

Sobel, A., and J. Sheth. 2000. *Clients for life: How great professionals develop breakthrough relationships.* New York: Simon & Schuster.

Chapter 27

Cynthia, G.L. 2012. *Entrepreneurship: Ideas in action.* 5th ed. Mason, OH: South-Western Cengage Learning.

Frazer Robinson, J. 2003. *It's all about customers! The perfect way to grow your business through marketing, sales and service.* London: Kogan Page.

Friedmann, S. 2009. *The complete idiot's guide to target marketing.* New York: Alpha Books.

Hall, R. 2003. *Starting a small business: A step-by-step guide to help you plan and start a business.* West Conshohocken, PA: Infinity Publishing.

Hayes, J.W. 2012. *Becoming the expert: Enhancing your business reputation through thought leadership marketing.* London: Brightword Publishing.

Hiam, A. 2014. *Marketing for dummies.* 4th ed. Somerset, NJ: Wiley.

Humbatov, S. 2015. *Brand management and social media: In service industry.* Hamburg: Anchor Academic Publishing.

Kuzmeski, M. 2010. *And the clients went wild! (Revised and updated): How savvy professionals win all the business they want.* Somerset, NJ: Wiley.

Neuman, J. 2007. *The complete Internet marketer. A practical guide to everything you need to know about marketing online.* USA: With-A-Clue Press.

Price, J., and M. Bratcher. 2010. *The BioMechanics Method corrective exercise specialist certification program.* San Diego, CA: The BioMechanics Press.

Price, J., and M. Bratcher. 2012. *Corrective exercise business professional educational course.* San Diego, CA: The BioMechanics Press.

Rieva, L. 2001. *Start your own business: The only start-up book you'll ever need.* 2nd ed. Irvine, CA: Entrepreneur Press.

Silk, A.J. 2006. *What is marketing?* Boston: Harvard Business School Press.

Schultz, M., and J.E. Doerr. 2011. *Rainmaking conversations: Influence, persuade, and sell in any situation.* Somerset, NJ: Wiley.

Shepherd, J., and N.L. Augenti. 2012. *How to start a home-based online retail business.* 2nd ed. Guilford, CT: Globe Pequot Press.

Urquhart-Brown, S. 2008. *The accidental entrepreneur: The 50 things I wish someone had told me about starting a business.* New York: American Management Association.

Chapter 28

Aluise, J.J. 1980. *The physician as manager.* 2nd ed. New York: Springer Verlag.

Blakemore, P. 2011. *Networking for lawyers.* Reading, UK: PEP Partnership LLP.

Brocato, J.B. 2010. *A service provider's guide to starting a unique business networking group.* Chicago, IL: Intense Publishing.

Bryant, C.X., and D.J. Green, eds. 2010. *ACE personal trainer manual: The ultimate resource for fitness professionals.* 4th ed. San Diego, CA: American Council on Exercise.

Bryant, C.X., D.J. Green, and S. Newton-Merrill, eds. 2013. *ACE health coach manual: The ultimate guide to wellness, fitness, and lifestyle change.* San Diego, CA: American Council on Exercise.

Burg, B. 2006. *Endless referrals.* 3rd ed. New York: McGraw-Hill.

Ciletti, D. 2011. *Marketing yourself.* Columbus, OH: South-Western Cengage Learning.

DiNubile, N.A., and W. Patrick. 2005. *FrameWork: Your 7-step program for healthy muscles, bones, and joints.* New York: Rodale.

Fisher, D. 2001. *Professional networking for dummies.* Hoboken, NJ: Wiley.

Howley, E.T., and D.L. Thompson, eds. 2016. *Fitness professional's handbook.* 7th ed. Champaign, IL: Human Kinetics.

Knoote-Parke, A. 2009. *Brand it purple: Stand out in a crowd.* St Agnes, Australia: Tish N Enigma Books.

Levinson, J.C., and M. Mann. 2007. *Guerrilla networking: A proven battle plan to attract the very people you want to meet.* New York: Morgan James.

Phillips, S. 2014. *The complete guide to professional networking: The secrets of online and offline success.* Philadelphia: Kogan Page.

Price, J., and M. Bratcher. 2010. *The BioMechanics Method corrective exercise specialist certification program.* San Diego, CA: The BioMechanics Press.

Price, J., and M. Bratcher. 2012. *The BioMechanics Method corrective exercise business professional educational course.* San Diego, CA: The BioMechanics Press.

Thomas, S. 2014. *Business networking for dummies.* Chichester, UK: Wiley.

Index

Note: The italicized *f* following page numbers refers to figures.

About the Author

Justin Price is the creator of The BioMechanics Method, a systematic process used to assess and correct the underlying causes of musculoskeletal pain and dysfunction. Thousands of health and fitness professionals in more than 60 countries have earned The BioMechanics Method Corrective Exercise Specialist (TBMM-CES) credential—the highest-rated corrective exercise program in the industry.

Known as one of the top musculoskeletal assessment and corrective exercise experts in the world, Price was named the Personal Trainer of the Year by the IDEA Health & Fitness Association in 2006. He is a subject matter expert on corrective exercise for the American Council on Exercise, BOSU, TRX (Fitness Anywhere), Personal Training on the Net, and PTA Global.

Price has also authored *The Complete Idiot's Guide to Functional Training Illustrated* and *The Amazing Tennis Ball Back Pain Cure*. He has been an expert consultant for *Arthritis Today*, BBC, *Chicago Tribune*, Discovery Health, Fox News, *Los Angeles Times*, *Men's Health*, MSNBC, *New York Times*, *Newsweek*, *Time*, *Wall Street Journal*, WebMD, and *Women's Health & Fitness*.

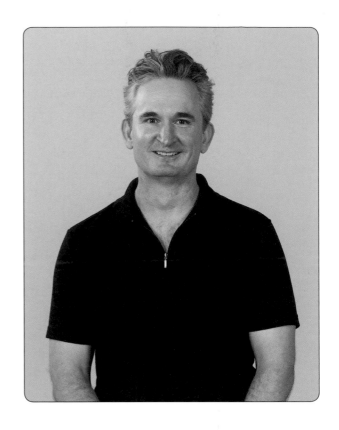